LANGE Q&A

MRI EXAMINATION

NOTICE

Medicine is an ever-changing science. As new research and clinical experience broaden our knowledge, changes in treatment and drug therapy are required. The authors and the publisher of this work have checked with sources believed to be reliable in their efforts to provide information that is complete and generally in accord with the standards accepted at the time of publication. However, in view of the possibility of human error or changes in medical sciences, neither the authors nor the publisher nor any other party who has been involved in the preparation or publication of this work warrants that the information contained herein is in every respect accurate or complete, and they disclaim all responsibility for any errors or omissions or for the results obtained from use of the information contained in this work. Readers are encouraged to confirm the information contained herein with other sources. For example and in particular, readers are advised to check the product information sheet included in the package of each drug they plan to administer to be certain that the information contained in this work is accurate and that changes have not been made in the recommended dose or in the contraindications for administration. This recommendation is of particular importance in connection with new or infrequently used drugs.

LANGE Q&A
MRI EXAMINATION

Barry Southers, M.Ed., RT(R)(MR)(FSMRT)
MRI Program Director
Associate Professor, MRI Section
Advanced Medical Imaging Technology Program
University of Cincinnati
Cincinnati, Ohio

Tiffany Roman, MA Ed, RT(R)(CT)(MRI)
Program Director and Associate Professor of Radiologic Imaging Technology
University of Cincinnati
Cincinnati, Ohio

Clinical Solutions Delivery Consultant, MR
Philips Healthcare
Cincinnati, Ohio

Maureen Hood, Ph.D., RN, RT(MR), FISMRT, FAHA
Department of Radiology & Radiological Sciences
Director, Biomedical Research Imaging Core
Assistant Professor
Uniformed Services University
Bethesda, Maryland

John Posh, B.S., RT(R)(MR)
Director of Global Training and Education, MRI Safety Officer
Aspect Imaging
Nashville, Tennessee

Adjunct Faculty
Department of Medical Imaging, College of Health Sciences
Rush University
Chicago, Illinois

Adjunct Faculty
School of Medical Imaging Sciences
John Patrick University
South Bend, Indiana

Owner, Posh Education
Bethlehem, Pennsylvania

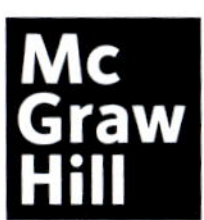

Lange Q&A MRI Examination

1 2 3 4 5 6 7 8 9 DSS 30 29 28 27 26 25

ISBN 978-0-07-184369-0
MHID 0-07-184369-8

The book was set in Minion Pro by KnowledgeWorks Global Ltd.
The editors were Sydney Keen Vitale and Christina M. Thomas.
The production supervisor was Richard Ruzycka.
Project management was provided by Abhishek Singh, KnowledgeWorks Global Ltd.
The cover designer was W2 Design.

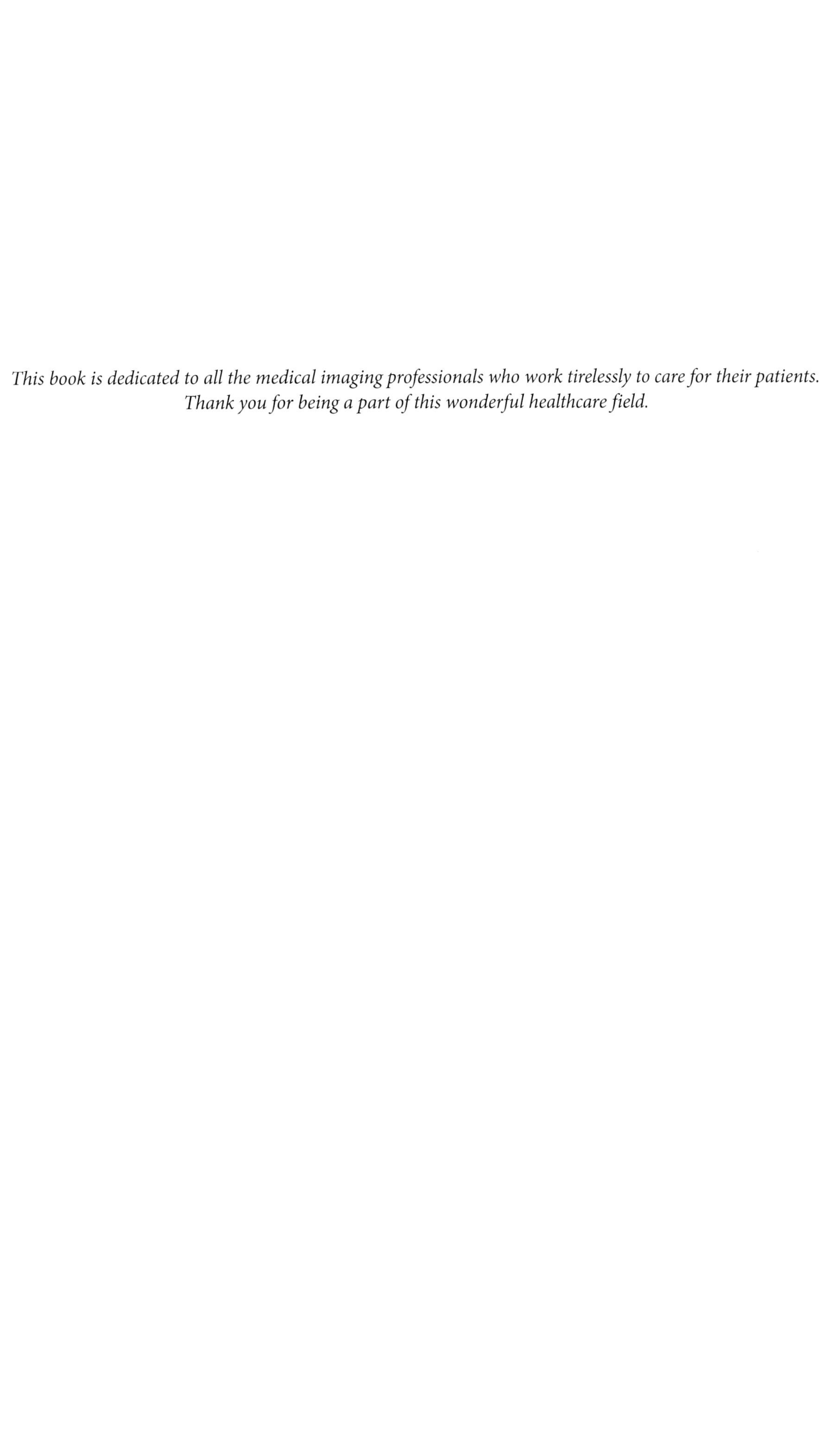

This book is dedicated to all the medical imaging professionals who work tirelessly to care for their patients. Thank you for being a part of this wonderful healthcare field.

CONTENTS

ACKNOWLEDGMENTS

The authors would like to thank Ms. Gail Kohls, RT, for her assistance in searching for and obtaining the images in this book. We would also like to thank Dr. Kevin DeMarco for his supervision of the clinical aspects of questions.

We hope this book helps technologists and radiographers who are getting into the field of MRI to improve their knowledge and thought processes regarding the vast field of magnetic resonance.

PREFACE

In my 27 years of being in the field of magnetic resonance imaging (MRI), I have seen countless changes—from technological advances in pulse sequences, to increased coil sensitivity and rapid imaging techniques. The field is ever-changing, indeed. However, the basic physics remains the same—place a patient in the magnet, manipulate their hydrogen protons, collect signals, and Fourier transform this collected analog data into digital images. No matter the advancements we have developed as a field, the basic premises remain the same.

My colleagues and I began working on this project a grueling 8 years ago with the grossly underestimated timeline of 2 years to publication. Several years and countless updates later, we are finally here. Our primary goal for this project was to fill a need in medical imaging by adding to the small, yet vital, group of MRI Registry Examination textbooks available to MRI professionals. This textbook will serve as an important supplemental MRI education resource for both users new to the field and experienced professionals wishing to refresh themselves with the magical field that we call MRI.

Our research initially started by using the ARRT MRI Registry content specifications as a guide. We met many times to hash out the details, changed our direction a few times, and then finally agreed upon the current content. Then, our group of authors divided up the topics and got to work. All of us diligently worked to ensure all valuable topics were covered to provide a comprehensive Q&A textbook for everyone—regardless of experience level. We all have our strengths and differing writing styles, and those qualities were invaluable when collectively working on such a large project as this one.

On a personal note, a motivator for me was remembering how I studied and prepared to take my MRI Certification Exam many years ago. I made sloppy note cards, Q&A PowerPoints, and quizzed myself daily for weeks on end. I wish I would have had a resource like this when I was studying! I regularly thought to myself, "There has to be a better way." Lo and behold, decades later, we have found a better way to prepare for the exam and ultimately provide the reader with a comprehensive addition to your studying arsenal.

As mentioned above, the basic principles of MRI physics remain the same even though our field is always evolving. That is something we kept in mind when writing this book. Whether it be next week, next year, or even 20 years from now, we hope this book will continually prove to be a useful tool to you.

In closing, we truly appreciate you—the reader. Thank you for purchasing this text and entrusting us to help you achieve your goals—whether it be to pass the MRI Registry Examination or simply to refresh yourself on all things MRI. We are proud of this venture and sincerely hope this book will serve as a helpful supplement for many years to come.

Happy reading!

Barry Southers

ARRT Mock Boards

Content Category A. Patient Care

1-1. Consent can NEVER be:

A. Implied

B. Verbal

C. **Assumed**

D. None of the above

Discussion: Consent can never be assumed. Consent can be implied. For example, asking a patient to come with you for the procedure, and the patient willingly coming along, implies consent. The patient verbalizing that they consent for the procedure is not always necessary. Lastly, there is a presumption of consent for noninvasive procedures when the patient schedules the test, arrives for the test, and prepares for the test.

1-2. Once consent is given, it cannot be withdrawn until:

A. The procedure is complete

B. Submitted in writing

C. Witnessed by a physician

D. **Consent can be withdrawn at any time**

Discussion: Consent can be withdrawn at any time. A patient having four MRIs with and without contrast with 3 minutes to go can stop the exam and there is nothing you can do about it. We can encourage the patient to complete the test, we can remind them that they came this far and there are only a few more minutes to go, but in the end, when they say "I'm done. I want to stop," we stop. Once a patient says, "I don't want to continue," they have effectively withdrawn consent, and any further action on our part can be construed as either assault or battery.

1-3. "The commission of an act that a prudent person would not have done or the omission of an act that a prudent person would have fulfilled, resulting in injury or harm to another person" is the definition of:

A. Assault

B. Battery

C. **Negligence**

D. Malpractice

Discussion: The standard here is what a prudent person would or would not do. There is no distinction for training or education. It is merely the baseline of common sense.

1-4. "Professional negligence that is the proximate cause of injury or harm resulting from a lack or professional knowledge, experience, or skill that can be expected from others in the profession or from a failure to exercise reasonable care or judgment in the application of the professional knowledge, experience, or skill" is the definition of:

A. Assault

B. Battery

C. Negligence

D. **Malpractice**

Discussion: When negligence stems from a lack of professional knowledge, experience, or skill that should be expected by anyone in that profession, negligence rises to the level of malpractice.

1-5. Patients with a GFR above 60 can:

A. Be given IV contrast as clinically appropriate

B. Receive the test without contrast to avoid further kidney damage

C. Be given an alternative and safer agent

D. None of the above

Discussion: Glomerular filtration rate (GFR) is the most comprehensive measure of kidney function. The higher the number, the greater the function of the kidneys. Patients with a GFR above 60 can be given contrast as clinically indicated. It should be noted that GFR is no longer necessary before contrast administration with class 2 agents. For some facilities, class 1 and 3 agents are still only given with a GFR above 60 or at lower doses with lower GFRs.

1-6. The percentage of patients reported to have reactions to gadolinium contrast agents is:

A. Less than 1%

B. 10%

C. 5%

D. 20%

Discussion: The overall percentage of patients reported to have conscious reactions to gadolinium-based contrast agents is less than 1%. This includes all reactions from mild nausea and headaches through anaphylaxis.

1-7. Patients who are at an increased risk of reaction to MRI contrast are patients with:

A. A history of asthma and/or allergies

B. Prior contrast reactions

C. No known medical history

D. Both A and B

E. A, B, and C

Discussion: Patients with a history of asthma, allergies, or prior contrast reactions already grader, statistical risk of reaction to MRI contrast agents. Patients with no history of allergic reactions of any kind or at the same risk as other patients.

1-8. It is good practice for all patients who undergo MRI to be monitored:

A. visually and/or verbally

B. With ECG

C. For respiratory status

D. No monitoring needed

Discussion: All patients during MRI should be monitored visually and/or verbally. This means we watch the patient visually through the window for any movement or signs of distress. We also communicate with the patient via the intercom periodically throughout the exam to make sure the patient is okay and not in need of assistance. It should also be noted that all patients should be given the emergency call ball.

1-9. If a patient needs to be monitored with an electrical/mechanical device, it is critical that the MRI safety of the device be established by:

A. FDA device clearance

B. Prior testing

C. Manufacturer's declaration

D. All of the above

Discussion: No device should be used for any part of patient care unless that device has been labeled by the FDA as acceptable for use in MRI, tested for safety in MRI, and labeled by the manufacturer as safe for use in MRI. Additionally, while suitable for use in MRI, there may be conditions placed on any device, such as magnetic field exposure restrictions, etc.

1-10. Patient identification is important because it:

A. Assures the correct patient receives the correct test

B. Establishes initial rapport with the patient

C. Assesses the patient's comprehension level

D. All of the above

Discussion: Patient identification serves a variety of purposes. In the simplest sense, it ensures that we are performing the procedure on the proper patient. But when done properly, it also helps to establish an initial rapport with the patient and assess the patient's level of comprehension regarding what is being done. This is especially important for studies that involve any kind of intervention or medication where a change in the patient's comprehension level could indicate a medical complication.

1-11. In a normal adult, a heart rate above 100 is considered:

A. Normal

B. Tachycardia

C. Bradycardia

D. Not relevant in radiology

Discussion: "Tachy" is the medical prefix for "above." Tachycardia means above normal heart rate.

1-12. When compared to oral temperature, rectal temperature can be:

A. 0.5–1.0 degree lower

B. 0.5–1.0 degree higher

C. 1.0–2.0 degrees higher

D. None of the above

Discussion: Rectal temperatures, a more accurate indication of body core temperature, traditionally run 0.5 to 1.0 degree higher than oral temperature.

1-13. Elevated body temperature can be associated with:

A. Infection

B. Convulsions

C. Drug reaction

D. All of the above

Discussion: Elevated body temperature can be associated with a variety of conditions. Infections traditionally increase body temperature as part of the immune response, convulsions can raise body temperature due to increased muscle activity, and drug reactions can increase body temperature for a variety of reasons.

1-14. A pulse oximetry reading of 85% and below is considered:

A. Mild hypoxia

B. Moderate hypoxia

C. Severe hypoxia

D. None of the above

Discussion: Pulse oximetry measures the concentration of oxygen in the blood. While this measurement varies over the course of the day and with patient condition, a pulse oximetry reading of 85% or below is considered severe hypoxia and constitutes a medical emergency.

1-15. The lab value that best assesses kidney function because it considers age, race, and gender is:

A. BUN

B. Creatinine

C. GFR

D. None of the above

Discussion: While BUN and creatinine were the standard for many years, they did not factor in the patient's age, race, and gender. For this reason, glomerular filtration rate (GFR) is the new standard.

1-16. The three methods of communication used daily in MRI include:

A. Formal, informal, and legal

B. Verbal, nonverbal, and written

C. Medical, social, and legal

D. None of the above

Discussion: Both verbal and nonverbal communication are used on a daily basis in healthcare. Verbal communication involves asking questions regarding medical history and receiving answers from the patient. These answers can be oral (spoken) or nonoral (written responses or sign language). Nonverbal communication includes things like nodding, laughing, crying, body language, and gestures.

1-17. Which of the following could be barriers to effective communication:

A. Physical condition

B. Mental status

C. Ethnicity

D. Time of day

E. A, B, and C

Discussion: Lots of things can be barriers to effective communication. The patient's condition including hearing impairment, altered mental capacity, and emotional status plays a role in communication effectiveness. Additionally, cultural barriers such as degree of personal space, eye contact, and hand gestures and body posture can enhance or hinder communication. While time of day can play a factor in some medical conditions such as Alzheimer's, it in and of itself is not a barrier to effective communication.

1-18. Explaining the procedure to the patient before beginning aids in:

A. Assessing the patient's understanding of what is being done

B. Gaining the patient's cooperation

C. Determining the extent of the patient's injuries

D. Both A and B

Discussion: Explaining the procedure is often the first complex conversation many healthcare providers have with their patients. This is important because it allows you to assess the comprehension of the patient regarding what is being done to them and aids in getting their cooperation. While altered mental status can be evident from a conversation, it is not enough to determine the extent of an injury.

1-19. Infections contracted by patients while in the hospital are called:

A. Nosocomial (old term, now hospital acquired)

B. Payday for lawyers

C. Aseptic

D. None of the above

Discussion: Infections acquired in the hospital by patients are called hospital acquired. The old term for these infections was nosocomial, but that terminology has been phased out.

1-20. Infections contracted by healthcare workers while in the hospital are called:

A. Professionally acquired

B. Payday for lawyers

C. Aseptic

D. None of the above

Discussion: An infection contracted by a healthcare worker in the hospital is referred to as professionally acquired. These used to be called nosocomial infections, but that terminology did not distinguish between patients and healthcare practitioners.

1-21. The two types of aseptic techniques practiced are:

A. Surgical and medical asepsis

B. Medical and clean asepsis

C. Chemical and thermal

D. None of the above

Discussion: There are two basic types of aseptic technique practiced in most MRI departments. Medical asepsis is the removal of most pathogens and is accomplished via handwashing or the application of antimicrobial gel. Surgical asepsis, also known as sterilization, is the removal of all pathogens via heat, steam, or chemicals. While surgical asepsis is not actually done in the MRI department, it is not uncommon for surgical kits, trays, and instruments to be used in MRI during procedures.

1-22. Which of the following is *not* used in MRI to monitor patients:

A. ECG

B. Blood pressure

C. Blood oxygen level

D. EEG

Discussion: ECG is used to monitor the patient's heart rhythm, blood pressure can be monitored during the MRI via noninvasively, and blood oxygen level can be monitored via pulse oximetry. EEG, while a very important test for many patients, is not routinely be done during MRI at this time.

1-23. What items might be worn by the technologist for direct contact with a patient, such as when starting an IV?

A. Gloves

B. Masks

C. Gowns

D. All of the above

Discussion: Gloves must be worn for any contact with a patient if there is even a remote chance of contact with blood or body fluids, such as when starting an IV.

1-24. When positioning ECG leads for cardiac gating, if no R wave is seen on the ECG, the technologist should:

A. Stop the scan

B. Continue with the scan

C. Increase the R-to-R interval

D. Reposition the leads

Discussion: When positioning cardiac leads, if no R wave is seen, the first step is to simply reposition leads to try and get a better tracing. Since all this is done before the scan starts, stopping the scan or continuing to scan are not acceptable solutions.

1-25. What does hematocrit refer to?

A. Serum levels

B. Plasma levels

C. Red blood cell levels

D. Platelet levels

Discussion: Hematocrit is a measure of red blood cell concentration in the blood. It is not generally one of the values we test in MRI as it is generally more useful in interventional procedures. However, given the rise of interventional MRI procedures, it is something technologists must know.

1-26. What condition is present when the patient's diastolic pressure is greater than 100 mm Hg?

A. Hypotension

B. Hypertension

C. Low blood pressure

D. None of the above

Discussion: Elevated blood pressure above 100 mm Hg diastolic is the definition of hypertension or high blood pressure. Conversely, hypotension means below normal blood pressure.

1-27. What is the definition of a paraplegic:

A. A patient who is paralyzed from the waist down

B. A patient who is paralyzed from the waist up

C. A patient who is paralyzed in all four extremities

D. None of the above

Discussion: Paraplegia means impairment or alteration of the motor functions of the lower extremities.

1-28. Hand washing is a form of:

A. Medical asepsis

B. Surgical asepsis

C. Sterilization

D. None of the above

Discussion: Handwashing is a form of medical asepsis, meaning most pathogens are removed from the skin. Surgical asepsis refers to sterilization, which is very difficult to do without more detailed scrubbing and chemical cleansers, such as those used in the operating room.

1-29. The concept that the employer is responsible for the employee is described by which of the following?

A. Res ipsa loquitur

B. Stare decisis

C. Respondeat superior

D. None of the above

Discussion: Respondeat superior translates to "let the master answer." It sums up the concept that the employer is responsible for the actions of the employee, provided that the employee acts within the boundaries of their employment. It should also be noted that respondeat superior does not apply to independent contractors, but only regular employees in most jurisdictions.

1-30. If a patient is in isolation with contact precautions, which of the following protective personnel apparel should be worn?

A. **Gowns and gloves**

B. Mask and gown

C. Cap and gloves

D. Gown and booties

Discussion: Contact precautions are in place for diseases that are spread via direct contact such as *C. difficile*, *E. coli*, and scabies. To prevent direct contact, gowns and gloves are required.

1-31. If a patient is falling in front of you, from what part of the body should you catch?

A. From the chest

B. From the waist

C. **From the chest and the waist**

D. None of the above

Discussion: Catching a falling patient is one of the greatest risk factors for injury in technologists. If a patient is falling, it is essential to catch them from the chest and waist and utilize proper body mechanics to guide them to the floor as gently as possible.

1-32. Chest pain is also known as:

A. Myocardial infarction

B. **Angina pectoris**

C. Tetralogy of Fallot

D. A bad thing

Discussion: Angina pectoris is another name for chest pain, one of the first symptoms of cardiac infarction.

1-33. Impairment of motor function of the lower extremities is called:

A. Quadriplegia

B. **Paraplegia**

C. Hemiplegia

D. Monoplegia

Discussion: Paraplegia means impairment or alteration of the motor functions of the lower extremities.

1-34. Loss of motor function on one side of the body is called:

A. Paraplegia

B. Quadriplegia

C. **Hemiplegia**

D. Orthoplegia

Discussion: Hemiplegia refers to a loss of motor function on one side of the body.

1-35. Normal atmosphere has an oxygen concentration of approximately:

A. 15%

B. 18%

C. **21%**

D. 28%

Discussion: Normal atmospheric air has an oxygen concentration of approximately 21%. This number can fluctuate with weather and altitude, but the fluctuation range is relatively small.

1-36. The basement threshold for oxygen levels in MRI is generally set at:

A. 13.5%

B. 17.5%

C. **19.5%**

D. 26.5%

Discussion: All superconducting MRIs are equipped with oxygen sensors in the room as a safety system due to the presence of helium. If below 19.5% oxygen concentration, the oxygen sensor will trigger an alarm.

1-37. The effects of exposure to low oxygen levels can lead to:

A. Impaired perception and judgement

B. Confusion

C. Loss of the ability to self-rescue

D. **All of the above**

Discussion: When oxygen levels fall too low, the patient will suffer from hypoxia. Impaired perception and judgment, confusion, and the loss of the ability to self-rescue can happen very quickly in this situation.

1-38. At oxygen concentrations below ________, unconsciousness can occur in 10 seconds and death due to heart failure can occur in 2–4 minutes.

A. 10%

B. 8%

C. **6%**

D. 4%

Discussion: If the oxygen concentration in the room falls low enough, below 6%, severe hypoxia can result in unconsciousness in approximately 10 seconds and death due to heart failure in approximately 2 to 4 minutes.

1-39. To ensure the proper test is performed on the proper patient for the proper reason, it is important to:

A. Identify the patient verbally

B. Match the name on the request with the patient's name

C. Compare the written request to the clinical indications

D. **All of the above**

Discussion: One of the most fundamental tenants of imaging professionals is to not perform a test on the wrong patient. As such, it is very important to identify the patient properly using their name and one other identifier such as date of birth. Additionally, to make sure the patient undergoes the proper test, we match the name on the request with the name of the patient. Lastly, to make sure the test ordered is in fact the appropriate test, we compare the written request with the clinical indications. It is not uncommon for patients to say, "The pain is in my leg. Why are you imaging my back?" This is a legitimate question as patients might not understand the concept of referred nerve pain, etc. What becomes more complicated is if a male patient shows up with the request for an MRI of the pelvis for endometriosis. In this situation, it is very important to determine if the order is inappropriate, or if the patient is biologically female and simply identifying as male.

1-40. The Patient's Bill of Rights grants the following right(s) to recipients of medical care in the United States:

A. The right to privacy

B. The right to appoint a healthcare proxy

C. The right to access information

D. The right of participation (in care and research)

E. **All of the above**

Discussion: All patients have the right to privacy, the right to appoint a healthcare proxy to make decisions for them should they become incapacitated, the right to access their own information, and the right to participate in their care, and if applicable, any research programs they could be eligible for. Nowhere in the Bill of Rights does anything guaranteed the right to an attorney.

1-41. The ________ serves as a guide by which ARRT Certificate Holders and candidates may evaluate their professional conduct as it relates to patients, healthcare consumers, employers, colleagues, and other members of the healthcare team.

A. Code of conduct

B. **Code of ethics**

C. Standards of professional jurisprudence

D. This is not defined by the ARRT

Discussion: The ARRT code of ethics is the governing standard of conduct for imaging professionals.

1-42. The legal doctrine that states "the thing speaks for itself" is known as:

A. Caveat emptor

B. Semper ubi sub ubi

C. **Res ipsa loquitur**

D. Doctrine of clear voice

Discussion: Res ipsa loquitur means "the thing speaks for itself." If the cause of an injury is under the exclusive control of the person presumed responsible for the injury, then the thing speaks for itself. Caveat emptor means "buyer beware" and governs commercial transactions. Semper ubi sub ubi means "always wear underwear." Doctrine of clear voice is fictitious.

1-43. Res ipsa loquitur means that:

A. **One can be presumed to be negligent if one had exclusive control over the thing that caused injury**.

B. Negligence can be implied if someone tells you so

C. Negligence can only be proven if the thing says so

D. None of the above

Discussion: Res ipsa loquitur means "the thing speaks for itself." If the cause of an injury is under the exclusive control of the person presumed responsible for the injury, then the thing speaks for itself.

1-44. The legal doctrine that states the employer is responsible for the actions of his/her employer during the normal course of their employment is:

A. Res ipsa loquitur

B. Doctrine of divine coverage

C. Captain of the ship doctrine

D. **Respondeat superior**

Discussion: Respondeat superior translates into "let the master answer." This means the employer is responsible for the behavior of the employee, provided the employee is acting within the boundaries of their employment. Employees under the influence of drugs or alcohol, or functioning outside of their job responsibilities or scope of training, may not be included in this.

1-45. Consent can be given by:

A. An aware and competent person over 18

B. An emancipated minor

C. Parents and legal guardians of minors

D. Those appointed as healthcare proxies for others

E. **All of the above**

Discussion: Consent can be given by anyone aware and over 18, an emancipated minor, parents and legal guardians of minors, and anyone formally appointed as a healthcare proxy for someone else. A friend simply helping out, while they may be knowledgeable of the patient's history and wishes, cannot provide consent.

1-46. Consent can be:

A. Verbal

B. Written

C. Implied

D. **All of the above**

Discussion: Consent can never be assumed. Verbal consent, written consent, and implied consent are all used on a daily basis. But it is never safe to assume consent has been given.

1-47. Touching a patient without permission, doing the wrong examination, or examining the wrong patients are all examples of:

A. Neglect

B. **Battery**

C. Assault

D. Slander

Discussion: Touching a patient without permission, doing the wrong examination, and doing an examination on the wrong patient are all examples of battery, which, depending on the severity, is likely a felony and can result in revocation of your professional license and possible criminal charges.

1-48. Touching or threatening to touch in an injurious way is:

A. Neglect

B. **Battery**

C. Assault

D. Slander

Discussion: Assault is any conduct that places another person in a position where they feel they may be injured or battered. This is relevant in imaging because any threat of negative consequences can be perceived as assault. The patient who doesn't want to test and is refusing can be educated and negotiated with. That patient can never be threatened with negative consequences such as, "If you don't do this, you'll need surgery" or "The doctor wants this and if you don't do it, he'll be mad." In each of these examples, the patient is being threatened with negative consequences if they do not do something and that is the definition of assault.

1-49. Defamation of character verbally is known as:

A. Libel

B. Slander

C. Assault

D. Invasion of privacy

Discussion: Slander is defined as defamation of character verbally. It includes things like making disparaging comments about a patient in an elevator or public space where such comments could be overheard. It is generally accepted practice that patients are not to be spoken about outside of the clinical area and never in negative terms.

1-50. Defamation of character in writing is known as:

A. Libel

B. Slander

C. Assault

D. Invasion of privacy

Discussion: Making negative comments regarding a patient's character in writing is the definition of libel. This is especially important in the healthcare setting, as multiple people in multiple departments have access to the patient's written medical record, and disparaging or negative comments cannot generally be removed.

1-51. Accessing protected health information for family, friends, and others you have not personally participated in the care of is:

A. Invasion of privacy

B. A violation of HIPAA

C. A really good way to get fired

D. All of the above

Discussion: HIPAA violations are taken very seriously by hospitals. Healthcare practitioners are well within their rights to access to medical records of any patient for which they are providing care either directly or tangentially. However, an individual having no role in the care of a patient is absolutely violating the patient's rights if they access any protected health information. When it comes to family and friends, we as healthcare professionals, except in mitigating circumstances, are not permitted to provide direct care.

1-52. For malpractice to be present, which of the following must be proven:

A. The patient sustained loss, damage, or injury

B. A person or institution is at fault

C. The loss, damage, or injury is the result of negligence or improper practice

D. All of the above

Discussion: Malpractice requires three things. There must be a sustained loss, damage, or injury, a person or institution must be deemed at fault, and that loss, damage, or injury must be the result of some sort of negligent or improper practice. Whether the loss was intentional is not a factor.

1-53. The cycle of infection involves which of the following?

A. Pathogen, reservoir of infection, susceptible host, method of transmission

B. Pathogen, reservoir of infection, host, method of transmission

C. Fomite, vector, susceptible host, method of transmission

D. Pathogen, vector, vehicle, method of transmission

Discussion: The cycle of infection involves several components. There must be a pathogen and a reservoir for that pathogen to thrive and multiply. There must also be a susceptible host and some sort of method of transmission from the reservoir to the host.

1-54. A pathogen is a(n):

A. Microorganism capable of causing disease

B. Infectious organism

C. Bacteria, virus, fungus, prion, or parasitic protozoa

D. All of the above

Discussion: Pathogens can be defined as microorganisms capable of causing disease or infectious organisms, or they can be listed by their type, such as bacteria, viruses, fungi, prion, or parasitic protozoa.

1-55. The most important portion of any infection control program is:

A. Hand sanitizer in all clinical areas

B. Hand washing

C. Latex gloves

D. All of the above

Discussion: The most important component of any infection control program is hand washing. Washing hands with warm water and soap for a minimum of 20 seconds is extremely effective at controlling the spread of hospital and professionally acquired infections. Hand sanitizers can be substituted but only if the hands are not visibly soiled.

1-56. Alcohol-based hand sanitizers may be used in place of hand washing if:

A. Hand sanitizer is of medical grade

B. Hand sanitizer contains over 79% alcohol by volume

C. The hands are not visibly soiled

D. Hand sanitizers may never be used to replace hand washing

Discussion: Alcohol-based hand sanitizers may be used in place of hand washing if the hands are not visibly soiled. Any visible blood or body fluids on the hands requires the hands to be washed with warm water and soap for a minimum of 20 seconds and dried completely.

1-57. What is the process to safely recap a needle?

A. Slide the needle into the cap while on the table

B. Flip the cap onto the needle

C. Gently align the cap and slowly advance until it clicks

D. It is never safe to recap needles

Discussion: There is no safe process to recap a needle. Needles should never be recapped. The needle, regardless of what it was used for, should be disposed of in a properly labeled sharps container, which must be present anywhere sharps are used.

1-58. Hand washing and alcohol-based hand rubs are types of:

A. Medical asepsis

B. Surgical asepsis

C. Medical sepsis

D. Surgical sepsis

Discussion: Both hand washing and alcohol-based hand rubs are types of medical asepsis, meaning they remove most pathogens from the hands.

1-59. Boiling, steam, gas, radiation, chemicals, and dry heat are types of:

A. Medical asepsis

B. Surgical asepsis

C. Medical sepsis

D. Surgical sepsis

Discussion: Boiling, steam, gas, radiation, chemicals, and dry heat are all types of surgical asepsis and are used to sterilize or remove all pathogens from objects.

1-60. When removing dirty linens from the bed, it is important to:

A. Shake out the linens to make sure there are no needles

B. Roll the linens to the center and fold over

C. Pull the linens from one side and drop to the floor

D. None of the above

Discussion: When removing dirty linens from the bed, it is very important to roll them in to the center and fold them over. Never pull the linens from one side and drop them to the floor, and never shake out the linens. Both of these processes can result in pathogens being distributed in the air.

1-61. Gloves, gowns, booties, face masks, goggles, and N95 respirators are all types of:

A. Safety gear (SG)

B. Barrier protection (BP)

C. Personal protective equipment (PPE)

D. Individual protective stuff (IPS)

Discussion: Gloves, gowns, booties, facemasks, and goggles are all types of personal protective equipment or PPE. While they are types of safety gear, this is not an accepted term. While they might provide barrier protection, this is not an accepted term.

1-62. In the United States, patient privacy is protected by:

A. *H*ealth *I*nsurance *P*ortability and *A*ccountability *A*ct (HIPAA)

B. *H*ealth *I*nsurance *P*rivacy *A*ct (HIPA)

C. *H*ealth *I*nformation *P*ortability and *A*ccountability *A*ct (HIPAA)

D. *H*ealth *I*nsurance *P*rofitability *A*ct (HIPA)

Discussion: The Health Insurance Portability and Accountability Act (HIPAA) of 1996 is the primary governing standard for patient privacy. HIPAA established national standards for all electronic healthcare transactions regarding a patient's health information, including what constitutes a unique identifier, who can access personal health information, and how that information can be used.

1-63. Explanation of the procedure, pre- and postprocedure instructions, and communication during the procedure are all examples of what?

A. Patient education

B. Patient counselling

C. Patient prep

D. Patient compliance measures

Discussion: Explaining the procedure in any pre- and postprocedure instructions, as well as any communication during the procedure, are all examples of patient education.

1-64. What is being done, why it is being done, and how long it should take are all examples of things that should be done during which category of patient education?

A. Explanation of the procedure

B. Pre- and postprocedure instructions

C. Communications during the procedures

D. Discharge instructions

Discussion: Given the importance of explaining the procedure to the patient, it makes sense to include details about what is being done, why it is being done, and how long it should take. An informed patient is generally a more cooperative patient.

1-65. Pre- and postprocedure instructions should include:

A. Patient preparation

B. Patient discharge instructions

C. Copies of necessary paperwork

D. Both A and B

Discussion: Pre- and postprocedure instructions are important for a variety of reasons. They ensure the patient is properly prepped, and can take care of themselves after discharge. While copies of all necessary paperwork are important, they're not really instructional.

1-66. The key element of communicating during a procedure is:

A. Patient education

B. Patient counselling

C. Providing proper instruction

D. Listening to the patient

Discussion: The big part of communication during the procedure is listening to the patient. What words they are using and how they are using them can be an indicator of anxiety or stress.

1-67. Knowing your patient's fall risk, keeping work areas clear of hazards, always using side rails and safety straps, and never leaving patients unattended are all important for:

A. Patient fall prevention

B. OSHA gold level certification

C. FDA certification

D. Keeping the Joint Commission happy

Discussion: Patient fall prevention is everyone's responsibility. It is important to understand every patient's fall risk. Additionally, keeping work areas clean of hazards, using side rails and safety straps, and never leaving patients unattended are all very important steps in preventing patient falls.

1-68. This vital sign is a measure of the concentration of oxygen in a patient's blood:

A. Pulse oximetry

B. Blood pressure

C. CPAP

D. ECMO

Discussion: The concentration of oxygen in a patient's blood is measured via pulse oximetry.

1-69. Wheelchairs, stretchers, beds, and cribs or isolates are all potential methods for:

A. Keeping the patient comfortable while in the MRI department

B. Transferring the patient to and from the MRI department

C. Keeping patient safe while in the hall outside the department

D. Both A and B

Discussion: Wheelchairs, stretchers, beds, and cribs or isolates are all methods for transferring the patient to and from the MRI department. While they are designed to be as comfortable as possible, they are not comfort measures. While they are designed to be a safe as possible, they are not safety measures.

1-70. Sheet transfers, slider boards, and mechanical assistive devices are all potential methods for:

A. Keeping the patient comfortable while in the MRI department

B. Transferring the patient to and from imaging equipment

C. Keeping patient safe while in the hall outside the department

D. Restraining combative patients

Discussion: Transferring the patient to and from the imaging equipment can be done via a variety of techniques such as sheet transfers, slider boards, and mechanical assistive devices.

1-71. Proper body mechanics in MRI consist of three basic categories, which are:

A. The base of support, the center of gravity, and the line of gravity

B. The base of support, the spinal axis, and the hip angle

C. The center of gravity, the line of gravity, and the hip angle

D. The spinal axis, the center of gravity, and the line of gravity

Discussion: The three main categories of proper body mechanics include the base of support, the center of gravity, which should be oriented over base of support, and the line of gravity, which connects the center of gravity with the base of support.

1-72. The vertical line connecting the center of gravity in the base of support is known as the:

A. Spinal axis

B. Line of gravity

C. Center of gravity

D. Base of support

Discussion: The imaginary vertical line connecting to the center of gravity support is known as the line of gravity. While this frequently corresponds with the orientation of the spine, it is not referred to as the spinal axis.

1-73. This should be centered over the base of support:

A. Spinal axis

B. Line of gravity

C. Center of gravity

D. Base of support

Discussion: The base of support is defined as the portion of our body that touches the floor. Keeping the body's center of gravity centered over the base of support ensures proper body mechanics when moving or lifting.

1-74. With respect to lifting, which of the following is true:

A. Keep a wide base of support

B. Lift with the back

C. Lift with the knees

D. Both A and C

Discussion: Proper body mechanics, especially when lifting, require a wide base of support, coupled with lifting with the knees. It is important to never lift with the back, as this puts undue strain on the spine.

1-75. With respect to drug delivery systems, the two ways to ensure constant delivery of medication to the patient are:

A. The infusion pump can be taken in the room if it is labeled as MRI safe

B. Infusion tubing can be lengthened and routed through a wave guide

C. The nurse can remain in the room and supervise the floor infusion pump

D. Both A and B

Discussion: Ensuring constant medication is delivered to the patient while in the MRI room can often be a challenge. The two acceptable ways of doing so are by using MRI conditional infusion pumps inside the room or running a lengthened extension tubing through a proper wave guide.

1-76. Temperature, pulse, respiration, blood pressure, pulse oximetry, and ECG are all ________ and part of routine patient monitoring.

A. Critical values

B. Vital signs

C. Health physiology indicators

D. Nursing duties only

Discussion: Temperature, pulse, respiration, blood pressure, pulse oximetry, and ECG are all vital signs. All these values may or may not be critical and may or may not be indicators of health physiology depending on the patient's condition. Additionally, vital signs are the responsibility of all healthcare providers, not just nurses.

1-77. A normal pulse rate for an adult is generally:

A. 40 to 60 bpm

B. 60 to 100 bpm

C. 80 to 100 bpm

D. 100 to 120 bpm

Discussion: Normal adults have a pulse rate between 60 and 100 bpm.

1-78. Bradycardia means the patient has a:

A. Higher than normal pulse rate

B. Lower than normal pulse rate

C. Very aggressive pulse rate

D. Very soft pulse rate

Discussion: "Brady" is the medical prefix for "below." Bradycardia means lower than normal pulse rate.

1-79. Tachycardia means the patient has a:

A. Higher than normal pulse rate

B. Lower than normal pulse rate

C. Very aggressive pulse rate

D. Very soft pulse rate

Discussion: "Tachy" is the medical prefix for "above." Tachycardia means above normal pulse rate.

1-80. As a general rule, pediatric pulse rates are ________ when compared to adults.

A. Softer

B. Slower

C. Faster

D. Easier to detect

Discussion: While pediatric pulses might be softer, they are almost always faster. Additionally, pediatric pulse rates are almost never easier to detect.

1-81. A normal pulse rate for an infant is generally:

A. 40 to 60 bpm

B. 60 to 100 bpm

C. 80 to 100 bpm

D. 100 to 120 bpm

Discussion: Normal infant pulse rates are generally in the range of 100 to 120 bpm. The actual rate depends on the physiologic status and overall health of the patient.

1-82. A normal pulse rate for neonates is generally:

A. 40 to 60 bpm

B. 60 to 100 bpm

C. 80 to 100 bpm

D. 120 to 160 bpm

Discussion: Normal neonatal pulse rates are generally in the range of 120 to 160 bpm. The actual rate depends on the physiologic status and overall health of the patient.

1-83. The most common places to manually take a pulse are:

A. The radial pulse in the wrist

B. The carotid pulse in the neck

C. The femoral pulse in the groin

D. The popliteal pulse in the knee

E. Both A and B

Discussion: While a patient's pulse can be taken anywhere an artery can be palpated in theory, the two commonly accepted pulse points used in imaging are the radial pulse in the wrist in the carotid pulse in the neck. The popliteal pulse in the knee is often hard to detect, and the femoral pulse in the groin is rarely used outside of interventional radiology.

1-84. The respiratory rate in a normal adult is generally:

A. 5 to 10 breaths per minute

B. 12 to 20 breaths per minute

C. 15 to 25 breaths per minute

D. 20 to 30 breaths per minute

Discussion: Normal adult respirations occur 12 to 20 times per minute. Increased respiratory rate is considered tachypnea, and decreased respiratory rate is considered bradypnea.

1-85. When compared with adults, the respiratory rate in children is generally:

A. Higher

B. Louder

C. Lower

D. Harder to detect

Discussion: The average respiratory rate in adults is 10 to 20 breaths per minute. As patient age decreases, the respiratory rate generally increases.

1-86. The respiratory rate in a normal child is generally:

A. 5 to 10 breaths per minute

B. 12 to 20 breaths per minute

C. 15 to 30 breaths per minute

D. 25 to 35 breaths per minute

Discussion: The average child respiratory rate is between 15 and 30 breaths per minute. This rate slows in adulthood and increases with decreasing age.

1-87. The respiratory rate in a normal infant is generally:

A. 5 to 10 breaths per minute

B. 12 to 20 breaths per minute

C. 15 to 25 breaths per minute

D. 25 to 50 breaths per minute

Discussion: The average infant respiratory rate is between 25 and 50 breaths per minute. This rate slows in adulthood and increases with decreasing age.

1-88. The respiratory rate in a normal neonate is generally:

A. 5 to 10 breaths per minute

B. 12 to 20 breaths per minute

C. 15 to 25 breaths per minute

D. 40 to 60 breaths per minute

Discussion: The average neonate respiratory rate is between 40 and 60 breaths per minute. This rate slows in adulthood and increases with decreasing age.

1-89. This blood pressure number represents the pumping pressure of the heart:

A. Systole

B. Diastole

C. Tidal volume

D. Outflow volume

Discussion: Systolic pressure (systole) is a measure of the contractile force of the heart and, thus, equals the pumping pressure. Diastole is a measure of the resting pressure of the heart, i.e., the minimum continuous pressure on the arterial system.

1-90. This blood pressure number represents the minimum continuous pressure on the arterial system:

A. Systole

B. Diastole

C. Tidal volume

D. Outflow volume

Discussion: Diastole is a measure of the resting pressure of the heart, i.e., the minimum continuous pressure on the arterial system.

1-91. In a normal adult, the acceptable range for blood pressure is:

A. 90–120 mm Hg systolic, 60–80 mm Hg diastolic

B. 110–130 mm Hg systolic, 75–100 mm Hg diastolic

C. 60–90 mm Hg systolic, 40–60 mm Hg diastolic

D. Not relevant in radiology

Discussion: 90 to 120 mm Hg systolic (pumping pressure) over 60 to 80 mm Hg of diastolic pressure (resting pressure) is considered a normal adult blood pressure.

1-92. Technologists should always be prepared for ________, which can include allergic reactions, cardiac or respiratory arrest, RF burns, or other issues.

A. Challenging patients

B. Unforeseen imaging findings

C. Medical emergencies

D. Imaging problems

Discussion: Challenging patients, unforeseen imaging findings, and imaging problems are all encountered on a regular basis and can be solved in a variety of ways. Medical emergencies, however, are something a technologist must always be prepared for, because when encountered, they must be dealt with immediately. Technologists lack the luxury of time.

1-93. In the event of a medical emergency in MRI, all assessment and intervention should only be undertaken in:

A. Zone II

B. Zone III or II

C. Zone IV or III

D. Any zone is acceptable

Discussion: Because of the equipment needed by first responders for medical resuscitation, the patient must be evacuated to Zone III or II before any intervention is attempted.

1-94. The overall percentage of patients reported to have reactions to gadolinium contrast agents is:

A. Less than 1%

B. 5%

C. 15%

D. 20%

Discussion: 1% includes mild reactions such as nausea, hives, headache, etc., up to severe reactions such as anaphylaxis.

1-95. What is the one zone in which medical intervention to medical emergencies should never take place?

A. Zone I

B. Zone II

C. Zone III

D. Zone IV

Discussion: Zone IV. Because of the equipment needed by first responders for medical resuscitation, the patient must be evacuated to Zone III or II before any intervention is attempted.

1-96. Why is it that medical emergencies in MRI present a greater risk to first responders than medical emergencies in other departments in radiology?

A. MRI departments tend to be in the basement away from common corridors

B. MRI units have very strong magnetic fields that could create projectiles of the many small ferrous objects carried by first responders

C. The MRI room really does not have enough light to see during a code

D. There is not enough space in the MRI room for a code

Discussion: The specialized environment of MRI necessitates that no medical resuscitation should ever take place in Zone IV. The ferrous materials and resuscitation equipment required by first responders pose an increased risk to both the patient and staff.

1-97. Because of the complexities of medical emergencies in MRI, in addition to comprehensive policies ________ should be carried out on an annual basis.

A. Testing the emergency response system

B. Making sure department doors are never locked when patients are there

C. Conducting "mock code" drills

D. Both A and C

Discussion: Mock codes are an excellent way to maintain readiness for medical emergencies in the MRI department. They should be conducted annually for medical emergencies, fire emergencies, and any other emergencies likely to be encountered in the department.

1-98. The most common cause of allergic reaction in MRI is:

A. The administration of contrast material

B. Exposure to latex

C. Peanuts from the cafeteria

D. Special chemicals used to clean the MRI

Discussion: By far, the most common cause of allergic reactions in MRI is the administration of contrast material, though this is very rare. Latex is rarely used in hospital gloves and materials, so that issue is not much of a problem anymore.

1-99. Medical treatment is rarely required for ________.

A. Mild allergic reactions

B. Severe allergic reactions

C. Anaphylaxis

D. Allergic shock

Discussion: Most mild reactions rarely require treatment. A patient who feels nauseous might benefit from a cool washcloth on their forehead but rarely requires medical intervention.

1-100. When it comes to allergic reactions, which of the following is true?

A. They always result in a medical rapid response

B. They always require CPR

C. The severity of the reaction dictates the level of response

D. It is always radiology nursing's responsibility to deal with it

Discussion: When it comes to allergic reactions, the severity dictates the response. Reactions can range from simple dizziness and nausea to full-blown anaphylaxis, also known as allergic shock. Most mild reactions rarely require treatment. A patient who feels nauseous might benefit from a cool washcloth on their forehead but rarely requires medical intervention.

1-101. The three most common drugs used to treat an anaphylactic reaction are:

A. Diphenhydramine, epinephrine, and methyl iodide

B. Diphenhydramine, epidural, and methylprednisolone

C. Dramamine, epinephrine, and methylprednisolone

D. Diphenhydramine, epinephrine, and methylprednisolone

Discussion: Diphenhydramine disrupts the histamine response and prevents swelling of mucous membranes, epinephrine stimulates the sympathetic nervous system and keeps the heart beating, and methylprednisolone reduces swelling of the bronchial tree, enabling the patient to breath.

1-102. Which of the following emergency response drugs stimulate the sympathetic nervous system?

A. Benadryl

B. Adrenaline

C. Solu-Medrol

D. Dramamine

Discussion: Adrenaline, also known as epinephrine, stimulates the sympathetic nervous system and keeps the heart beating.

1-103. Which of the following drugs is sometimes administered prior to the test, in conjunction with steroids, in patients with a history of allergic reaction to contrast?

A. Benadryl

B. Adrenaline

C. Solu-Medrol

D. Dramamine

Discussion: Benadryl, also known as diphenhydramine, disrupts the histamine response and can lessen the chance of an allergic reaction to contrast.

1-104. The first step to be taken with a potential cardiac or respiratory arrest is to:

- **A. Perform an initial "shake and shout" to determine if the patient is truly unresponsive**
- B. Initiate a code blue
- C. Initiate a medical rapid response
- D. Begin CPR

Discussion: CPR should not be initiated until it has been determined that the patient is unresponsive. This is done via the "shake and shout." Only when it is determined the patient is unresponsive should the medical rapid response/code blue be activated and CPR initiated.

1-105. If available, which of the following could be deployed before the arrival of the code team?

- A. A ventilator
- B. Intra-aortic balloon pump
- **C. External defibrillator**
- D. External pacemaker

Discussion: If available, an external defibrillator can be applied to the patient and deployed prior to the arrival of the internal code team. External pacemakers, intra-aortic balloon pumps, and ventilators require special training and cannot be used by lay staff.

1-106. The most important role in aiding a patient experiencing a seizure is:

- A. Insert something in their mouth so they don't bite their tongue
- **B. Prevent them from harming themselves**
- C. Restrain them so they can't bang into furniture
- D. Get an IV started so medication can be administered quickly

Discussion: When a patient or other individual is having a seizure, the most important thing to do is prevent them from harming themselves. Do not attempt to stick anything in their mouth; that is old thinking and causes more harm. It is also inappropriate to restrain them because restraints are unlawful without a physician's order and difficult to apply to a seizing patient. Starting an IV should never be attempted on a seizing patient. The risk of needle stick is far too great and the likelihood of success far too low.

1-107. ________ used in MRI can lead to focal hotspots in the patient's tissues.

- A. Rapidly switching gradient magnetic fields
- B. High-power static magnetic fields
- **C. High-frequency radio waves**
- D. Physiologic monitoring equipment

Discussion: High-frequency radio waves can be deposited into the tissues leading to focal hotspots. Rapidly switching gradient fields are primarily responsible for acoustic noise, peripheral nerve stimulation, and active implant impairment. Physiologic monitoring equipment receives information from the patient and gives nothing back as a general rule.

1-108. Important precautions to take to prevent RF burns include:

- A. Padding the patient to prevent skin-to-bore contact
- B. Padding the patient to prevent skin-to-skin contact
- C. Positioning the patient to eliminate conductive body loops
- D. Precooling the patient with ice bags
- **E. A, B and C**

Discussion: Padding and positioning are two of the most important aspects of patient safety. Patients should never contact the bore, have skin-to-skin contact, or any conductive body loops. Precooling the patient with ice bags would be ineffective against a rapid rise in local temperature.

1-109. ________ is the agency of the government responsible for ensuring workplace safety.

A. **OSHA**

B. FDA

C. NIH

D. CDC

Discussion: The Occupational Safety and Health Administration (OSHA) is the government agency responsible for ensuring safety in the workplace. The FDA oversees medical devices and drugs, the NIH conducts research into living systems and the diseases that affect them, and the CDC monitors biostatistics on diseases in the nation.

1-110. OSHA requires that eye-wash stations be accessible in areas where:

A. Patients are scanned

B. Intravenous contrast is used

C. Traditional sinks are inconvenient

D. **Hazardous or corrosive chemicals are used**

Discussion: To enhance worker safety, OSHA requires that eye-wash stations be accessible in any areas where hazardous or corrosive chemicals are used.

1-111. If an eye-wash station is unavailable:

A. **Any running water will suffice**

B. Use saline from a flush syringe

C. Rub the eyes with a clean dry cloth

D. Lie down with the eyes closed for 15 minutes

Discussion: In the event of a chemical splash to the eye and an eye-wash station is unavailable, any running water will suffice.

1-112. When a chemical splash to the eye occurs, it is imperative to:

A. Wipe away all of the splash chemical as soon as possible with a clean dry cloth

B. **Flush the eye with running water from an eye-wash station or sink for 5 minutes**

C. Call poison control and see what you should do

D. Immediately file an incident report with the EPA

Discussion: In the event of a chemical to the eye, it is imperative to flush the eye with running water from an eye-wash station or sink for a minimum of 5 minutes. Never try and wipe chemicals out of the eye with a dry cloth. Filing an incident report is important, but not before proper medical treatment to the eye is obtained.

1-113. ________ gloves are impervious to most chemical substances and are preferred when handling hazardous or corrosive chemicals.

A. **Nitrile**

B. Polypropylene

C. Vinyl

D. Latex

Discussion: When handling corrosive or caustic chemicals, nitrile gloves are preferred because they are impervious to most chemicals.

1-114. The safe disposal of hazardous waste is controlled by this government agency:

A. OSHA

B. The Centers for Disease Control and Prevention

C. **Environmental Protection Agency**

D. Greenpeace

Discussion: The Environmental Protection Agency controls and governs the disposal of all hazardous and toxic waste.

1-115. Chemical spills in the department are dangerous for the following reason:

A. Risk or danger of injury from falls

B. Exposure to potentially hazardous chemicals

C. They can ruin the floor

D. **Both A and B**

Discussion: Chemical spills in the department are dangerous because they expose patients and staff to potentially hazardous chemicals. In addition, the spill increases the risk of injury from slips and falls. While spilled chemicals can ruin the floor, it is not really considered a danger.

1-116. Specialized equipment kept in a department for dealing with spill incidents is called:

A. Bucket and mop

B. Spill kit

C. Janitor supplies

D. EPA go bag

Discussion: The specialized equipment kept in a department to deal with spills is called a spill kit. This kit may include janitorial supplies and a bucket and mop, but it also includes other specialized equipment for dealing with chemical spills.

1-117. All containers used in a healthcare facility are required to be labeled with this:

A. The contents of the container

B. Any hazards posed by the contents of the container

C. A Mr. Yuck sticker

D. Both A and B

Discussion: Any container used in a healthcare facility, regardless of the contents, is required to be labeled with both the contents of the container and any hazardous conditions posed by the contents.

1-118. The ________ lists the hazardous ingredients of a product, its flammability, its effect on human health, safe-handling instructions, and emergency and first aid instructions.

A. EPA report

B. Material safety data sheet (MSDS)

C. Oh crap document

D. OSHA reactivity report

Discussion: The list of the hazardous ingredients of a product, its flammability, its effect on human health, its safe-handling instructions, and emergency and first aid instructions are all listed on the document called the material safety data sheet (MSDS).

1-119. Microorganisms capable of causing disease are called:

A. Toxins

B. Chemical agents

C. Pathogens

D. Pathologics

Discussion: Any microorganism capable of causing disease is referred to as a pathogen.

1-120. The mouth, nose, urethra, vagina, and anus area are all:

A. Portals of infection

B. Portals to disease

C. Portals of exit

D. Frequently contacted in MRI

Discussion: The mouth, nose, urethra, vagina, and anus are all portals of exit. This means these are all ways a pathogen can leave the body of an infected person.

1-121. People with reduced resistance to infection are termed:

A. Vectors

B. Reservoirs of infection

C. Susceptible hosts

D. Immunolimited

Discussion: Those with reduced resistance to infection are often referred to as susceptible hosts. Reduced resistance can be natural or the result of a disease process, medical treatment, or exposure to unique pathogens.

1-122. As a method of disease transmission, direct contact means:

A. Physical touch

B. Droplets landing on your skin

C. Getting physically bitten by a diseased insect

D. Particles directly contacting your eye

Discussion: With respect to disease transmission, direct contact means physically touching the patient.

1-123. Droplets, vehicles, fomites, and vectors are all methods of:

A. Direct transmission

B. Indirect transmission

C. Portals of entry

D. Portals of exit

Discussion: Indirect transmission can occur between an infected individual and a susceptible host by droplets, vehicles, fomites, or vectors.

1-124. The asepsis technique that reduces the number of pathogens is:

A. Medical asepsis

B. Surgical asepsis

C. Sterilization

D. Medical cleansing

Discussion: The definition of medical asepsis is the reduction in the number of pathogens.

1-125. Hand washing or the use of alcohol-based hand gels is a type of:

A. Medical asepsis

B. Surgical asepsis

C. Sterilization

D. Medical cleansing

Discussion: Both handwashing and the use of alcohol-based hand gels are types of medical asepsis. They can be used interchangeably as long as the hands are not visibly soiled.

1-126. Alcohol-based hand gels are acceptable as long as hands are not:

A. Chapped or cracked

B. Visibly soiled

C. Infected

D. Both A and B

Discussion: Alcohol-based hand gels are acceptable as long as the hands are not visibly soiled. If blood or body fluids are visible on the skin, the hands should be washed with warm water and soap for a minimum of 20 seconds.

1-127. Gowns, gloves, masks, and face shields are all types of:

A. Professional proactive equipment (PPE)

B. Professional protection equipment (PPE)

C. Personal protective equipment (PPE)

D. FDA level two gear

Discussion: Gloves, gowns, masks, and face shields are all types of personal protective equipment (PPE).

1-128. Gloves should be changed and hands washed after:

A. Every failed IV attempt

B. Every patient

C. Every time the hands go below the waist

D. Both A and B

Discussion: Gloves should be changed and hands washed after every patient. Gloves should never be worn while going from department to department or in and out of patient rooms.

1-129. *C. diff*, *E. coli*, and scabies are pathogens that require ________ precautions.

A. Hand-washing

B. Contact

C. Airborne

D. Droplet

Discussion: *C. diff*, *E. coli*, and scabies are all pathogens that require contact precautions.

1-130. Meningitis, pneumonia, and pertussis are pathogens that require ________ precautions.

A. Airborne

B. Contact

C. Droplet

D. Hand-washing

Discussion: Meningitis, pneumonia, and pertussis are pathogens that all require droplet precautions.

1-131. Measles, varicella, and tuberculosis are pathogens that require ________ precautions.

A. Hand-washing

B. Contact

C. Airborne

D. Droplet

Discussion: Measles, varicella, and tuberculosis are pathogens that all require airborne precautions.

1-132. The ________ monitors and studies the types of infections occurring in the nation.

A. CDC

B. FDA

C. NIH

D. OSHA

Discussion: The governmental agency responsible for monitoring and studying the types of infections occurring in the nation is the Centers for Disease Control and Prevention (CDC).

1-133. ________ is the agency of the government responsible for ensuring workplace safety.

A. OSHA

B. FDA

C. NIH

D. CDC

Discussion: The governmental agency responsible for ensuring safety in the workplace is the Occupational Safety and Health Administration (OSHA).

1-134. If a patient has been sedated with Valium, he/she should be monitored by:

A. Pulse oximeter

B. Cardiac gating

C. Respiratory gating

D. All of the above

Discussion: The type of monitoring to be used for any patient depends on the patient's condition. If the patient has been given a sedative, such as Valium, that could impact respiratory rate, and thus the respiratory function should be monitored. This is done by measuring oxygen concentration in the blood by pulse oximetry. Respiratory gating is not used for monitoring the patient but for controlling physiologic respiratory motion during the data-acquisition process.

1-135. Patients who may require additional monitoring during an MRI procedure include:

A. Unresponsive and uncommunicative patients

B. Sedated, psychiatric, and pediatric patients

C. Patients who have weak voices and/or impaired hearing

D. Both A and B

E. A, B, and C

Discussion: While all patients should be monitored verbally and visually, some patients require additional monitoring. Those patients include anyone who might be unresponsive or uncommunicative, or someone who has been sedated, has a weak voice, is hearing impaired, and is a psychiatric or pediatric patient. The type of additional monitoring varies and could include things such as pulse oximetry, noninvasive blood pressure, and ECG.

1-136. Diaphoresis is a medical term that means:

A. Profuse coughing

B. Profuse sweating

C. Profuse vomiting

D. Increased heart rate

Discussion: Diaphoresis is a medical term that means profuse sweating. It is the body's way of trying to dissipate heat and regulate body temperature.

1-137. All of the following are routes used to take a body's temperature except:

A. Brachial

B. Axillary

C. Temporal

D. Oral

Discussion: The five routes commonly used to measure the body's core temperature are axillary, temporal, tympanic, rectal, and oral.

1-138. ________ is considered a normal adult resting pulse rate.

A. 40–100 bpm

B. 60–100 bpm

C. 70–100 bpm

D. 90–100 bpm

Discussion: Pulse rates measure the rapidity of each heart contraction in beats per minute. Normal adult resting pulse rates range from 60–100 bpm.

1-139. The systolic pressure of a healthy adult would not exceed:

A. 90 mm Hg

B. 100 mm Hg

C. 120 mm Hg

D. 130 mm Hg

Discussion: Normal blood pressure for a healthy adult would not exceed a systolic pressure of 120 mm Hg.

1-140. Pulse rates exceeding 100 bpm are termed:

A. Hypocardia

B. Bradycardia

C. Hypercardia

D. Tachycardia

Discussion: Pulse rates/heart contractions exceeding 100 bpm are termed tachycardia.

1-141. A branch of science that applies the laws of physics to living creatures is:

A. Biometrics

B. Biomechanics

C. Biology

D. Biodynamics

Discussion: The branch of science that applies the laws of physics to living creatures is called biomechanics. Biomechanics looks at the action of forces on the body in both rest and motion.

1-142. The following are all a technologist's priority during a medical emergency except:

A. Make sure the airway is open

B. Remove the patient from the magnetic field

C. Take measures to prevent shock

D. Administer medications to the patient

Discussion: An MRI technologist should be able to contribute to the well-being of the patient in their care. Technologists should keep these priorities in mind when working with patients during medical emergencies. These things should be a priority of the technologist: ensure an open airway, control bleeding, take measures to prevent or treat shock, remove patient from the magnetic field, attend to wounds or fractures, provide emotional support, and continually reevaluate. It is not within the scope of practice of a technologist to administer any medication to patients.

1-143. Restlessness, apprehension, tachycardia, decreasing blood pressure, and cold and clammy skin are indications of which of the following medical emergencies?

A. Contrast media reaction

B. Shock

C. Cardiac arrest

D. Diabetic crisis

Discussion: Signs and symptoms that a patient might be going into shock include restlessness, apprehension, tachycardia, decreasing blood pressure, cold and clammy skin, and pallor. If a patient starts to exhibit this situation, the patient should be immediately removed from the magnetic field and the patient's medical team alerted.

1-144. A tube used for gastric decompression is called:

A. Nasogastric tube

B. J-tube

C. Endotracheal tube

D. Feeding tube

Discussion: Nasogastric tubes are rubber or plastic tubes inserted through the patient's nasopharynx into the stomach. It is used to decompress the patient's stomach and to remove flatus and fluids.

1-145. Urinary collection bags should be kept where during imaging procedures?

A. Above the patient's head

B. Below the patient's heart

C. Below the patient's bladder

D. Urinary collection bags should be removed prior to MRI

Discussion: A patient's urine collection bag should be kept as low as possible, below the level of the patient's bladder, to prevent reflux of urine back into the bladder, which can lead to urinary tract infections.

ARRT Mock Boards

Content Category B. Safety

2-1. Which persons should be educated about the effects of the static magnetic field, especially in high-field superconducting magnets?

- **A.** The nursing staff and the code team
- **B.** The housekeeping staff and the fire department
- **C.** The anesthesiology and respiratory therapy department
- **D.** Both A and B
- **E.** **A, B, and C**

Discussion: It is important that anyone entering or potentially entering the MRI environment be educated about the dangers associated with the static magnetic field, especially as it pertains to projectiles and implants in foreign bodies.

2-2. Family members and ancillary personnel accompanying the patient into the scan room _________.

- **A.** need not be screened as they are not to undergo MR imaging
- **B.** can enter the scan room to check on the patient but cannot stay for the procedure
- **C.** **should be screened as if they are having the procedure themselves**
- **D.** must wear a lead apron during the procedure

Discussion: The patient and anyone accompanying the patient into Zone IV must be screened as if they are having a procedure themselves. The atlas, your magnitude, or anyone remaining in Zone IV during active scanning could potentially be exposed to the static, time-varying, and RF-magnetic fields.

2-3. Why is RF shielding used in MRI?

- **A.** To minimize patient heating
- **B.** To confine the magnetic field to the scan room
- **C.** **To attenuate external RF**
- **D.** To maintain magnetic homogeneity

Discussion: RF shielding, sometimes called a Faraday cage, is used to attenuate external RF, which could interfere with the imaging process. For effective imaging, precise transmission of RF energy at a precise frequency is transmitted into the patient. Any extraneous RF could interfere with this process, cause artifacts, and degrade image quality.

2-4. Cool scan-room temperatures are preferred because they:

- **A.** Reduce cryogen boil-off
- **B.** Increase RF transmission
- **C.** Keep the gradients cool
- **D.** **Reduce patient heating**

Discussion: Because MRI deposits energy in the tissues, some heating is inevitable. By maintaining a cooler scan room, patient heating is reduced and patient comfort is increased. For patients who are too cool, a blanket can always be added.

2-5. Which of the following is not a property of helium gas?

- **A.** Metallic taste
- **B.** **Smells like rotten eggs**
- **C.** Extremely cold
- **D.** Displaces oxygen

Discussion: Helium gas is extremely cold, displaces oxygen, and does have a slight metallic taste when inhaled. The smell of rotten eggs is not a property of helium gas; in general, it is often added artificially to help detect leaks. This is not generally done for helium.

2-6. When imaging an infant below 8 kg, a warning window pops up stating that you cannot use presaturation pulses. The reason for this is:

A. Decibel levels will be too high

B. SAR levels will be too high

C. Gradient heating will be too high

D. Homogeneity is not good enough

Discussion: Specific absorption rate (SAR) is a mass-normalized rate of RF deposition into the patient's tissues, as estimated by the scanner software. With low-mass patients such as children and infants, the RF deposition can often exceed the absorption capacity based on FDA limits. Spatial presaturation pulses are additional RF pulses applied prior to the imaging sequence to oversaturate, or eliminate, signal from a specific anatomic area. Sometimes these additional sequences simply add too much RF and cannot be used.

2-7. Which of the following does not have an FDA limit?

A. SAR

B. Db/T

C. Static field strength

D. Scan time

Discussion: The FDA sets limits on the static magnetic field strength (B_0), RF power (B_1) in the form of SAR/B1+rms, and gradient switching in the form of the nebulous painful peripheral nerve stimulation. The FDA does not regulate scan time.

2-8. The FDA limit for SAR is:

A. 2.0 W/kg whole-body average in normal operating mode per 15 minutes

B. 3.2 W/kg head average in normal operating mode per 10 minutes

C. 4.0 W/kg whole-body average in first level controlled operating mode per 15 minutes

D. 3.2 W/kg whole-body average in first level controlled operating mode per 10 minutes

E. All of the above

Discussion: The FDA sets limits on the RF power in the form of SAR limitations. These limitations are based on body part exposed as well as the operating level used by the scanner. Normal operating mode is the default position and with it comes the most restrictive SAR limitations of 2.0 W/kg whole-body average and 3.2 W/kg head average over 15 and 10 minutes, respectively. Changing to first level controlled operating mode increases the SAR limits to 4.0 W/kg whole-body average per 15 minute scanning. Head SAR limitations do not change between normal operating mode and first level controlled mode.

2-9. The following items are usually allowed to enter the scan room in high-magnetic-field systems:

A. Surgical stainless steel hemostats

B. Surgical stainless steel scissors

C. Bronze tools

D. All of the above

Discussion: Surgical stainless steel may or may not be ferrous. Bronze tools have traditionally been considered safe for use in MRI, so it should be noted that more modern tools made from stainless alloys are preferred. This question is dated but still valid.

2-10. Absolute contraindications for MRI include:

A. Cardiac pacemaker

B. Pregnancy

C. Ferrous intracranial aneurysm clips

D. Both A and C

Discussion: This question has gotten complicated. While ferrous intracranial aneurysm clips are fairly straightforward, pacemakers have gotten quite complex. The question does not refer to MRI conditional pacemakers and, in general terms, standard pacemakers are still contraindicated as a matter of policy for most facilities. This is not to say many facilities don't scan them, but this is not the norm.

2-11. Patients with a GFR above 60 can:

A. Be given IV contrast as clinically appropriate

B. Receive the test without contrast to avoid further kidney damage

C. Be given an alternative and safer agent

D. None of the above

Discussion: GFR (glomerular filtration rate) is the most commonly accepted measure for kidney function. Above 60 is considered very healthy kidneys and, therefore, no limits are placed on contrast administration. It should be noted that contrast administration also depends on the group of agents being administered, with some groups requiring blood testing and other groups, due to their safety profile, not requiring the need for prior blood tests, such as GFR.

2-12. A trauma patient arrives in the department for an emergent MRI of the cervical spine to assess spinal cord damage. Which of the following is the safest method for screening the patient?

A. The exam is emergent, so screening is not critical

B. Ask the patient and her family about her medical history

C. Visually inspect her chest and abdomen for scars

D. Proceed and hope for the best

Discussion: The first step in screening any patient is to ask the patient screening questions. Trauma patients are often able to answer questions regarding their own history, and this should always be the first step. If the patient is unresponsive, unable to communicate, or otherwise unable to be questioned, then we move on to family members, screening, radiographs, etc.

2-13. Before a patient enters the MRI environment, they should be screened for:

A. Prior injuries

B. Prior surgical implants

C. Pregnancy

D. All of the above

Discussion: It is important to understand the medical history of any patient presenting for MRI. Prior injuries may involve the placement of surgical metal, surgical implants may be unsafe for MRI, and pregnancy may preclude the use of contrast.

2-14. When used for MR imaging, cables from RF coils and ECG leads should be _________.

A. thermally and electrically isolated

B. laying along the patient's right arm along the bore

C. formed into loops within the imager

D. neatly coiled and ready for use

Discussion: Isolating all cables, leads, and conductors, both thermally and electrically, prevents them from causing harm to the patient should they heat.

2-15. The cable of a surface coil poses a danger to the patient when it:

A. Is frayed and in disrepair

B. Touches the patient

C. Forms a loop

D. All of the above

Discussion: As a general rule, cables are conductors. As such, if they are frayed or in disrepair, touch the patient, or form a loop, they present burn danger.

2-16. Passive magnetic shielding can be achieved by lining the MRI room with _________.

A. copper

B. steel

C. lead

D. None of the above

Discussion: Passive magnetic shielding means adding a barrier to the magnetic field to keep it contained as close as possible to Zone IV. Traditional passive magnetic shielding is done with steel in the walls or concrete. Copper is used for RF shielding. Lead generally applies to radiographic rooms.

2-17. During a quench, patients and operators should be evacuated from the room to avoid _________.

A. asphyxiation and frostbite

B. subarachnoid hemorrhage

C. ruptured tympanic membranes

D. Both A and C

E. All of the above

Discussion: During a quench, is it possible for helium gas to be released into the room should the quench fail. As such, patients should be evacuated as helium displaces oxygen, which could lead to asphyxiation, is very cold and could lead to frostbite, and can increase pressure in the room, which could cause ruptured tympanic membranes. Though the pressure increase can be significant, subarachnoid hemorrhage is not possible.

2-18. The predominant biological effect of radio frequency fields is ________.

A. induced voltages

B. tissue heating

C. hypothermia

D. All of the above

Discussion: The predominant biological effect of radio frequency fields is tissue heating due to resistive losses.

2-19. In the United States, the FDA limits the allowable amount of radio frequency absorption to ________.

A. 0.4 W/kg

B. 4 W/kg

C. 2 W/kg

D. There is no FDA limit

Discussion: The original FDA limit was 0.4 W/kg. That number was increased to the current 4.0 W/kg. It should be noted that 4.0 W/kg is for first-level monitoring of the whole body only. The head is limited to 3.2 W/kg per 15 minutes in both normal mode and first-level operating mode.

2-20. A deliberate quench can be used to:

A. Temper the magnet to improve image quality

B. Rapidly remove the gradient fields

C. Prevent RF burns

D. Rapidly remove the main magnetic field

Discussion: The only reason to ever quench a magnet deliberately is to rapidly remove the main magnetic field. The quench has no effect on RF or gradient fields. A deliberate quench should only be done when someone is trapped and is an immediate danger.

2-21. The unit of measure of radio frequency absorption is known as the:

A. Sensitive Acquisition Range (SAR)

B. Specific Absorption Rate (SAR)

C. Susceptibility Attack Region (SAR)

D. None of the above

Discussion: SAR, the specific absorption rate, is the mass-normalized rate of energy deposition in the tissues, as estimated by the scanner software.

2-22. Radio frequency absorption is measured in ________.

A. watts per pound

B. volts per pound

C. watts per kilogram

D. volts per kilogram

Discussion: SAR is measured in watts per kilogram. There are no other units used.

2-23. Radio frequency energy is:

A. High-energy ionizing radiation

B. High-energy nonionizing radiation

C. Low-energy nonionizing radiation

D. Low-energy ionizing radiation

Discussion: The RF energy used in MRI is low-energy, nonionizing radiation.

2-24. The unit of measure for hardware output of radio-frequency energy is:

A. SAR

B. SED

C. B1+rms

D. ALARA

Discussion: B1+rms (root mean squared) is a measure of the RF output of the scanner. Unlike SAR, B1+rms is not estimated and is more accurate and precise.

2-25. The accumulated dose of RF energy in the tissues over time is calculated as:

A. SAR

B. **SED**

C. B1+rms

D. ALARA

Discussion: SED is SAR multiplied by the actual scan time. It is an accurate representation of the cumulative dose of RF delivered to the patient over the course of the exam.

2-26. The total cumulative dose of RF as calculated for each patient is known as:

A. **Specific energy dose**

B. Solenoid energy dose

C. Survivable energy dose

D. Cumulative dose is not calculated; it is measured with the RF probe

Discussion: SED (specific energy dose) is SAR multiplied by the actual scan time. It is an accurate representation of the cumulative dose of RF delivered to the patient over the course of the exam.

2-27. The unit of measure for specific energy dose is:

A. **Joules/kg**

B. Gauss/cm

C. Tesla/meter/sec

D. Watts/kg

Discussion: SED, or specific energy dose, is measured in joules per kilogram. The recommendation from the International Electrotechnical Commission, and most manufacturers, is that SED should be limited to 14,400 J/kg.

2-28. The International Electrotechnical Commission sets the limit of energy dose per patient per 24 hours to:

A. 5,280 J/kg

B. 4.0 J/kg

C. **14,400 J/kg**

D. There is no 24-hour limit

Discussion: SED, or specific energy dose, is measured in joules per kilogram. The recommendation from the International Electrotechnical Commission, and most manufacturers, is that SED should be limited to 14,400 J/kg.

2-29. The field strength at isocenter is measured in units of _________.

A. Gauss

B. **Tesla**

C. Watts

D. SAR

Discussion: The magnetic field at isocenter of the magnet is measured in tesla.

2-30. A magnetic field strength of 1 tesla is equal to:

A. 1,000 G

B. **10,000 G**

C. 100,000 G

D. 1 G

Discussion: 1 tesla is equal to 10,000 gauss.

2-31. The unusable magnetic field outside the scanner is call the:

A. **Fringe field**

B. Stray field

C. Scatter field

D. Faraday field

Discussion: The magnetic field used for imaging is found exclusively inside the bore of the scanner. The magnetic field that extends beyond the scanner, and which is clinically unusable, is called the fringe field.

2-32. Magnetic field strength outside the imager is usually measured in:

A. **Gauss**

B. Tesla

C. Watts

D. SAR

Discussion: The MRI fringe field, the magnetic field outside of the scan bore, is measured in gauss.

2-33. The attractive force that a projectile will experience is dependent upon:

A. The ferromagnetic properties of the object

B. The mass of the object

C. The field strength of the MRI unit

D. **All of the above**

Discussion: The more ferromagnetic an object, the greater the potential attractive force. The greater the mass of the object, the greater the potential attractive force. The larger the field strength of the magnet, the greater the potential attractive force.

2-34. The greatest concern about fringe field exists with which type of scanner?

A. Mid-field superconducting

B. Low-field resistive

C. High-field superconducting

D. Low-field permanent

Discussion: Superconducting magnets have the strongest magnetic field (B_0) and, therefore, the greatest potential for fringe field. The actual fringe field present varies with the type of magnetic shielding used, i.e., active versus passive, etc.

2-35. The most generally accepted method for screening patients for the presence of intraocular ferrous foreign bodies is:

A. CT

B. MRI

C. Plain film

D. Visual examination

Discussion: A detailed and proper history is the best way to determine patients who may be at risk for intraocular foreign bodies. That said, when a screening tool is required, plane films (radiographs) are the best tool. CT is overkill and MRI is inappropriate until the orbits are clear. While a two-view orbit has been the norm for many years, the American College of Radiology has recently changed its recommendation to a single-view orbit.

2-36. The percentage of patients reported to have adverse reactions to gadolinium contrast agents is:

A. 0.07–2.4%

B. 10%

C. 5%

D. 20%

Discussion: According to the 2021 American College of Radiology manual and contrast media page 79, the overall adverse rate of reactions for gadolinium-based contrast media administered at clinical doses ranges from 0.07% to 2.4%.

2-37. Patients who are at an increased risk of mild reactions to gadolinium are patients with:

A. A history of asthma and or allergies

B. Prior contrast reactions

C. No known medical history

D. Both A and B

E. a, b, and c

Discussion: According to the 2021 American College of Radiology manual and contrast media page 79, patients with a history of prior adverse reaction to gadolinium-based contrast media are at approximately eight times higher risk. Patients with asthma or other allergies have an increased risk, though that increased risk is mild.

2-38. For optimum operation of the MRI systems, the ambient temperature and relative humidity should remain between:

A. 30°F and 50°F/30% and 50%

B. 65°F and 75°F/50% and 70%

C. 70°F and 50°F/90% and 50%

D. None specified

Discussion: For efficient operation and to minimize static electricity, the optimum range of temperature and humidity should be 65–75°F and 50–70% ambient humidity.

2-39. The FDA limit for the static field is __________.

(For clinical imaging of patients to include: babies over 1 month of age, children, and adults.)

A. 2.0 T

B. 3.0 T

C. 4.0 T

D. 8.0 T

Discussion: 8 T is approved for babies 1 month of age up through adults. 4 T is approved for infants and neonates under 1 month of age as of July 2004, when the Food and Drug Administration (FDA) changed the limits.

2-40. Patient screening in MRI should be performed:

A. Once (complete the form only)

B. Once by anyone

C. More than once, by anyone

D. More than once, by trained professionals

Discussion: Screening is a multistep process that should be completed several times by trained professionals. While early screening at the time of scheduling can be done by non-MRI personnel, the ultimate and final screening before entering Zone IV must be done by level 2 personnel only.

2-41. It is __________ for all patients to be provided with hearing protection in the form of __________.

A. Required/headphones or earplugs

B. Recommended/headphones or earplugs

C. Required/head coil

D. Recommended/helmet

Discussion: It is recommended that all patients be provided hearing protection in the form of headphones or earplugs. At 1.5 T and below, headphones or earplugs are acceptable; at 3 T and above, headphones *and* earplugs are generally recommended. There is no requirement for hearing protection; this is merely a best practice.

2-42. The FDA limit for the static field is __________ for infants and children up to 1 month.

A. 2 T

B. 3 T

C. 4 T

D. 8 T

Discussion: 8 T is approved for babies 1 month of age up through adults. 4 T is approved for infants and neonates under 1 month of age.

2-43. The general public is limited to a magnetic field of:

A. 5 gauss

B. 10 gauss

C. 15 gauss

D. There is no limit

Discussion: 5 gauss has been the fringe field exposure limit for many years. However, in 2022, that number was increased to 9 gauss. If 9 gauss is one of the choices, then 9 gauss is the correct answer, but it may take a few years for that number to work its way into the boards.

2-44. The gradient magnetic fields __________.

A. augment the main magnetic field

B. can produce noise sufficient to cause temporary hearing loss

C. change rapidly during the scanning process

D. All of the above

Discussion: The primary function of the gradients is spatial localization. They do this by augmenting the main magnetic field in the X, Y, and Z directions. They are cycled on and off rapidly during the imaging sequence and one of the main consequences of this is acoustic noise.

2-45. The "effect" whereby the patient experiences a visual stimulation that gives the impression of seeing "stars in their eyes" is known as:

A. Magnetohydrodynamic effect

B. Magnet-hydrodynamic effect

C. Magnet-hemodynamic effect

D. Magnetophosphenes

Discussion: Magnetophosphenes are flashes of light caused by electromagnetically induced stimulation of the retina of the eye. Hydrodynamic effect is the elevated ST segment on the patient's ECG in response to induced currents in the magnetic field.

2-46. The FDA limit on time-varying magnetic fields is:

A. 10 G/cm

B. 6 T/sec

C. 1 G/cm

D. Below the level of painful peripheral nerve stimulation

Discussion: Though not very scientific or precise, the FDA limit of gradient fields is below the level of painful peripheral nerve stimulation.

2-47. Time-varied magnetic field (TVMF) effects include all of the following EXCEPT:

A. Heat and increased body temperature

B. Acoustic noise and hearing loss

C. Peripheral nerve stimulation and tingling

D. Magnetophosphenes and stars in the eyes

Discussion: Acoustic noise, hearing loss, and peripheral nerve stimulation and tingling are all potential effects of time-varying/gradient magnetic fields. Increased heat and body temperature are generally associated with the B_1 or RF magnetic field.

2-48. TVMF/gradient magnetic fields affect patient safety because they can:

A. Induce current in any local conductor

B. Produce significant RF energy

C. Cause short-term memory loss

D. All of the above

Discussion: Time-varying magnetic fields (TVMF) can induce occurrence in any conductor. They also have the potential to disrupt active implants.

2-49. RF shielding can be achieved by lining the scanner room walls with:

A. Copper

B. Steel

C. Lead

D. None of the above

Discussion: Most vendors achieve RF shielding with rolled copper sheeting. It is possible to shield RF with galvanized steel, but that is far less common.

2-50. Two areas of the body that do not dissipate heat from SAR efficiently are:

A. Face and neck

B. Brain and abdomen

C. Eyes and testicles

D. None of the above

Discussion: While most tissues in the body have excellent thermoregulatory ability, the eyes and the testicles both have poor capillary networks at the core and, therefore, do not dissipate heat efficiently.

2-51. The liquid cryogen commonly used to maintain the field strength in a superconducting MRI unit is:

A. Helium

B. Hydrogen

C. Nitrogen

D. None of the above

Discussion: Helium is the most commonly used cryogen for cooling superconducting magnets. While some older magnets used to have dual chambers for helium and nitrogen, this is not found in modern systems. Hydrogen is far too volatile and explosive.

2-52. Safety concerns associated with a superconducting electromagnet versus a permanent magnet are:

A. Higher fringe fields due to the system configuration

B. Colder temperature in the scan room due to the presence of cryogens

C. There is no difference in safety concerns between the two MRI systems

D. Sighting issues due to its heavier weight

Discussion: When compared with a permanent magnet, the primary safety concern of superconducting magnets is the higher fringe field due to the larger magnetic field strength. It should be noted that the fringe field varies with the type of magnetic shielding. While cryogens are indeed cold, under normal operating conditions, they are never found in the scan room.

2-53. The cryogens of the MRI system are used:

A. In conjunction with a constant source of power to maintain the MRI units field strength

B. To decrease the resistance in the loops of wire so that a constant source of power is not required to maintain the main magnetic field

C. As a cooling system to counteract the biological effects of radio frequency absorption in the patient

D. To cool the shim system as well as maintain the system's main magnetic field strength

Discussion: The function of the cryogens is to decrease the resistance in the loops of wire so that a constant source of power is not required to maintain the main magnetic field. This, of course, only applies to superconducting electromagnets.

2-54. Active shielding:

A. Uses steel to reduce the fringe field

B. Uses additional coils to reduce the fringe field

C. Uses both steel and coils to reduce the fringe field

D. Uses current to maintain the shim system

Discussion: Active shielding uses additional coils, called bucking coils, to oppose the static magnetic field, thereby reducing the fringe field.

2-55. In MRI, there are safety considerations associated with __________ type(s) of magnetic field(s) including __________.

A. one/main magnet or static magnetic field

B. two/main magnet or static magnetic field, and the radio frequency (RF) field

C. three/main magnet or static magnetic field, the radio frequency (RF) field, and time-varied magnetic field (TVMF)/the gradient field

D. four/main magnet or static magnetic field, the radio frequency (RF) field, time-varied magnetic field (TVMF)/the gradient field, and the shim field

Discussion: The static magnetic field has safety considerations for translational and rotational forces, the radio frequency field has safety concerns for tissue heating in resonant circuitry, and the time-varied/gradient magnetic field has safety concerns for acoustic noise and damaging activation implants. The shim field has no safety concerns.

2-56. When a superconducting system rapidly and uncontrollably loses liquid helium and, subsequently, the magnetic field, this effect is known as a:

A. Quench

B. Shim

C. Ramp up

D. Prescan

Discussion: A quench is a rapid and uncontrolled boil off of cryogens in a superconducting magnet. Liquid helium is approximately –473°F and expands 760:1. While this massive volume of gas normally vents through the quench pipe to the outside atmosphere without issue, the quench pipe has failed and helium gas vents into the room.

2-57. The "effect" that occurs as projectiles fly through the air, toward the magnet, is known as the:

A. Missile effect

B. Hemodynamic effect

C. Hydrodynamic effect

D. Magnetophosphene effect

Discussion: The missile affect describes what happens to ferromagnetic objects inadvertently brought into the static magnetic field.

2-58. The safety considerations associated with a quench in a high-field superconducting magnet could include all of the following EXCEPT:

A. Asphyxia

B. Frostbite

C. Increased pressure

D. Magnetohydrodynamic effect

Discussion: During a quench, cryogenic gases are vented to the outside atmosphere. Should the quench pipe fail, it is entirely possible for those gases to escape into Zone IV. Should this happen, there is a risk of asphyxiation due to oxygen displacement, frostbite due to the extreme cold temperatures, and increased pressure due to the large volume of gases being vented into the closed room. The magnetohydrodynamic affect is a consequence of performing an ECG in the magnetic field and poses no safety concerns.

2-59. Radio frequency effects include:

A. Heat and increased body temperature

B. Acoustic damage and hearing loss

C. Peripheral nerve stimulation and tingling

D. Magnetophosphenes and stars in the eyes

Discussion: The primary effect of RF energy deposited in the body is heating and increased body temperature. Acoustic damage and hearing loss, peripheral nerve stimulation and tingling, and magnetophosphenes are primarily associated with the gradient magnetic field.

2-60. RF heating is more of a concern in _________ imaging sequences.

A. gradient echo

B. echo planar imaging

C. spin echo

D. fast spin echo

Discussion: RF heating is a consequence of the B_1 field. As such, it is more of a concern with sequences that use the most RF, such as a fast spin echo. A fast spin echo uses a 90° RF pulse followed by multiple 180° RF pulses. Each 180° pulse is approximately four times the amount of RF found in a 90° pulse. The more 180° pulses found in the sequence, i.e., the eco train length (ETL), the greater the potential for RF heating.

2-61. The FDA limits the effect of RF absorption, in normal operating mode, as an increase in core body temperature to _________.

A. 0.5–1.0°C

B. 1.5–2.0°C

C. 2.5–3.0°F

D. There is no limit

Discussion: The FDA limits RF output and absorption in several ways (SAR, SED, B_1+rms), but the effect of the RF absorption is limited to a 0.5°C increase in core body temperature in normal operating mode. First-level control mode and second-level control mode have different limits.

2-62. As the flip angle is doubled, RF deposition increases by a factor of:

A. One

B. Two

C. Three

D. Four

Discussion: Doubling the flip angle increases RF deposition by a factor of four. This is the reason fast spin echo sequences have greater power deposition than traditional spin echo or gradient-based sequences.

2-63. Imaging systems with lesser concern for fringe fields are:

A. Midfield superconducting imagers

B. Midfield resistive imagers

C. High-field superconducting imagers that are shielded

D. Low-field permanent imagers

Discussion: The imaging systems with lesser concern for fringe fields are those that use low-field permanent magnets. This is because low-field magnets have the lowest magnetic strength and, therefore, the lowest fringe field.

2-64. An acceptable method for the detection of intraocular ferrous foreign bodies is:

A. CT

B. MRI

C. Plain film

D. Visual examination

Discussion: When imaging is indicated to rule out intraocular ferrous foreign bodies, plain films are generally the preferred method. It should be noted that in 2022, the FDA changed the recommendation from two-view orbit film to single-view. This was done primarily in response to the fact that most screening orbit films failed to reveal ferrous foreign bodies. Visual examination by a trained ophthalmologist with a proper slit lamp is acceptable, but not widely available.

2-65. Which of the following scan sequences is of greater concern for TVMF effects?

A. FSE

B. EPI

C. GE

D. SE

Discussion: TVMF effects are the effects associated with time-varying or gradient magnetic fields. Therefore, these effects are greater with sequences that use more frequent and rapid-gradient switching. The most heavily gradient-intense sequences are those based on echo planar/diffusion-weighted imaging (EPI).

2-66. Of the following implants, which would be considered acceptable to scan by MRI?

A. Ferrous intracranial aneurysm clips

B. Neurostimulators

C. Cardiac pacemakers

D. Heart valves

Discussion: Heart valves are generally considered safe for MRI as the force exerted by the MRI is generally far less than that exerted by the beating heart. Ferrous intracranial aneurysm clips are never safe, and neurostimulators and cardiac pacemakers may or may not be safe depending on their type, labeling, and manufacturer's intent.

2-67. What could cause a patient to be burned during an MRI procedure?

A. A hip replacement

B. Braids in a patient's hair

C. Improperly placed cardiac leads

D. None of the above

Discussion: Hip replacements, though generally metallic, rarely pose a problem for MRI beyond their impact on image quality. Braids in a patient's hair, even when wet, are not a safety concern. Improperly placed cardiac leads, however, have been associated with burns in numerous patients.

2-68. At what decibel does instantaneous acoustic hearing loss occur?

A. 60–90 dB

B. 90–120 dB

C. 20–40 dB

D. 120–140 dB

Discussion: Instantaneous reversible hearing loss occurs at 120–140 dB. Most modern scanners are capable of reaching this level. The actual sound-pressure levels depend on the sequence and parameters used.

2-69. MRI facilities should be divided into __________ zones for safety.

A. 3

B. 4

C. 5

D. 2

Discussion: MRI facilities should be conceptually divided into four zones. While four zones are ideal, it is not always possible given available space. Special attention should be paid in Zones II–IV.

2-70. __________ is the zone that is freely accessible to the general public.

A. I

B. II

C. III

D. IV

Discussion: Zone I is freely accessible to anyone, including the general public. It includes the entirety of the world. In essence, every MRI on the planet shares the same Zone I space. For this reason, Zone I is largely irrelevant.

2-71. __________ is the zone that interfaces between the general public and the controlled space.

A. I

B. II

C. III

D. IV

Discussion: Zone II is the interface between freely accessible Zone I and the more controlled Zone III. It generally includes areas such as the reception area and changing rooms.

2-72. __________ is the area in which free access to unscreened non-MR personnel and ferromagnetic objects can result in serious injury or death.

A. I

B. II

C. III

D. IV

Discussion: Zone III is the interface between Zone II and the access-restricted Zone IV. Zone III generally includes inpatient holding areas, gowned waiting areas, and the technologist control room.

2-73. __________ is the zone that is highly access restricted to only level 2 personnel or those under direct supervision of level 2 personnel.

A. I

B. II

C. III

D. **IV**

Discussion: Zone IV is analogous to the scan room. It is where access is strictly restricted to those personnel with advanced and specific training in MRI safety, who can enter and exit freely as well as supervise others.

2-74. Zones III and IV are typically access controlled with devices that can:

A. Distinguish between MRI techs and MRI nurses

B. Distinguish between level 2 and level 3 personnel

C. **Distinguish between MR personnel and non-MR personnel**

D. Zones III and IV are not access controlled

Discussion: While locks can be quite effective, they are unable to distinguish between MR personnel and non-MR personnel, and will allow access to anyone with a key. Combination locks are slightly more effective, but still fairly agnostic. RFID readers, key cards, and biometric devices that can be programmed to allow access to personnel with the appropriate level of training are the best access-control devices.

2-75. In which zone should patients be screened and changed for their MRI procedure?

A. Zone I

B. **Zone II**

C. Zone III

D. Zone IV

Discussion: All persons and objects entering Zone III should be physically screened for the presence of ferromagnetic materials, which, irrespective of size, can become threats in proximity to the MR. It is preferred for patient privacy and protection that patients be screened and changed in Zone II.

2-76. To effectively research an implant, which of the following information is needed?

A. Device name and manufacturer

B. Device make and model

C. Device implant date

D. **All of the above**

Discussion: Researching an implant can be quite complex. Optimum information can be obtained only once device name and manufacturer information is known, as well as the device make and model and date of implant.

2-77. A device that is acceptable for use in Zone IV because it is nonferromagnetic and nonconductive can be labelled as:

A. MR compatible

B. **MR safe**

C. MR conditional

D. MR groovy

Discussion: MR compatible is an outdated term and is no longer used. MR safe means a device can be used in the MRI environment without restrictions or conditions. MR conditional means a device is safe for use in MRI when the stated conditions are followed. MR groovy does not apply.

2-78. A device that can be scanned when in a patient, as long as certain conditions are followed, can be labeled as:

A. MR compatible

B. MR safe

C. **MR conditional**

D. MR groovy

Discussion: MR compatible is an outdated term and is no longer used. MR safe means a device can be used in the MRI environment without restrictions or conditions. MR conditional means a device is safe for use in MRI when the stated conditions are followed. MR groovy does not apply.

2-79. Certain transdermal drug delivery patches can pose a danger in MRI, especially if they are:

A. Newly placed

B. For schedule 4 narcotics

C. Foil-backed

D. None of the above

Discussion: Cloth-backed patches are generally considered safe, even when in the RF field. Foil-backed patches can heat when exposed to RF. It is generally recommended to remove foil-backed patches for the MRI exam when they will be in the RF field. The decision to remove any medication patch must be made by a medical practitioner.

2-80. __________ are defined as personnel who can safely and independently enter Zone IV and clear others to do so as well.

A. Level 1 personnel

B. Level 2 personnel

C. Level 3 personnel

D. All personnel

Discussion: Level 1 personnel have the least MRI training and are aware of the basic dangers associated with the magnetic field. They cannot independently enter Zone IV, nor can they certify others to do so. Level 2 personnel have the proper training needed to independently enter Zone IV and to certify others to do so.

2-81. __________ contrast agents have no associated cases, no NSF, and pose the lowest risk for patients.

A. Group I

B. Group II

C. Group III

D. All agents pose the same risk

Discussion: Group I and III agents have both been reported to be associated with NSF. There have been no NSF cases reported with Group II agents. It should be noted that this refers to NSF only; the risk of non-NSF reactions is the same for all agents.

2-82. When should you give hearing protection to patients undergoing an MRI study?

A. Only for 3 tesla scanners and above

B. Only for patients under the age of 16

C. Hearing protection is not needed in modern scanners

D. Always

Discussion: High-intensity acoustic noise can be produced by MRI scanners, primarily by the gradient coils. Low-field systems have been measured from 82–103 dB, 1.5 tesla scanners are in the range of 114–115 dB, and 3 tesla scanners can produce 126–131 dB of noise. According to the National Institute of Deafness and Other Communication Disorders, sound level and exposure time are factors in hearing loss and whether the hearing loss will be permanent. Noise under 75 dB is unlikely to cause hearing loss, but long or repeated exposure to sounds at or above 85 dB can cause permanent hearing loss.

2-83. The rapidly changing switching gradient fields (dB/dt) can induce unwanted electrical fields throughout the human body that can result in sensory perception or muscle contraction. What is this phenomenon called?

A. Nerve entrapment

B. Peripheral nerve stimulation

C. Internal nerve stimulation

D. Peripheral nervous disorder

Discussion: Peripheral nerve stimulation (PNS) happens when conductive nerves are exposed to rapidly changing (time varying) magnetic fields (gradients). Potential for PNS depends on the strength of the gradient and the rate of change. PNS can happen in both sensory and motor nerves.

2-84. Which parameter causes the most heating in MRI?

A. Spatial gradients

B. Pulsed radio frequency

C. Gradient switching

D. Shimming

Discussion: The primary effect of RF energy on biologic tissues is heating due to resistive losses.

2-85. The magnetohydrodynamic effect is:

A. Observed elevated R wave on an ECG during an MRI scan

B. Observed elevated T wave on an ECG during an MRI scan

C. Observed a-fib on an ECG during an MRI scan

D. Observed asystole on an ECG during an MRI scan

Discussion: When a conductive fluid (i.e., blood) moves across a magnetic field, a current can be induced in the conductor according to Faraday's law. The blood leaving the heart to the aorta travels at approximately 180 cm/s. This rapid movement of a conductor coupled with the high-static magnetic field of most MRI scanners results in a phenomenon called the magnetohydrodynamic effect. It is seen as an elevation in the ST segment (T wave) on the patient's ECG. This phenomenon is clinically silent and poses no risk to the patient whatsoever. It should be noted, however, that an elevated T wave in the absence of a magnetic field can indicate myocardial infarction, ischemic heart disease, or an electrolyte imbalance.

2-86. Peripheral nerve stimulation, magnetophosphenes, and acoustic noise can be effects of:

A. Static magnetic fields

B. Electromagnetic fields

C. Time-varying magnetic fields

D. Radio frequency fields

Discussion: Time-varying magnetic fields induce a voltage within the conductor or within the human body. The health concerns are related to the strength of the gradient field as well as the rate of change.

2-87. __________ law of induction states that changing magnetic fields induce an electrical voltage in any conducting medium.

A. Maxwell's

B. Ohm's

C. Faraday's

D. Ampere's

Discussion: Faraday's law of induction states that changing magnetic fields induce an electrical voltage in any conducting medium.

2-88. Types of sequences associated with peripheral nerve stimulation include all of the following except:

A. Perfusion

B. Diffusion

C. BOLD

D. FSE

Discussion: Time-varying magnetic field effects depend on the strength, speed, and duration of the gradient pulses. Particular pulse sequences such as perfusion, diffusion, and BOLD pose an increased risk due to the increase in gradient amplitude and speed.

2-89. The force that causes ferromagnetic materials and devices to twist or torque when entering the bore of the magnet is:

A. Rotational force

B. Translational force

C. Projectile force

D. Electrical force

Discussion: The force that causes ferromagnetic materials and devices to move/twist/torque, etc., when in the proximity of a static magnetic field is called the rotational force. Rotational forces, as the name implies, cause a device or implant to rotate or twist. The extent of this rotational force depends on the ferrous makeup of the object, the geometry of the object, and the strength of the static magnetic field (B_0). Round objects, such as BBs, experience very little if any rotational force, while elongated objects experience greater force. Rotational forces are exclusively associated with the static magnetic field.

2-90. The force responsible for ferromagnetic objects being violently attracted to the MRI scanner is:

A. Rotational force

B. Translational force

C. Projectile force

D. Electrical force

Discussion: The force that causes ferromagnetic materials and devices to be attracted to the MRI scanner is called translational force. Translational force, as the name implies, causes a device or implant to translate from one point to another. The extent of this translational force depends on the ferrous makeup of the object, the strength of the static magnetic field (B_0), and the proximity of the object to the magnetic field. Translational effects are inversely proportional to the distance from the scanner. As the distance to the scanner is halved, attractive force increases by a factor of four. Translational forces are exclusively associated with the static magnetic field.

2-91. MRI screening can include all of the following except:

A. Ferromagnetic detectors

B. Fluoroscopy

C. Hand-held magnets

D. Talking to the patient

Discussion: Patient screening prior to MRI is a detailed and comprehensive process. It frequently includes an interview with the patient along with associated paperwork documenting the process, and may include the use of tools to improve the screening process like hand-held magnets and ferromagnetic detectors. Fluoroscopy is never used as a screening tool except under extreme and unique circumstances.

2-92. For what reason(s) is it advisable to have patients remove all readily removable metallic items and change into attire provided by the MRI clinic?

A. Some metal items could become a hazard to the patient in the MRI scanner

B. Some clothing contains metal fasteners, which can cause artifacts

C. Some clothing contains metallic fibers, which can be a burn risk

D. All of the above

Discussion: All persons undergoing an MRI procedure must be screened and have all readily removable metallic items and devices on or in them (e.g., jewelry, pagers, smartphones, watches, body piercings [if removable], contraceptive diaphragms, metallic drug-delivery patches) removed. Certain cosmetics contain metallic particles (such as eye makeup) and should also be removed. Reports have now also demonstrated that certain clothing items contain metallic components or threads that have resulted in burns.

2-93. What item can be brought into the MRI scanner room without checking it for safety?

A. Glasses

B. Tools

C. Floor mops

D. None of the above

Discussion: The standard of care for MRI safety means that qualified personnel check every item that enters the MRI scanner room (Zone IV).

2-94. Extra caution should be exercised when giving gadolinium chelates to persons with end-stage renal failure due to what potential adverse consequence?

A. Nephrogenic diabetes insipidus

B. Nephrogenic systemic fibrosis

C. Decreased urge to void

D. Increased urge to void

Discussion: Gadolinium-based contrast agents (GBCAs) have been associated nephrogenic systemic fibrosis in patients with acute kidney injury or severe chronic kidney disease. However, not all GBCAs are the same. Group I and III GBCAa should be avoided in at-risk groups. For inpatients, eGFR should be obtained within 48 hours of administration of Group I and III agents. Group II agents may be given as clinically appropriate.

2-95. What is the definition of MRI safe?

A. An item that has been demonstrated to pose no known hazards in a specified MRI environment with specified conditions of use

B. An item that poses no known hazards in all MRI environments

C. An item that is tested to pose no hazard in the current MRI environment

D. An item that poses no known hazards in the current MRI environment

Discussion: Terminology for labeling is from the American Society for Testing and Materials (ASTM) International and is being utilized by the FDA. For an item to be labeled as MRI safe, it must pose no known hazards in all MRI environments. MRI safe items include nonconducting, nonmetallic, nonmagnetic items, such as a plastic basin.

2-96. What is the best way to prevent conductive loops from forming in a patient's body?

A. Insulating the patient with blankets

B. Insulating the patient with sheets

C. Using nonconductive padding between body parts that may touch (e.g., legs, arms)

D. Using nonconductive padding between the patient and the bore of the wall

Discussion: The human body is full of polar molecules, free ions in solution, and ion channels, which means that our bodies are capable of electrical activity. This means patients can form electrically conductive loops within their bodies. If the loops are large enough and the contact area is small enough, burns can occur. Sheets and blankets are not made of sufficient material or thickness to prevent conduction. Nonconductive padding is the best way to prevent burns.

2-97. Monitoring sedated individuals can be performed safely in the MRI suite as long as the monitoring is performed:

A. Using the same equipment that the rest of the hospital staff is accustomed to

B. Using MRI-specific monitoring equipment

C. After checking the patient's body for any non-MRI-approved devices, cables, or patches

D. Both B and C

Discussion: No patient should ever be scanned without going through the screening process. If patients arrived to the MRI suite with monitoring equipment being used, all of the non-MRI equipment must be changed over to the MRI-approved monitoring equipment, including any ECG patches, pulse oximeters, etc., to minimize the chance of a thermal burn.

2-98. Which of the following have been attributed to causing death in MRI?

A. Cardiac pacemaker

B. Ferrous intracranial aneurysm clip

C. Ferromagnetic projectile

D. Drug infusion pump

E. All of the above

Discussion: Cardiac pacemakers, ferrous intracranial aneurysm clips, drug infusion pumps, and ferromagnetic projectiles have all been responsible for patient deaths in MRI environments.

2-99. Safety considerations of ultra-high imaging systems would include all of the following except:

A. Protocol optimization on humans and animals

B. Lack of testing of implants and devices

C. Increase in SAR and RF power

D. Lack of clinical experience

Discussion: The use of ultra-high field systems is increasing since the FDA approved clinical 7T scanners in 2017. These scanners have all the same safety concerns as lower-field scanners plus a few additional concerns, such as increased SAR/RF power deposition, lack of testing for implants, and limited clinical experience. Protocol optimization, while challenging from an image-quality standpoint, is not a safety consideration.

2-100. Wires in the bore of the MRI scanner should be positioned where to prevent burns?

A. Along the bore wall, but with a sheet between the patient and wires to prevent conductive loops

B. Away from the bore wall, but with padding between the patient and wires to prevent conductive loops

C. Away from the bore wall, but along the patient's side to prevent conductive loops

D. Along the bore wall, but with a pillow between the patient and wires to prevent conductive loops

Discussion: Any loops of conducting material in the bore of an MRI scanner must be identified to help reduce the chance of a burn. Equipment with cables attached to the patient needs to be accounted for and placed carefully in the MRI scanner. Wires in the bore of the scanner can act as an antenna and increase the heating chance. Positioning cables in close proximity to the inside wall of the MRI bore will increase the possibility of thermal injury (a consequence of the inhomogeneity of the electric field component). As the power and frequency of the pulsed RF field increase with the field strength of the magnet, thermal injuries may be more likely with high-field RF systems.

2-101. What is the ACR's recommendation on pregnant women receiving gadolinium-based contrast agents (GBCA)?

A. Case-by-case basis, and only if there is significant benefit to the patient or fetus to outweigh the unknown risk to the fetus of free gadolinium ions.

B. Case-by-case basis, and only if there is significant benefit to the patient or fetus to outweigh the moderate risks to the fetus from free gadolinium ions.

C. Use GBCAs routinely as prescribed by referring provider.

D. Use GBCAs routinely when medically necessary.

Discussion: GBCAs have been found to be teratogenic in animal studies, albeit at high and repeated doses. Human studies thus far have not found harmful effects. Since there is still not enough data on humans who have received GBCA during pregnancy, it is clear that gadolinium should not be administered in pregnancy unless there is an absolutely essential clinical indication, especially early during the pregnancy. The ACR recommends that each case be reviewed carefully. Informed consent should be obtained.

2-102. One potential consequence of metallic implants includes:

A. No effect

B. Misinterpretation of MR images

C. Implants will appear symmetrically on all sequences

D. Patients with metallic implants cannot be scanned

Discussion: Artifacts are not considered a safety concern per se; however, misinterpretation and/or misdiagnosis of MR images can lead to serious consequences for patients. The size of the metallic implant, metal used, and the pulse sequence will all impact the severity of the artifact.

2-103. Radio frequency (RF) antenna effects are defined as:

A. Stray voltage induced in the RF shield by outside RF sources

B. Current induced in elongated conductors within the RF field

C. Excitation of one coil channel by the neighboring coil channel

D. Tendency of a receiver coil to vibrate, while pulsing RF

Discussion: Wires, catheters, IV lines and other elongated conductors can act like antennas. These "antennas" can have a current induced in them by the pulsed radio frequency (RF) fields. If not properly dissipated, this current can rapidly build up a high degree of heat. The ideal antenna effect is created when the conductor length is approximately one-half of the RF wavelength, or 26 cm at 1.5 T or 13 cm at 3 T.

2-104. When assessing a ferrous foreign body for potential risks, which of the following should be considered?

A. The location of the foreign body

B. The shape of the foreign body

C. The length of time the foreign body has been in place

D. All of the above

Discussion: The location of the foreign body is important because some tissues are more susceptible to injury than others. Brain tissue, for example, does not form scar tissue the way muscle tissue does. This could lead to an implant, even after having been in place for a long time, to still be freely movable and likely to damage delicate brain tissue. That same foreign body in dense muscle, unless extremely large, would be unlikely to contain enough mass to be movable, as scar tissue (fibrosis) would secure it tightly in place.

2-105. All of the following are currently acceptable terms used to describe the safety of devices in the MR field except:

A. MR safe

B. MR conditional

C. MR unsafe

D. MR compatible

E. MR untested/unlabeled

Discussion: MR safe, MR conditional, and MR unsafe are all in the current ASTM lexicon for labeling devices for use in MRI. MR untested/unlabeled is a new designation under review and refers to devices that have not had formal testing and, therefore, remain unlabeled as to their suitability for use in MRI. Any untested/unlabeled device should trigger a risk–benefit assessment by a qualified MRI safety expert. MRI untested/unlabeled devices include things such as sternal wires, artificial joints, and wire braces. MR compatible is an outdated term and is no longer acceptable for describing devices and their use in MRI, though this label can still be found on devices tested before 2005 when the term was phased out.

2-106. An implanted device that contains its own power source is considered to be a/an:

A. Active implant

B. Passive implant

C. Untested/unlabeled implant

D. Conditional implant

Discussion: An implanted device that contains its own power source is considered to be an active implant. Active implants include things like implanted drug delivery systems, pacemakers, cardioversion, defibrillators, and deep-brain stimulators.

2-107. To be labeled as MRI safe, a device needs to:

A. Be able to be turned off while in the MRI

B. Contain no ferrous metal components

C. Contain no metallic components whatsoever

D. None of the above

Discussion: To warrant the label of MRI safe, a device/object cannot contain any metallic components whatsoever.

2-108. Heating can be caused by all of the following except:

A. Static magnetic field strength

B. Frequency of the pulsed RF

C. Patient condition

D. Patient size

Discussion: Heating within the patient is related to three things: field strength, frequency, and patient size. As frequency increases, so does absorbed energy, so tissue heating becomes highly frequency-dependent.

Physical Principles of Image Formation

3-1. To achieve resonance, a range of frequencies is applied by the RF excitation pulse during slice selection. This is called the _________.

A. receiver gain

B. transmit bandwidth

C. transmitter gain

D. receiver bandwidth

Reference: MRI in Practice, 5th Ed., page 139

3-2. The abbreviation for the primary, or main, magnetic field is _________ and the abbreviation for the secondary, or RF, field is _________.

A. $B_{1,}$ B_0

B. $B_{0,}$ B_2

C. $B_{2,}$ B_0

D. $B_{0,}$ B_1

Reference: MRI in Practice, 5th Ed., pages 6, 14

3-3. Decreasing FOV size will have what effect on resolution?

A. Decrease spatial resolution

B. Increase spatial resolution

C. No change in spatial resolution

D. Fluctuate spatial resolution

Discussion: By decreasing FOV (i.e., 20 cm to 15 cm), your voxel volume will decrease, thus improving spatial resolution.

Reference: MRI in Practice, pages 126–127

3-4. _________ materials demonstrate a weak attraction to an external magnetic field.

A. Diamagnetic

B. Paramagnetic

C. Ferromagnetic

D. Most

Reference: MRI in Practice, 5th Ed., page 313

3-5. Truncation artifacts can be reduced by which of the following?

A. Undersampling data in the phase encoding direction

B. Increasing FOV

C. Using spin echo sequences

D. Increasing phase encoding steps

Reference: MRI in Practice, page 250

3-6. Which type of magnets were the first generation of MR systems?

A. Iron-core electromagnets

B. Permanent magnets

C. Superconducting magnets

D. Air-core resistive magnets

Discussion: Air-core resistive magnets were typically comprised of four large coils wound with copper or aluminum bands.

Reference: MRI From Picture to Proton, page 169

3-7. The range of frequencies sampled or digitized is called the __________.

A. transmit bandwidth

B. transmitter gain

C. **receiver bandwidth**

D. receiver gain

Reference: MRI in Practice, 5th Ed., page 172

3-8. Duty cycle refers to:

A. The time it takes for a gradient to reach maximum amplitude and what the amplitude is

B. **The percentage of time the gradient is allowed to be on**

C. The time it takes for a gradient to reach maximum amplitude

D. The steepness or strength of a gradient

Reference: MRI in Practice, page 326

3-9. A remedy for reducing aliasing in the phase-encoding direction is to:

A. Decrease pixel size

B. **Incorporate antialiasing techniques**

C. Increase number of slices

D. Increase slice gap

Discussion: Antialiasing, also called no-phase wrap, oversampling, or antifoldover, is a sampling method to increase the number of phase-encoding steps by increasing the FOV in the phase direction, thus, not allowing a duplication of sampled phase values outside the FOV. This may result in an increase in scan time.

Reference: MRI in Practice, page 240

3-10. In axial head imaging, frequency encoding typically is performed along what direction?

A. **Anterior-posterior**

B. Head-foot

C. Superior-inferior

D. Combination of all three

Discussion: The long axis in this case is in the anterior-posterior direction, so frequency encoding is typically performed in this direction.

Reference: MRI in Practice, pages 68–69

3-11. What is the magic angle?

A. 45°

B. 69°

C. **55°**

D. 37°

Discussion: The magic angle artifact occurs when a collagen-containing structure, such as a tendon, lies at a 54.74°, or 55°, angle to the main magnetic field.

Reference: MRI in Practice, pages 257–258

3-12. Gradient amplitude refers to:

A. The time it takes for a gradient to reach maximum amplitude and what the amplitude is

B. The percentage of time the gradient is allowed to be on

C. The time it takes for a gradient to reach maximum amplitude

D. **The steepness or strength of a gradient**

Reference: MRI in Practice, page 326

3-13. The use of monitoring equipment in the scanner room can cause an artifact known as:

A. Moiré pattern

B. **Zipper**

C. Ghosting

D. Wraparound

Reference: MRI From Picture to Proton, page 103

3-14. Slew rate refers to:

A. **The time it takes for a gradient to reach maximum amplitude and what the amplitude is**

B. The percentage of time the gradient is allowed to be on

C. The time it takes for a gradient to reach maximum amplitude

D. The steepness or strength of a gradient

Reference: MRI in Practice, page 326

3-15. The image below demonstrates what type of artifact?

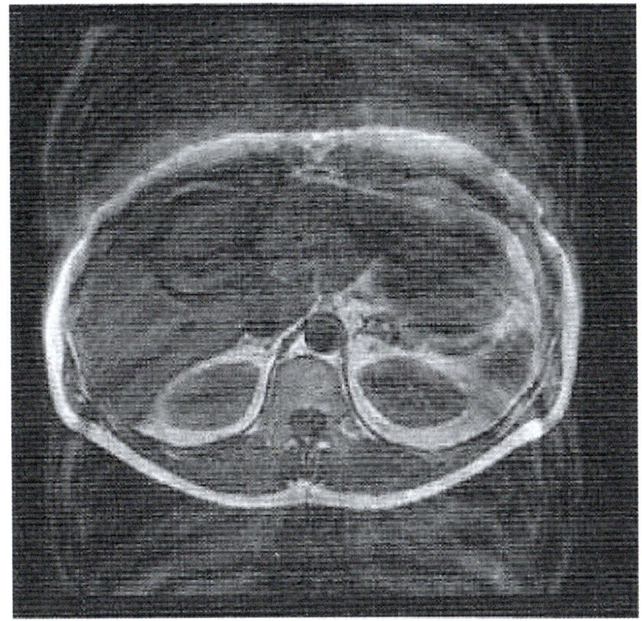

Source: Reproduced with permission from McRobbie DW, Moore EA, Graves MJ, Prince MR. *From Picture to Proton*, 2nd ed. Cambridge University Press; 2006.

A. Phase mismapping

B. Zipper

C. Truncation

D. Gibbs

Reference: Image from MRI From Picture to Proton, page 80

3-16. Assuming FOV does not change, decreasing the phase matrix will have what effect on SNR?

A. Decrease SNR

B. Increase SNR

C. No change on SNR

D. Fluctuate SNR

Discussion: By decreasing the phase matrix (i.e., 256 to 128), your voxel volume will increase, thus increasing SNR.

Reference: MRI in Practice, pages 105–107

3-17. Rise time refers to:

A. The time it takes for a gradient to reach maximum amplitude and what the amplitude is

B. The percentage of time the gradient is allowed to be on

C. The time it takes for a gradient to reach maximum amplitude

D. The steepness or strength of a gradient

Reference: MRI in Practice, page 326

3-18. What method will reduce chemical shift artifacts?

A. Scanning at a lower field strength

B. Scanning at a higher field strength

C. Gating

D. Increasing FOV

Discussion: Scanning at a lower field strength will reduce chemical shift as the precessional frequency differences between fat and water are shorter at lower field strengths.

Reference: MRI in Practice, page 244

3-19. This equation ($\omega_0 = B_0 \times \gamma$) is called what?

A. Planck's equation

B. Vector equation

C. Larmor equation

D. SNR equation

Reference: MRI in Practice, page 9

3-20. In sagittal imaging, phase encoding typically is performed along what direction?

A. Anterior-posterior

B. Head-foot

C. Superior-inferior

D. Combination of all three

Discussion: The short axis in this case is in the anterior-posterior direction, so phase encoding is typically performed in this direction.

Reference: MRI in Practice, page 71

3-21. In this equation ($\omega_0 = B_0 \times \gamma$), what does ω_0 represent?

A. Magnetic field strength

B. Gyromagnetic ratio

C. **Precessional frequency**

D. Vector frequency

Reference: MRI in Practice, page 9

3-22. In this equation ($\omega_0 = B_0 \times \gamma$), what does γ represent?

A. Magnetic field strength

B. **Gyromagnetic ratio**

C. Precessional frequency

D. Vector frequency

Reference: MRI in Practice, page 9

3-23. How does the gradient field affect the resonant frequency of protons?

A. **The resonant frequency will be different at different locations along the gradient axis.**

B. The resonant frequency remains constant due to the Larmor frequency; therefore, gradient magnetic fields do not affect precessional frequencies at all.

C. The resonant frequency remains unchanged due to the gradient slope.

D. The resonant frequency will continuously decrease over time.

3-24. The polarity of an applied gradients is determined by __________.

A. the strength of B_0

B. the chemical shift

C. the gyromagnetic ratio

D. **the direction of current**

Reference: MRI in Practice, 5th Ed., page 129

3-25. The parameter that controls how much T2-weighting is present on the resultant image is:

A. Flip angle

B. Repetition time

C. **Echo time**

D. NEX

Reference: MRI in Practice, 5th Ed., page 44

3-26. The mass number of an element is the __________.

A. number of electrons around the nucleus

B. number of protons in the nucleus

C. sum of electrons, protons, and neutrons

D. **sum of protons and neutrons in the nucleus**

Reference: MRI in Practice, page 2

3-27. Which of the following is an MR active nuclei?

A. H^2

B. P^{32}

C. O^{16}

D. **F^{19}**

Reference: MRI in Practice, page 4

3-28. The parameter that controls how much T1-weighting is present on the resultant image is:

A. Flip angle

B. **Repetition time**

C. Echo time

D. NEX

Reference: MRI in Practice, 5th Ed., page 42

3-29. If you know the gyromagnetic ratio of H^1 is 42.58 MHz/T, and you are scanning on a 2T scanner, what is the precessional frequency of H^1 at that field strength?

A. 170.32 MHz

B. **85.16 MHz**

C. 42.57 MHz

D. 63.87 MHz

Discussion: To determine the precessional frequency, multiply the gyromagnetic ratio by the field strength. In this case, you would multiply 42.57 by 2 to get 85.16.

Reference: MRI in Practice, page 4

3-30. Protons that line up with the external magnetic field are called _________ or _________ nuclei.

A. Antiparallel, spin-up

B. Parallel, spin-up

C. Antiparallel, spin-down

D. Parallel, spin-down

Reference: MRI in Practice, page 6

3-31. The MR system must be able to locate signal spatially in three dimensions. What is this the definition of?

A. Resonance

B. Encoding

C. Shimming

D. Spin-spin interaction

Reference: MRI in Practice, page 60

3-32. In coronal imaging, frequency encoding typically is performed along what direction?

A. Anterior-posterior

B. Head-foot

C. Superior-inferior

D. Combination of all three

Discussion: The long axis in this case is in the superior-inferior direction, so frequency encoding is typically performed in this direction.

Reference: MRI in Practice, page 68

3-33. The transmit bandwidth is related to the slope of the _________.

A. frequency encoding gradient

B. slice select gradient

C. phase encoding gradient

D. a combination of slice select, frequency, and phase encoding gradients

Reference: MRI in Practice, page 65

3-34. Regarding rectangular FOV, which of the following statements is true?

A. Resolution will decrease

B. SNR will increase

C. Scan time will increase

D. Scan time will decrease

Discussion: Rectangular FOV is a time-saving technique to be utilized when the anatomy is rectangular.

Reference: MRI in Practice, page 98

3-35. Which of the following is not a parameter to determine scan time in volume imaging?

A. TR

B. Slice thickness

C. Phase encoding steps

D. NEX

Reference: MRI in Practice, page 112

3-36. Increasing slice thickness will have what effect on SNR?

A. Decrease SNR

B. Increase SNR

C. No change on SNR

D. Fluctuate SNR

Discussion: By increasing slice thickness, your voxel volume will increase, thus increasing SNR.

Reference: MRI in Practice, pages 105–107

3-37. Decreasing TR will have what effect on SNR?

A. Decrease SNR

B. Increase SNR

C. No change on SNR

D. Fluctuate SNR

Discussion: Decreasing TR does not allow a full recovery of longitudinal magnetization, so less will be flipped to the transverse plane, which will reduce SNR.

Reference: MRI in Practice, pages 105–107

3-38. Decreasing TR will have what effect on resolution?

A. Decrease spatial resolution

B. Increase spatial resolution

C. No change in spatial resolution

D. Fluctuate spatial resolution

Discussion: Altering TR does not have any effect on spatial resolution since TR does not affect pixel/voxel size.

Reference: MRI in Practice, pages 105–107

3-39. When protons lose energy from the RF pulse and return to equilibrium, this is known as _________.

A. T2 relaxation

B. spin-spin relaxation

C. spin-lattice relaxation

D. gradient moment nulling

Reference: MRI From Picture to Proton, page 151

3-40. Magnetic susceptibility artifacts can be reduced by:

A. Avoiding SE sequences

B. Decreasing TE

C. Increasing TR

D. Reducing bandwidth

Reference: MRI in Practice, pages 250–252

3-41. Moiré pattern artifacts can be reduced by:

A. Gradient echo sequences

B. Spin echo sequences

C. Increasing the number of frequency encodings

D. Decreasing FOV

Reference: MRI in Practice, pages 256–257

3-42. Shading artifacts can be caused by _________.

A. abnormal loading of coil

B. leak in RF shielding

C. adjacent slices are erroneously excited

D. periodicity of fat and water matches the TE selected

Reference: MRI in Practice, page 256

3-43. Replications of moving anatomy across the image in the phase-encoding direction is called:

A. Phase mismapping

B. Chemical shift

C. Shading

D. Moiré pattern

Discussion: Phase mismapping or ghosting is an artifact that produces replications of moving anatomy across the image in the phasing-encoding direction. It originates from anatomy that moves intermittently throughout the scan, i.e., chest wall due to respiration and swallowing.

3-44. Phase mismapping only happens along the phase gradient because:

A. The phase encoding gradient never changes

B. The amplitude of the phase gradient changes

C. There is no time delay between the phase encoding and readout

D. The phase encoding happens as the signal is read and digitized

Discussion: Phase mismapping only occurs along the phase gradient because the phase-encoding gradient has a different amplitude every TR, while frequency and slice select gradients remain the same. There is also a time delay between the phase encoding and readout.

3-45. Phase mismapping can be remedied by all of the following except:

A. Keeping the phase encoding gradient the same

B. Using presaturation pulses

C. Swapping the phase and frequency directions

D. Using respiratory compensation techniques

Discussion: Phase mismapping can be remedied by using several different techniques depending on the cause of the mismapping: swapping the phase and frequency so that the artifact will not interfere in the scan, using respiratory compensation and presaturation techniques, cardiac gating, and gradient moment nulling.

3-46. On a T1-weighted image, the timing parameters must be _________; otherwise differences in tissue contrast will not be demonstrated.

A. short

B. long

C. opposite

D. maximized

Reference: MRI in Practice, 5th Ed., page 42

3-47. Tissues with a long T2 time will demonstrate as _________ on T2-weighted imaging.

A. hyperintense

B. hypointense

C. isointense

D. no signal

Discussion: The longer a tissue's T2 time, the longer it will take for T2 signal decay, and as a result, tissue will demonstrate as hyperintense on T2-weighted imaging.

3-48. The term phase coherence refers to when the magnetic moments of hydrogen are _________.

A. precessing around B_0 at different rates

B. precessing around B_0 at the same place at a moment in time

C. precessing around B_0 at different places at a moment in time

D. spinning on their axis at the same time

Reference: MRI in Practice, 5th Ed., page 13

3-49. T2 time is the time it takes for _________.

A. 63% of magnetization to recover in the longitudinal plane

B. 37% of magnetization to recover in the longitudinal plane

C. 63% of magnetization to dephase in the transverse plane

D. 37% of magnetization to dephase in the transverse plane

Reference: MRI in Practice, 5th Ed., page 29

3-50. Resonance is achieved in MR imaging when what occurs?

A. Two equal gradient slopes are applied simultaneously

B. A radio-frequency pulse is applied at the same time as a gradient is applied

C. A radio-frequency pulse is applied at the same precessional frequency as the magnetic moments of hydrogen

D. When a radio-frequency pulse is equal to B_0

Reference: MRI in Practice, 5th Ed., page 15

3-51. When current passing through a gradient coil is applied clockwise, field strength will _________.

A. increase

B. decrease

C. stay the same

D. fluctuate

Discussion: Applying a clockwise current through a gradient coil will increase field strength and, thus, increase precessional frequency; applying a counterclockwise current through a gradient coil will decrease field strength and, thus, decrease precessional frequency.

Reference: MRI in Practice, 5th Ed., page 129

3-52. The timing parameters used in a proton density-weighted image are _________.

A. a short TR and short TE

B. a long TR and short TE

C. a long TR and long TE

D. a short TR and long TE

Discussion: To diminish both T1 and T2 contrast, a long TR (to reduce T1 contrast) and a short TE (to reduce T2 contrast) are utilized.

3-53. _________ materials demonstrate a mild repulsion to an external magnetic field.

A. Diamagnetic

B. Paramagnetic

C. Ferromagnetic

D. Most

Reference: MRI in Practice, 5th Ed., page 313

3-54. The *z gradient* alters the magnetic field along the *z-axis* of the magnet and from _________ in the patient.

A. right to left

B. front to back

C. head to foot

D. Combination of A and C

Reference: MRI in Practice, 5th Ed., page 134

3-55. The *x gradient* alters the magnetic field along the *x-axis* of the magnet and from _________ in the patient.

A. right to left

B. front to back

C. head to foot

D. Combination of A and B

Reference: MRI in Practice, 5th Ed., page 134

3-56. The *y gradient* alters the magnetic field along the *y-axis* of the magnet and from _________ in the patient.

A. right to left

B. front to back

C. head to foot

D. Combination of B and C

Reference: MRI in Practice, 5th Ed., page 134

3-57. To what temperature is helium cooled when turned into a liquid?

A. 4° Celsius

B. 4° Fahrenheit

C. 4 Kelvin (K)

D. 0 Kelvin (K)

Discussion: Helium will turn to a liquid at 4° above absolute zero, or 4 Kelvin (K).

Reference: MRI in Practice, 5th Ed., page 7

3-58. There are a larger number of protons that are in the _________ energy state, and these numbers will _________ as magnetic field strength increases.

A. lower, increase

B. higher, increase

C. lower, decrease

D. higher, decrease

Reference: MRI in Practice, 5th Ed., page 320

3-59. 1.5 tesla is the equivalent of _________ gauss.

A. 1,500

B. 15,000

C. 150,000

D. 150

Discussion: The ratio of tesla (T) to gauss (G) is 1:10,000, so 1.5 T is the equivalent of 15,000 gauss.

3-60. As the magnitude of coherent transverse magnetization decreases, an initial signal is induced in the receiver coil and is called:

A. T2 signal

B. T1 signal

C. Free induction decay signal

D. Signal amplitude

Reference: MRI in Practice, 5th Ed., page 20

3-61. The flip angle for a given tissue and a given T1 time that results in maximum signal for that tissue is the definition of what?

A. Faraday angle

B. Ohm angle

C. Lauterbur angle

D. Ernst angle

Reference: MRI in Practice, 5th Ed., page 101

3-62. Additional coils located at each end of the magnet that apply current in the opposite direction to the main magnet windings in order to reduce the magnetic field is a definition of:

A. Passive shielding

B. Fringe field

C. Active shielding

D. Copper shielding

Reference: MRI in Practice, 5th Ed., page 327

3-63. The movement of molecules due to random thermal motion can be imaged using MRI by performing what type of imaging?

A. Functional magnetic resonance imaging

B. Diffusion-weighted imaging

C. Perfusion imaging

D. Magnetic resonance spectroscopy

Reference: MRI in Practice, 5th Ed., page 52

3-64. What is the extrinsic contrast parameter that controls how much the ADC contributes to DWI?

A. TR

B. TE

C. b-value

D. Flip angle

Reference: MRI in Practice, 5th Ed., page 54

3-65. The parameter known as b-value or b-factor is expressed in units of __________.

A. mL/min/G

B. $\mathbf{s/mm^2}$

C. W/kg

D. cm/s

Reference: MRI in Practice, 5th Ed., page 54

3-66. The most common sequences used in black blood imaging are__________ which incorporate a presaturation technique.

A. fast spin echo

B. spin echo

C. EPI

D. gradient echo

Reference: MRI in Practice, 5th Ed., page 303

3-67. An acute infarct has a __________ ADC.

A. high

B. low

C. intermediate

D. no

Reference: MRI in Practice, 5th Ed., page 52

3-68. Signal intensity differences in a __________ image are based on the relative amount of mobile hydrogen protons per unit of tissue.

A. T1-weighted

B. DWI-weighted

C. T2-weighted

D. proton density-weighted

Reference: MRI in Practice, 5th Ed., page 41

3-69. The energy exchange caused by the magnetic fields of each nucleus interacting with surrounding nuclei is termed:

A. Spin-lattice relaxation

B. T2* decay

C. T1 relaxation

D. Spin-spin relaxation

Reference: MRI in Practice, 5th Ed., page 27

3-70. The T2* time is always __________ the T2 time.

A. longer than

B. shorter than

C. equal to

D. not related to

Reference: MRI in Practice, 5th Ed., page 30

3-71. If the polarity of the phase-encoding gradient is positive, the __________ lines of k-space will be filled.

A. top

B. bottom

C. left

D. right

Reference: MRI in Practice, 5th Ed., page 30

3-72. The __________ is applied at the time the MR system reads and digitizes the echo.

A. slice select gradient

B. phase-encoding gradient

C. frequency-encoding gradient

D. shim system

Reference: MRI in Practice, 5th Ed., page 167

3-73. The chemical shift frequency difference between fat and water, expressed in ppm, can be calculated by multiplying __________ and __________.

A. 3.5 ppm, B_0

B. 3.5 ppm, precessional frequency of a given field strength

C. 3.5 ppm, precessional frequency of fat

D. 3.5 ppm, gyromagnetic ratio

Reference: MRI in Practice, 5th Ed., page 262

3-74. Chemical shift __________ when field strength __________.

A. does not change, decreases

B. increases, increases

C. decreases, increases

D. increases, decreases

Reference: MRI in Practice, 5th Ed., page 228

3-75. Industry trends have increased superconducting magnet bore size to __________.

A. 60 cm

B. 70 cm

C. 80 cm

D. 90 cm

Discussion: Historically, superconducting magnet bore size has been 60 cm; however, this recently has been increased to 70 cm to accommodate larger patients.

Reference: Essentials of MRI Safety, page 11

3-76. To create larger precessional frequency differences between two points in a patient, __________ gradient slopes must be utilized.

A. shallow

B. steep

C. alternating

D. fast

Discussion: Steeper gradient slopes will create larger precessional frequency differences between two points.

Reference: MRI in Practice, 5th Ed., page 133

3-77. In spin echo sequences, the slice select gradient is switched on __________.

A. before the 90° RF excitation pulse

B. after the 90° RF excitation pulse

C. during the 90° RF excitation pulse

D. during the 90° RF excitation pulse and the 90° RF refocusing pulse

Reference: MRI in Practice, 5th Ed., page 136

3-78. The localization of signal along the __________ is called phase encoding.

A. short axis

B. long axis

C. y-axis

D. z-axis

Reference: MRI in Practice, 5th Ed., page 145

3-79. In conventional spin or gradient echo sequences, __________ is/are filled per TR period.

A. multiple lines

B. two lines

C. four lines

D. one line

Reference: MRI in Practice, 5th Ed., page 69

3-80. High signal information is stored in _________.

A. the center of k-space

B. the top half of k-space

C. the bottom half of k-space

D. the outer edges of k-space

Reference: MRI in Practice, 5th Ed., page 185

3-81. In _________, all lines of k-space are filled at once.

A. fast spin echo sequences

B. conventional spin echo sequences

C. inversion recovery sequences

D. gradient echo planar imaging sequences

Reference: MRI in Practice, 5th Ed., page 122

3-82. The B_1 magnetic field is oriented _________ to the B_0, or the main magnetic field.

A. parallel

B. perpendicular

C. 180°

D. at a 45° angle

Reference: MRI in Practice, 5th Ed., page 14

3-83. Niobium-titanium (Nb-Ti) alloy windings are primarily used in _________ magnet systems.

A. air-core

B. iron-core

C. permanent

D. superconducting

Reference: Essentials of MRI Safety, page 11

3-84. Superconducting magnet systems use a _________ to recondense helium gas to a liquid.

A. air conditioner

B. cold head

C. condenser

D. evaporator

Reference: Essentials of MRI Safety, page 12

3-85. The Larmor frequency, or precessional frequency, of hydrogen in a 1.5 T MRI scanner is:

A. 10 MHz

B. 42.58 MHz

C. 64 MHz

D. 128 MHz

Reference: Essentials of MRI Safety, page 25

3-86. Coil channels refer to the number of _________ in a coil.

A. power supplies

B. receive elements

C. preamps

D. None of the above

Discussion: The term coil channels, in practical use, is synonymous with the number of receive elements in a coil. While the configuration can vary from single loop to multiloop, and linear to quadrature, the overall number of channels, strictly speaking, refers to the number of receive elements.

Reference: MRI in Practice, 5th Ed., page 122

3-87. ____ refers to the position of magnetic moments along the precessional path at any point in time.

A. Frequency

B. Phase

C. Gyromagnetic ratio

D. Dephasing

Discussion: Phase refers to the location (position) of spins along the precessional path.

Reference: MRI in Practice, 5th Ed., page 13

3-88. What is/are the primary function(s) of an MRI coil?

A. Transmit RF to the patient

B. Receive the signal from the patient

C. Both A and B

D. None of the above

Discussion: While there are many coiled designs and configurations, the two basic functions are the transmission of RF energy into the patient and the receiving of signal induced by the changing bulk magnetic field.

Reference: MRI in Practice, 5th Ed., pages 339–343

3-89. Which of the following is correct with respect to image contrast parameters?

A. Intrinsic, controlled by us

B. Extrinsic, controlled by us

C. Intrinsic, not controlled by us

D. Extrinsic, not controlled by us

E. Both A and D

F. Both B and C

Discussion: Intrinsic contrast parameters (mechanisms) including T1, T2, PD, flow, and motion (ADC) are inherent to the body tissues and as such are beyond the control of the technologist. Extrinsic parameters including TR, TE, RF, flip angle, TI, ech, train length, value, and VENC are parameters that are well within the control of the professional technologist and are commonly modified to alter image contrast.

Reference: MRI in Practice, 5th Ed., page 25

3-90. Compared to other modalities, MRI has better:

A. Soft-tissue resolution

B. Soft-tissue contrast

C. Soft-tissue SNR

D. None of the above

Discussion: Image contrast is defined as the ability to distinguish between adjacent structures. High soft-tissue contrast is the foundational benefit of MRI over other imaging modalities.

Reference: MRI in Practice, 5th Ed., pages 24–25

3-91. Fat has _________ T1 and T2 times compared to water.

A. short

B. long

C. equal

D. None of the above

Discussion: The T1 and T2 times of fat are 5–10 times shorter than that of water.

Reference: MRI in Practice, 5th Ed., pages 26–30

3-92. What are the two types of motion seen in MRI?

A. Periodic and aperiodic

B. Patient and electronic

C. Physiologic and pathologic

D. All of the above

Discussion: Periodic motion has a repetitive pattern and includes things like the respiratory and cardiac cycles. The repetitive pattern allows for compensation via tracking the respiratory and cardiac cycles in a process called gating. Aperiodic motion has no pattern and includes things like patient motion, peristalsis, and swallowing.

3-93. Chemical shift is mapped in the frequency direction and is measured in _________.

A. pixel/hertz

B. hertz/pixel

C. frequencies

D. None of the above

Discussion: Chemical shift is the difference in precessional frequencies between fat and water. Water precesses faster than fat by 220 Hz (cycles per second). When these processional differences are mapped across the imaging matrix, there is a finite number of frequencies in each pixel as defined by the number of pixels (frequency Matrix) and the range of frequencies sampled (receiver bandwidth). Chemical shift is measured in hertz per pixel.

Reference: MRI in Practice, 5th Ed., page 228

3-94. Chemical shift can never be _________.

A. eliminated

B. minimized

C. maximized

D. None of the above

Discussion: Because differences in precessional rates are inherent to the chemical makeup of fat and water, their effects can never be eliminated. The impact of those facts, however, can be minimized by maximizing the amount of frequencies per pixel. This is achieved by using a very wide receiver bandwidth.

Reference: MRI in Practice, 5th Ed., page 228

3-95. Chemical shift _________ with an increase in Precessional bandwidth and image matrix.

A. increases

B. decreases

C. depends on field strength

D. None of the above

Discussion: Increasing receiver bandwidth increases the range of frequencies sampled during the read out and, therefore, the number of frequencies contained within each pixel of the reconstructed images. The greater the receiver bandwidth, the lower the overall chemical shift.

Reference: MRI in Practice, 5th Ed., pages 228, 264

3-96. Fat and water are in phase at _________ TE at 1.5 T.

A. 2.1 ms

B. 4.2 ms

C. 6.3 ms

D. None of the above

Discussion: At 1.5 T, fat and water are in phase every 4.2 ms. While, classified as an artifact, this info is out of phase periodicity is clinically useful for classifying fatty tissues.

Reference: MRI in Practice, 5th Ed., pages 261–268

3-97. K-space is where _________ is stored during the data collection process.

A. the image

B. raw data

C. contrast weighting

D. Nyquist data

Discussion: K-space is not the image. It is merely a storage space where raw data, an aggregate of phase in frequency information, is stored.

Reference: MRI in Practice, 5th Ed., page 159

3-98. Once all data is collected, it is turned into an image by applying a _________.

A. fast Fourier transform (FFT)

B. Boltzmann equation

C. Avogadro's number

D. None of the above

Discussion: Even when completely filled, k-space is still not an image. To transform the raw data (k-space data) into image data, a mathematical equation called a fast Fourier transform is applied.

Reference: MRI in Practice, 5th Ed., pages 158–159

3-99. The gradient that is on during the production of the echo is called the:

A. Phase-encoding gradient

B. Slice select gradient

C. Frequency-encoding gradient/readout gradient

D. None of the above

Discussion: The frequency encoding gradient, also called the readout gradient, is on at the same time as the production of the echo, or when the echo is read. This occurs in all MR sequences.

Reference: MRI in Practice, 5th Ed.

3-100. RF shielding can be achieved by lining the scanner room walls with:

A. Copper

B. Steel

C. Lead

D. None of the above

Discussion: The RF used during the imaging process is very precise and controlled. To prevent outside radio waves from altering, disturbing, or disrupting this precise RF, the room must be shielded to keep any stray radio waves out. This is done most commonly with copper. Other methods of RF shielding (aluminum, galvanized steel, or silicone carbon steel panels) are available, but are far less common.

Reference: MRI in Practice, 5th Ed., pages 337–338

3-101. Which one of the following pulse sequences would have the longest scan time?

A. TR 300 ms, TE 30 ms, RCV BW 20 kHz, phase matrix 256, 30 slices, 4 NSA

B. TR 150 ms, TE 2 ms, RCV BW 15 kHz, phase matrix 224, 20 slices, 6 NSA

C. TR 1,500 ms, TE 20 ms, RCV BW 32 kHz, phase matrix 192, 10 slices, 2 NSA, ETL 8

D. TR 6,000 ms, TE 180 ms, RCV BW 15 kHz, phase matrix 192, 15 slices, 1 NSA, ETL 12

Discussion: When approaching questions regarding scan time, it is important to read the question carefully. Does the question specifically mention the type of sequence used, i.e., spin echo versus fast spin echo, or mention anything about 3-D or volume imaging? This is important as those two distinctions will change the formula for scan time dramatically. Some questions will include parameters like echo train length (ETL) or number of slices, and those parameters may or may not be relevant depending on how the question is worded. Individual preferences vary, but many find it helpful to start out by converting milliseconds to seconds by dividing by 1,000, i.e., moving the decimal point four (4) places to the left, so 500 ms becomes 0.5 seconds, etc.

Reference: MIP (5)

TR	Matrix-p	NSA	ETL	# Slices	Msec	Sec	Min
300	256	4			307,200	307.2	5.12
150	224	6			201,600	201.6	3.36
1,500	192	2			72,000	72	1.2
6,000	192	1			81,000	81	1.35

3-102. Which one of the following volume pulse sequences would have the shortest scan time?

A. TR 500 ms, TE 30 ms, RCV BW 20 kHz, phase matrix 256, 30 slices, 2 NSA

B. TR 100 ms, TE 8 ms, RCV BW 15 kHz, phase matrix 256, 20 slices, 1 NSA

C. TR 300 ms, TE 20 ms, RCV BW 32 kHz, phase matrix 192, 10 slices, 2 NSA, ETL 8

D. TR 2,000 ms, TE 12 ms, RCV BW 15 kHz, phase matrix 192, 25 slices, 1 NSA, ETL 4

Discussion: When approaching questions regarding scan time, it is important to read the question carefully. Does the question specifically mention the type of sequence used, i.e., spin echo versus fast spin echo, or mention anything about 3-D or volume imaging? This is important as those two distinctions will change the formula for scan time dramatically. Some questions will include parameters like echo train length (ETL) or number of slices, and those parameters may or may not be relevant depending on how the question is worded. Individual preferences vary, but many find it helpful to start out by converting milliseconds to seconds by dividing by 1000, i.e., moving the decimal point four (4) places to the left, so 500 ms becomes 0.5 seconds, etc.

TR	Matrix-p	NSA	ETL	# Slices	Msec	Sec	Min
500	256	2		30	5,120,000	5,120	85.3
100	256	1		20	512,000	512	8.5
300	192	2	8	10	14,400	14.4	.024
2,000	192	1	4		96,000	96	1.6

3-103. Which one of the following pulse sequences would have the shortest scan time?

A. TR 500 ms, TE 10 ms, phase matrix 256, 2 NSA

B. TR 600 ms, TE 8 ms, phase matrix 224, 1 NSA

C. TR 700 ms, TE 20 ms, phase matrix 206, 2 NSA, ETL 2

D. TR 800 ms, TE 35 ms, phase matrix 192, 2 NSA, ETL 4

Discussion: When approaching questions regarding scan time, it is important to read the question carefully. Does the question specifically mention the type of sequence used, i.e., spin echo versus fast spin echo, or mention anything about 3-D or volume imaging? This is important as those two distinctions will change the formula for scan time dramatically. Some questions will include parameters like echo train length (ETL) or number of slices, and those parameters may or may not be relevant depending on how the question is worded. Individual preferences vary, but many find it helpful to start out by converting milliseconds to seconds by dividing by 1000, i.e., moving the decimal point four (4) places to the left, so 500 ms becomes 0.5 seconds, etc.

TR	Matrix-p	NSA	ETL	# Slices	Msec	Sec	Min
500	256	2			256,000	256	4.2
600	224	1			134,000	134.4	2.2
700	206	2	2		144,200	144.2	2.4
800	192	2	4		76,800	76.8	1.2

3-104. As echo train length (ETL) is increased, the effective TE fills less of the central portion of k-space resulting in:

A. Increased blurring

B. Increased spatial resolution

C. Increased scan time

D. Increased T2 contrast

Discussion: The effective TE is the primary image contrast driver in fast spin echo (FSE). With long echo train lengths (ETLs), the ratio of affective TEs to noneffective TEs decreases, leading to a greater range of contrast values populating the center of k-space. The effect of this is increased image blurring. Other factors playing a role in image blurring include receiver, bandwidth, and TE.

3-105. In a fast spin echo sequence, the effective TEs are the echoes that are encoded:

A. In the outer edges of k-space

B. With a high-amplitude phase-encoding gradient

C. With a low-amplitude phase-encoding gradient

D. With the first phase encoding steps

Discussion: In a fast spin echo sequence, each 180° RF pulse generates an echo with a unique TE. To avoid image blurring, the echoes fill k-space differently than other sequences. The effective or target TE is placed in the center of K-space while the noneffective TE echoes are sent to the periphery of k-space to add resolution. This means the effective TEs are encoded with the low-amplitude phase-encoding gradient that fills the central lines of K space.

Reference: MRI in Practice, 5th Ed., pages 70–71

3-106. Presaturation pulses usually occur:

A. Prior to the excitation pulse

B. After the 180 degree RF pulse

C. Between the 90 degree and the 180 degree RF pulse

D. Prior to the TE

Discussion: Spatial presaturation pulses designed to nullify signal from a specific anatomical location are applied prior to the initial expectation pulse.

Reference: MRI in Practice, 5th Ed., page 228

3-107. Increasing the TE:

A. Allows for more T1 information on the image

B. Allows for more T2 information the image

C. Has no affect on the image contrast

D. Allows for more T1 and T2 information on the image

Discussion: TE controls the amount of spin-spin dephasing permitted in an image and is also known as T2 decay. Increasing TE increases T2 contrast.

Reference: MRI in Practice, 5th Ed., pages 44–46

3-108. In an inversion recovery pulse sequence, image contrast is controlled by:

A. TR and TE

B. TI

C. TI and TE

D. TR, TE, and TI

Discussion: TR and TE are the primary determinants of image contrast for most sequences. When using inversion recovery, TI takes the leading role in contrast determination, though TR and TE still play an important role.

Reference: MRI in Practice, 5th Ed., pages 80–81

3-109. What factors control the flip angle?

A. The static field and the RF duration

B. The static field and the gradient field

C. The gradient field and the RF field

D. The amplitude and duration of the pulsed RF field

Discussion: The factors controlling the flip angle are the amplitude and duration of the post-RF field. For a 90° RF pulse, the RF is turned on only long enough to flip the net magnetic vector 90° into the transverse plane. The exact amount of energy this requires, however, depends on other factors, such as static magnetic field strength and coil choice.

Reference: MRI in Practice, 5th Ed., page 17

3-110. To increase the voxel volume, which parameters would you change?

A. FOV, slice thickness, and imaging matrix

B. FOV, slice gap, and imaging matrix

C. Slice gap and slice thickness

D. Imaging matrix, slice gap, and slice thickness

Discussion: Voxels are three-dimensional boxes. The length and width are controlled by both the field of view (FOV) and matrix. The voxel depth is synonymous with slice thickness.

3-111. To rephase the signal from moving spins, gradient moment nulling uses a _________.

A. rapid gradient reversal

B. well-timed RF pulse

C. careful timing to the cardiac cycle

D. None of the above

Discussion: Gradient moment nulling, also known as flow compensation, uses a rapid gradient reversal of a bilobed balanced gradient to first dephase, then rephase flowing spins.

3-112. To nullify signal from a specific anatomic area for the purpose of eliminating artifacts, we can use additional RF pulses known as _________.

A. spectral presaturation pulses

B. spatial presaturation pulses

C. fat suppression

D. None of the above

Discussion: Additional RF pulses are designed to target specific anatomical areas to eliminate artifacts, also known as spatial presaturation pulses. Spectral presaturation pulses target specific frequencies, such as that of fat or silicone, to eliminate signal from those tissue frequencies only, regardless of location.

3-113. What effect will increasing the frequency matrix from 256 to 512 have on scan time?

A. Increase by 2X

B. Increase by 4X

C. Decrease by 2X

D. No change

Discussion: The basic scan time formula is: Repetition time (TR) × matrix (P) × number of signal averages (NSA) (NEX). Matrix (F), the frequency matrix, is important to spatial resolution and signal-to-noise ratio (SNR), but plays no role in scan time.

3-114. The 180° RF pulse that follows the initial 90° RF pulse in a spin echo sequence will produce an echo while correcting for _________.

A. slight magnetic field inhomogeneities

B. chemical shift

C. slight magnetic susceptibility effects

D. All of the above

Discussion: The 180° RF refocusing pulse is designed to produce the spin echo (Hahn echo) while correcting for <u>S</u>usceptibilities, <u>I</u>nhomogeneities, and <u>C</u>hemical shift. This is the reason that spin echo, and, more precisely, fast spin echo sequences are more effective at minimizing the impact of metallic implants and foreign bodies when compared to gradient echo sequences that lack a 180° pulse.

Reference: MRI in Practice, 5th Ed., pages 62, 73, 270–271

3-115. An inversion recovery sequence begins with a _________.

A. 90 degree RF pulse

B. short TI

C. short TE

D. 180 degree RF pulse

Discussion: Inversion recovery sequences, as the name implies, begin with an inversion pulse of 180°. Inversion proposals can be applied prior to a spin echo, fast spin echo, or gradient-based sequence.

Reference: MRI in Practice, 5th Ed., page 78

3-116. In a fast spin echo pulse sequence, if the echo train length is increased by a factor of four, ________.

A. the scan will be one time faster

B. the scan will be twice as fast

C. the scan will be three times as fast

D. the scan will be four times as fast

Discussion: Increasing the echo train length (ETL) by a factor of four (4) means acquiring four (4) times more signal per TR period. The effect of this is that we complete the data acquisition process four times faster, so the overall scan time is four times faster.

3-117. In a 3-D volume acquisition, the scan time is:

A. TR × NSA × BW × thickness

B. TR × NSA × phase encodings × slab thickness

C. TR × NSA × number of phase encodings × ETL

D. TR × NSA × number of phase encodings × number of slices

Discussion: The baseline formula for scan time is TR × phase matrix × NSA. With a 3-D or volume acquisition, the scan time is also multiplied by the number of slices due to the fact that the slice select gradient has to be cycled once per slice at the conclusion of the scan.

3-118. In a spin echo sequence, the time between the 90 degree RF pulse and the 180 degree RF pulse is the:

A. TE

B. TR

C. TI

D. ½ TE

Discussion: To allow equal time for dephasing/rephasing, the 180° RF refocusing pulse in a spin echo sequence occurs at ½ TE.

Reference: MRI in Practice, 5th Ed., pages 59–61, 64

3-119. The best pulse sequence to minimize susceptibility artifacts is:

A. Gradient echo

B. Spin echo

C. EPI

D. Fast spin echo

Discussion: From an imaging standpoint, susceptibility artifacts are minimized partially through the use of 180° refocusing pulses. As fast spin echo uses the most 180s, it is the best sequence for minimizing susceptibility artifacts.

Reference: MRI in Practice, 5th Ed., pages 270–272

3-120. Which would give you more chemical shift artifacts?

A. Permanent magnet

B. Superconducting magnet

C. Chemical shift has nothing to do with magnets

D. None of the above

Discussion: Chemical shift scales with field strength, and superconducting magnets have the highest magnetic fields and, therefore, the greatest chemical shift.

Reference: MIP (5) 264

3-121. Increasing the number of signal averages (NSA):

A. Increases SNR by the square root of the increase

B. Decreases the SNR by the square root of the decrease

C. Does not affect the SNR

D. Decreases the scan time

Discussion: Any increase in the number of single averages (NSA) (NEX) will increase the signal-to-noise ratio. The amount of the increase will be equal to the square root of the change. For example, doubling the NSA from two (2) to four (4) is the same as multiplying by two (2). The square root of two is 1.41 or 41%. It should be noted that while doubling, the NSA does by 41% more signal. It comes at a cost of doubling the scan time.

Reference: MRI in Practice, 5th Ed., page 213

3-122. Reducing the FOV:

A. Increases SNR

B. Decreases SNR

C. Has no affect on SNR

D. Increases the voxel size

Discussion: Reducing the field of view (FOV) reduces pixel size and, subsequently, voxel volume. Since SNR is proportional to voxel volume, any decrease involving the volume will have a proportional decrease in SNR.

Reference: MRI in Practice, 5th Ed., page 221

3-123. The timing of RF pulses during an MRI pulse sequence controls:

A. Image contrast

B. Voxel size

C. Spatial localization

D. None of the above

Discussion: The timing of the RF pulses refers to the TR, TE, and TI. It describes when they're on in the overall imaging process. The timing of TR, TE, and TI determines image contrast.

Reference: MRI in Practice, 5th Ed., page 20

Sequence Parameters and Options

4-1. Which of the following is not an example of extrinsic contrast parameters, or parameters the operator can change?

A. Repetition time (TR)

B. Flip angle

C. b-value

D. T2 relaxation time

Discussion: T2 relaxation time is the only listed parameter that is inherent to the human body and cannot be changed by the operator. All other parameters listed can be manipulated and/or changed to alter image contrast.

4-2. If you are performing an MRI scan with the parameters of 2000 ms TR and 30 ms TE on a spin echo sequence, what range of contrast would you expect to see on your resultant images?

A. T1-weighted

B. Proton density-weighted

C. Diffusion-weighted

D. T2-weighted

Discussion: Using a long TR (e.g., 2,000 ms) will limit T1 weighting on the images, while using a short TE (e.g., 30 ms) will limit T2 weighting. The result will be a more pronounced proton density signal.

4-3. What term describes how much the net magnetization is rotated away from B_0 via an RF (radio frequency) excitation pulse?

A. Flip angle

B. Magnetic vector

C. Vector sum

D. Receiver bandwidth

Discussion: The flip angle is the angle in which the net magnetization moves away from the longitudinal plane into the transverse plane. This is based upon the pulse sequence used.

4-4. The timing parameter demonstrating the time between the 90° pulse and 180° pulse on a spin echo sequence is called what?

A. Gamma

B. Omega

C. Tau

D. Rho

Discussion: Tau is the term given to the interpulse time between the 90° and 180° pulses. Tau is half of the TE. Tau is also commonly used as the term to describe the time from a 180° inversion pulse to the 90° excitation pulse.

4-5. Signal-to-noise ratio (SNR) _________ when moving to a magnet with a higher field strength.

A. will decrease

B. will increase

C. will not change

D. will vary

Discussion: The higher the field strength of a magnet, the more signal will be available to be flipped into the transverse plane. Subsequently, more signal equates to higher SNR.

4-6. What pulse-timing sequence defines when the MR signal will be read?

A. Repetition time (TR)

B. Flip angle

C. b-value

D. Echo time (TE)

Discussion: The echo time (TE) is the timing parameter that defines the time from the application of the 90° pulse to the peak of the MR signal. Adjusting the TE will either allow your MR signal to occur earlier (shorter TE) or later (longer TE).

4-7. What parameter is used solely in fast spin echo imaging to determine the number of echoes created?

A. Interecho spacing

B. Echo train length

C. TI

D. Flip angle

Discussion: Echo train length (ETL) determines how many echoes are produced per TR. This is also called turbo factor.

4-8. What pulse timing sequence defines the duration of the RF excitation pulse?

A. Repetition time (TR)

B. Flip angle

C. b-value

D. Echo time (TE)

Discussion: The repetition time (TR) is the timing parameter that defines the time from the application of the RF excitation pulse to the next RF excitation pulse. Adjusting the TR will either allow your MR pulse to be shorter (shorter TR) or longer (longer TR).

4-9. What factor listed below affects SNR and resolution?

A. Flip angle

B. Number of signal averages

C. Field of view (FOV)

D. Magnetic field strength

Discussion: Field of view (FOV) affects both SNR and resolution since adjusting FOV will adjust voxel/pixel size. All other listed parameters do not adjust voxel/pixel size.

4-10. Short values of TR (<1,000 ms) are common in images exhibiting _________.

A. T1-weighted contrast

B. T2-weighted contrast

C. proton density contrast

D. diffusion-weighted contrast

Discussion: A shorter TR is needed to maximize T1 weighting on your images. Longer TRs will reduce T1 weighting.

4-11. In fast spin echo imaging, if a 256 phase matrix is used, with 1 second TR, 2 signal averages, and an echo train length (ETL) of 4, what is the resultant scan time?

A. 64 seconds

B. 128 seconds

C. 256 seconds

D. 512 seconds

Discussion: The formula for determining fast spin echo scan time is:

TR × Number of phase encodings × Number of signal averages / ETL

To determine scan time in this example:

1,000 ms TR (1 second) × 256 × 2 / 4 = 128 seconds (or 2 minutes, 8 seconds)

4-12. Shorter values of TE (<50 ms) are common in images exhibiting _________ imaging.

A. proton density-weighted and T2-weighted

B. proton density-weighted and T1-weighted

C. only proton density-weighted

D. diffusion-weighted and T2-weighted

Discussion: Shorter TE values will reduce T2 weighting. By reducing T2 weighting, you can increase T1 and PD contrast on your images.

4-13. A _________ will help reduce magnetic susceptibility artifacts.

A. reduced TR

B. increased TR

C. reduced TE

D. increased TE

Discussion: Decreasing TE will help reduce magnetic susceptibility artifacts since it will allow less dephasing.

Reference: http://mri-q.com/susceptibility-artifact.html

4-14. A STIR sequence uses _________ inversion times.

A. short

B. long

C. medium

D. no

Discussion: STIR is an acronym for short tau inversion recovery. As mentioned in question #4, tau is commonly used as a term to describe inversion time (TI).

4-15. In a gradient echo pulse sequence, the T2* time is always _________ the T2 time.

A. more than

B. less than

C. the same as

D. not related to

Discussion: T2* is the term to describe T2 weighting in gradient echo sequences. It is always less than the T2 time due to the presence of magnetic field inhomogeneities and chemical shift in the signal.

4-16. Decreasing _________ will reduce the artifact called partial volume averaging.

A. FOV

B. receiver bandwidth

C. slice thickness

D. TR

Discussion: Reducing slice thickness will allow for better resolution and reduce partial volume averaging.

4-17. When you obtain equal voxel dimensions in a volume scan, you create a/an _________ voxel.

A. anisotropic

B. isotropic

C. parallel

D. rectangular

Discussion: Isotropic voxels are voxels with equal resolution in all dimensions. The formula for creating an isotropic voxel is: **FOV/frequency matrix** × **FOV/phase matrix** × **slice thickness**.

4-18. Increasing TR will:

A. Increase scan time

B. Increase slice thickness

C. Decrease resolution

D. Decrease SNR

Discussion: Increasing TR will increase scan time. It does not affect slice thickness and resolution and will increase SNR.

4-19. Chemical shift in the frequency encoding direction can be affected by what parameter?

A. TR

B. TE

C. Flip angle

D. Receiver bandwidth

Discussion: Reducing the receiver bandwidth will increase chemical shift artifact, so shorter receiver bandwidths should be avoided in areas where this is a concern.

Reference: http://mriquestions.com/chemical-shift-artifact.html

4-20. What flip angle, TR, and TE values must you use to produce a T2*-weighted image in gradient echo sequences?

A. Low flip angle, long TR, long TE

B. High flip angle, long TR, long TE

C. Low flip angle, long TR, short TE

D. High flip angle, short TR, short TE

Discussion: Using a low flip angle with a long TR and TE will produce T2*-weighting in gradient echo sequences.

Reference: MRI in Practice, page 165

4-21. To maximize spatial resolution, which of the following would be an option?

A. Increase slice thickness

B. Increase FOV

C. Decrease number of signal averages

D. Increase phase matrix

Discussion: Increasing phase matrix, or number of phase encoding steps, will increase spatial resolution since pixel/voxel dimensions will be smaller, thus resulting in increased resolution.

4-22. Which of the following is not a parameter in determining volume imaging scan time?

A. Slice thickness

B. TR

C. Number of phase-encoding steps

D. Number of signal averages

Discussion: Slice thickness has no bearing on volume imaging scan time; however, the number of slices does. To determine volume imaging acquisition time, use this formula:

TR × Number of phase encoding steps × Number of signal averages × Number of slices

4-23. Increasing the flip angle will have what effect on SNR?

A. Increase

B. Decrease

C. No change

D. None of the above

Discussion: Increasing the flip angle will allow for more magnetization to be flipped into the transverse plane. Subsequently, more signal in the transverse plane will increase signal and, thus, SNR.

4-24. To maximize SNR, which of the following would be an option?

A. Decrease receive bandwidth

B. Decrease FOV

C. Decrease number of signal averages

D. Increase phase matrix

Discussion: Decreasing receive bandwidth will increase SNR, since less noise will be present compared to overall signal when sampled.

4-25. If I have a scan with the parameters of 1,000 ms TR, 1 signal average, and 240 PE steps, what is the resultant scan time?

A. 4 minutes

B. 7 minutes

C. 10 minutes

D. 14 minutes

Discussion: Scan time is determined by this formula:

TR × Number of phase encoding steps × Number of signal averages

To determine scan time in this example:

1,000 ms (or 1 second) × 240 × 1 = 240 seconds.
240/60 = 4 minutes

4-26. In fast spin echo imaging, if a 256 phase matrix is used, with 1 second TR, 2 signal average, and an ETL of 8, how many phase-encoding steps are completed per each TR?

A. 4

B. 8

C. 16

D. 32

Discussion: The number of phase-encoding steps completed per TR is based upon the echo train length. In this example, we have an 8 ETL; hence, we have 8 phase-encoding steps completed per TR.

4-27. What effect does increasing TE have on image contrast?

A. Increases contrast based on T2 differences

B. Decreases contrast based on T2 differences

C. Increases contrast based on T1 differences

D. Decreases contrast based on T1 differences

Discussion: An increased TE will increase T2 contrast based on the differences created by T2 decay times of tissues. A longer TE will allow for more T2 decay and allow for more differences to be present.

4-28. If I want to increase spatial resolution by altering the image matrix, what would I need to do?

A. Increase image matrix

B. Decrease image matrix

C. Not change image matrix

D. Image matrix has no effect on spatial resolution

Discussion: Image matrix has a direct impact on spatial resolution. To increase spatial resolution, you need to have a smaller voxel size, so increasing the image matrix (specifically the phase matrix) will accomplish this.

4-29. Which example will have the highest SNR?

A. Scan with 10 ms TE

B. Scan with 20 ms TE

C. Scan with 30 ms TE

D. Scan with 40 ms TE

Discussion: The lower the TE, the higher the SNR. This is because the lower TE scan will have more transverse magnetization available to be rephased and create a signal. TE and SNR are inversely affected, so conversely, the higher the TE, the lower the SNR.

4-30. Which of the following is not a method to increase contrast-to-noise ratio (CNR)?

A. Use T2-weighted imaging

B. Use contrast agents

C. Use T1-weighted imaging

D. Use chemical saturation techniques

Discussion: Using T1-weighted imaging will not improve CNR, unless you use contrast agents and perform T1-weighted imaging postcontrast.

4-31. What effect does increasing TR have on image contrast?

A. Increases contrast based on T2 differences

B. Decreases contrast based on T2 differences

C. Increases contrast based on T1 differences

D. Decreases contrast based on T1 differences

Discussion: An increased TR will decrease T1 contrast based on the differences created by T1 relaxation times of tissues. A longer TR will allow for more T1 relaxation and allow for fewer differences to be present.

4-32. The period of time before each R wave in cardiac imaging is known as the __________.

A. trigger delay

B. trigger window

C. VENC encoding

D. R-R interval

Discussion: The trigger window is the waiting period before each R wave of the QRS complex.

4-33. What three parameters affect pulse sequence acquisition time?

A. Image matrix, FOV, TE

B. Slice thickness, TR, TE

C. FOV, TR, TE

D. Image matrix, TR, number of signal averages

Discussion: Image matrix, TR, and the number of signal averages all directly affect image acquisition time, specifically the phase matrix. To determine imaging acquisition time, use this formula:

TR × Number of phase encoding steps × Number of signal averages

4-34. A 3-D volumetric scan is primarily used for the ability to produce __________.

A. thin slices

B. long scan times

C. anisotropic voxels

D. T2 weighting

Discussion: 3-D volume scans have the ability to produce very thin slices with little to no gap while maintaining high SNR due to the entire volume being excited at once.

4-35. TE controls the amount of __________ when the signal is read.

A. T1 weighting

B. T2 weighting

C. PD weighting

D. diffusion weighting

Discussion: TE controls the amount of T2 weighting present on the imaging when the signal is read. Longer TE times allow more T2 weighting, and shorter TE times allow less T2 weighting.

Reference: MRI in Practice, page 103

4-36. Signal-to-noise ratio (SNR) _________ when the TR increases.

A. will decrease

B. will increase

C. will not change

D. will vary

Discussion: As TR increases, SNR increases. This is due to more transverse magnetization to recover before the next repetition.

4-37. Signal-to-noise ratio (SNR) _________ when the TE increases.

A. will decrease

B. will increase

C. will not change

D. will vary

Discussion: As TE increases, SNR decreases. This is due to longer TE times allowing more decay of transverse magnetization before the signal is collected and read.

4-38. Flow compensation is affected when using gradient moment nulling, thus causing flowing nuclei to appear _________.

A. hypointense

B. hyperintense

C. as aliasing

D. turbulent

Discussion: Gradient moment nulling alters the polarity of nuclei with the application of positive and negative gradient lobes. This creates a net-zero phase change and allows flowing nuclei to remain hyperintense.

Reference: MRI in Practice, page 210

4-39. Proton-density weighted imaging utilizes a _________ TR.

A. long

B. short

C. medium

D. no

Discussion: A long TR is used in proton-density weighted imaging to decrease T1 effects.

4-40. Which of the following will create the shortest scan time?

A. 500 ms TR, 30 ms TE, 224 × 224 matrix, 1 signal average

B. 500 ms TR, 30 ms TE, 256 × 256 matrix, 2 signal averages

C. 700 ms TR, 30 ms TE, 224 × 256 matrix, 1 signal average

D. 700 ms TR, 30 ms TE, 224 × 224 matrix, 2 signal averages

Discussion: Using a longer TR, higher matrix, and more signal averages will all increase scan time.

4-41. What method must be employed to differentiate a syrinx from a truncation artifact on a cervical spine scan?

A. Increase phase matrix

B. Use inferior and superior saturation pulses

C. Use gradient moment nulling

D. None of the above

Discussion: Increasing the phase matrix will reduce a truncation, or Gibbs, artifact. All other listed options will not reduce the artifact.

4-42. What pulse sequence listed below should be used to identify hemorrhage?

A. Proton density

B. T2-weighted FSE

C. STIR

D. Gradient echo

Discussion: Magnetic susceptibility artifacts are often apparent in the case of hemorrhage due to the presence of iron in the blood. Magnetic susceptibility artifacts are increased with gradient echo sequences due to the lack of 180° refocusing pulses.

4-43. Which method listed below is best to reduce scan time without directly affecting image contrast?

A. Decrease TR

B. Decrease phase matrix

C. Use gradient moment nulling

D. Decrease TE

Discussion: Reducing the phase matrix will reduce scan time and have no effect on overall image contrast.

4-44. Reducing the FOV by a factor of 2 reduces voxel volume by what factor?

A. $\sqrt{2}$

B. 2

C. 4

D. 8

Discussion: Reducing FOV by a factor of 2 will cut voxel volume in half in two dimensions (phase and frequency directions). This in turn will reduce the voxel size to ¼ the original size.

Reference: MRI in Practice, page 112

4-45. Increasing the TE from 80 ms to 120 ms on a spin echo sequence will create _________.

A. increased T1 weighting

B. better tissue contrast based on T2 tissue characteristics

C. fewer protons experiencing spin-spin interactions

D. a signal void

Discussion: Increasing TE will increase T2 contrast due to more transverse magnetization available.

4-46. How will image quality be affected when reducing TR?

A. SNR decreases

B. T2 contrast increases

C. Proton density weighting increases

D. Resolution decreases

Discussion: SNR decreases when TR is decreased due to less transverse magnetization available for the next repetition.

4-47. The Ernst angle is used to achieve _________ signal that can be produced with a _________ TR.

A. maximum; short

B. minimum; short

C. maximum; long

D. minimum; long

Discussion: Exciting an RF pulse with an Ernst angle will produce maximum signal that can be achieved with a short TR.

4-48. To minimize scan time, which of the following would be an option?

A. Decrease receiver bandwidth

B. Decrease FOV

C. Decrease number of signal averages

D. Increase phase matrix

Discussion: Decreasing the number of signal averages will directly lower scan time. The trade-off is lower SNR, however.

4-49. If you are performing an MRI scan with the parameters of 600 ms TR and 30 ms TE on a spin echo sequence, what range of contrast would you expect to see on your resultant images?

A. T1-weighted

B. Proton density-weighted

C. Diffusion-weighted

D. T2-weighted

Discussion: Using a short TR (i.e., 600 ms) will increase T1 weighting on the images, while using a short TE (i.e., 30 ms) will limit T2 weighting. The result will be more pronounced T1-weighted signal.

4-50. Which of the following pulse sequences is the most flow sensitive?

A. STIR

B. FLAIR

C. T2 FSE

D. T2 gradient echo

Discussion: Gradient echo pulse sequences are more flow sensitive than all spin echo pulse sequences. This is because gradient rephasing is not slice selective compared to spin echo.

Reference: MRI in Practice, page 165

4-51. Increasing slice thickness will have what effect on resolution?

A. Decrease it

B. Increase it

C. Have no effect on it

D. Will be dependent on TR selected

Discussion: Increasing slice thickness will create larger voxels and, in turn, will decrease image resolution.

4-52. Using a(n) _________ measurement time in a fast spin echo sequence increases spatial and contrast resolution.

A. increased

B. decreased

C. high

D. amplified

Discussion: In fast spin echo (FSE), superior spatial resolution with better contrast resolution can be obtained with a reduced measurement time.

4-53. T1-weighted images are beneficial in demonstrating anatomy because they have a _________ signal-to-noise ratio (SNR).

A. high

B. low

C. intermediate

D. T1 weighting does not affect SNR

Discussion: T1-weighted images are beneficial in demonstrating anatomy because they have a high SNR and, when contrast is used, they provide excellent enhancement of pathology.

4-54. By reducing _________, spatial resolution of an MRI image is reduced.

A. repetition time

B. NEX

C. scan time

D. phase encodings

Discussion: Reducing the number of phase encodings reduces the spatial resolution.

4-55. In fast spin echo (FSE), the number of 180° rephasing pulses performed per _________ corresponds to the number of echoes produced and number of k-spaces filled.

A. TR

B. TE

C. PD

D. TI

Discussion: In fast spin echo (FSE), the number of 180° rephrasing pulses performed per TR corresponds to the number of echoes produced and number of k-spaces filled. This number is referred to as echo train length or turbo factor. The higher the turbo factor or echo train length, the shorter the scan time. The echoes sampled with the effective TE will be placed in the center of k-space where they will have a greater impact on image contrast. None effective TE echoes will be placed in the periphery of K space where they have a lower impact on image contrast.

4-56. The Ernst angle consists of a flip angle of _________.

A. more than 90°

B. less than 90°

C. zero

Discussion: The Ernst angle is usually less than 90°.

4-57. Refocused gradient echo (GRE) pulse sequences produce a(n) _________ contrast and a _________ signal to noise than spoiled gradient echo (GRE) sequences.

A. better; poorer

B. poorer; better

C. enhanced; better

D. reduced; reduced

Discussion: In general, refocused gradient echo (GRE) pulse sequences produce a poorer contrast and a better signal to noise than spoiled gradient echo (GRE) sequences. At flip angles >20°, spoiled sequences have exceptional T1 weighting, and fluids like blood appear hypointense, refocused images will appear with less contrast, and fluids will be hyperintense.

4-58. Contrast resolution is improved when k-space is filled using spiral filling because:

A. Data is filled line-by-line during acquisition

B. Data is filled in the center during acquisition of the image

C. Data is filled per segment during acquisition of the image

D. Data is filled from the edges to the center during acquisition of the image

Discussion: During spiral imaging, the center of k-space is filled in more than the periphery of the image, improving contrast resolution.

4-59. What happens to SNR when the receiver bandwidth is increased?

A. SNR decreases

B. SNR increases

C. SNR does not change

D. None of the above

Discussion: SNR will decrease when receiver bandwidth is increased. This is due to more noise sampled compared to signal.

4-60. A pixel's SNR is proportional to __________.

A. the square root of the number of acquisitions (NEX)

B. the number of phase encoding steps

C. voxel volume

D. All of the above

Discussion: All the listed aspects will proportionally affect a pixel's SNR.

4-61. If slice thickness is reduced, what happens to image quality if all other parameters are unchanged?

A. Partial volume averaging decreases

B. SNR increases

C. Spatial resolution decreases

D. None of the above

Discussion: Partial volume averaging will decrease with thinner slices, while SNR will decrease, and spatial resolution will increase. This is all due to overall voxel size.

4-62. What type of MR angiography method relies on velocity-induced phase shifts to distinguish flowing nuclei from stationary nuclei?

A. Time of flight

B. MIP

C. VENC

D. Contrast-enhanced

Discussion: Changes in velocity cause phase shifts to occur; specifically, the objective is to cause a greater phase shift in flowing nuclei rather than in stationary nuclei (i.e., background tissue).

Reference: MRI in Practice, page 278

4-63. To minimize scan time, which of the following would be an option?

A. Decrease TR

B. Decrease slice thickness

C. Increase number of signal averages

D. Increase number of slices in volume acquisition

Discussion: Decreasing TR will directly lower scan time as well as increase T1 weighting. The trade-off is potentially fewer available slices, however.

4-64. What does proton density imaging measure?

A. Magnetic susceptibility

B. Specific absorption rate

C. Subset of hydrogen protons present in tissues

D. Magnetic field strength

Discussion: Proton density weighting imaging measures the overall density of hydrogen protons in the tissues being examined. Tissue structures measure differing densities on the imaging and are displayed as high and low signal.

4-65. In a 3-D imaging sequence, SNR increases when what parameter listed below is increased?

A. FOV

B. TE

C. TR

D. TI

Discussion: When FOV is increased, SNR will also increase on a 3-D sequence due to the overall imaging volume being excited at once rather than slice-selective excitation.

4-66. What effect does reducing the receiver bandwidth have on the length of time the frequency-encoding gradient is on for sampling?

A. **Increases sampling time**

B. Decreases sampling time

C. Is directly proportional to sampling time

D. Has no effect on sampling time

Discussion: Receiver bandwidth is inversely proportional to sampling time, so when receiver bandwidth is reduced, sampling time increases and vice versa. Here is an example:

Frequency matrix = 256

Sampling time (also called acquisition window) = 8 ms

256/8 ms = 32 kHz

Now, look if the sampling time is increased:

Frequency matrix = 256

Sampling time = 4 ms

256/4 ms = 64 kHz

Reference: MRI in Practice, page 77

4-67. Of the options listed below, which statement is true regarding increasing TR?

A. Spatial resolution will decrease

B. T1 weighting will increase

C. SNR will decrease

D. **Number of available slices will increase**

Discussion: Increasing TR will increase the overall number of available slices since there will be more time between each RF excitation pulse. Spatial resolution will not be affected. SNR will increase and T1 weighting will decrease.

4-68. Of the options listed below, which statement is true regarding decreasing TE?

A. Spatial resolution will decrease

B. **T2 weighting will increase**

C. SNR will decrease

D. Chemical shift will increase

Discussion: Increasing TE will increase the T2 weighting present since the TE determines how much T2 decay is allowed to occur when the MR signal is read. SNR will increase. Chemical shift and spatial resolution will not be affected.

4-69. The transmit bandwidth is applied when the __________ is on.

A. **slice select gradient**

B. phase-encoding gradient

C. frequency-encoding gradient

D. None of the above

Discussion: The transmit bandwidth is the range of frequencies to be excited when applying a RF excitation pulse, so this is applied when the slice select gradient is on (i.e., spin echo 90° and 180° pulses).

4-70. A 2-D sequential acquisition __________.

A. collects k-space data all at once

B. **collects k-space data for one slice before collecting the next slice**

C. collects k-space data for one line in a slice, then the same line in the next slice

D. is not related to data collection

Discussion: 2-D sequential acquisitions collect all data for one slice at a time (e.g., Slice 1) before collecting k-space data in the next line (e.g., Slice 2).

4-71. If you are performing an MRI scan with the parameters of 2,000 ms TR and 120 ms TE on a spin echo sequence, what range of contrast would you expect to see on your resultant images?

A. T1-weighted

B. Proton density-weighted

C. Diffusion-weighted

D. **T2-weighted**

Discussion: Using a long TR (i.e., 2,000 ms) will limit T1 weighting on the images, while using a short TE (i.e., 120 ms) will increase T2 weighting. The result will be more pronounced T2-weighted signal.

4-72. Applying two gradients simultaneously would be helpful in only which of the following processes?

A. No phase wrap

B. **Oblique slice acquisition**

C. Reducing eddy currents

D. Gradient reversal

Discussion: Oblique slice acquisitions require two gradients applied simultaneously to produce oblique slices.

4-73. Fat remains hyperintense on T2-weighted FSE sequences due to multiple 180° pulses. This is an effect called __________.

A. Moiré pattern

B. Browning effect

C. apodization

D. J-coupling

Discussion: Multiple 180° RF refocusing pulses in fast spin echo imaging reduce spin-spin interactions in fat, thus causing the fat signal to display as hyperintense. Conventional spin echo imaging only has one refocusing pulse and, thus, is not affected.

4-74. Utilizing a __________ TE will allow CSF to appear hyperintense on T2-weighted images.

A. long

B. short

C. medium

D. variable

Discussion: Since CSF has a long T2 relaxation time, incorporating a long TE will allow for T2 contrast differences between tissues, including a hyperintense signal from CSF.

4-75. Echo train length, or ETL, is:

A. The number of k-space lines

B. The number of 180° refocusing pulses per TR period

C. The number of 90° excitation pulses per TR period

D. The number of echoes produced by dephasing

Discussion: In a fast spin echo sequence (FSE), the overall number of 180° pulses refers to the echo train length. For example, if an FSE sequence has four 180° refocusing pulses, the ETL is four (4).

4-76. Since echoes produced during a fast spin echo (FSE) pulse sequence will have variable image weighting, a/an __________ must be selected to provide the necessary image contrast for a scan.

A. minimum TE

B. sliding TE

C. multi-TE

D. effective TE

4-77. STIR sequences will demonstrate bone contusions as a(n) __________ signal.

A. hypointense

B. hyperintense

C. mixed

D. isointense

Discussion: STIR sequences are fat-suppression sequences, so the signal from fat (marrow) will be hypointense, while other signals will appear hyperintense.

4-78. Which of the following would produce more T2 weighting?

A. 4 ETL FSE

B. 8 ETL FSE

C. 12 ETL FSE

D. 16 ETL FSE

Discussion: Utilizing a longer ETL will produce more T2 weighting since there will be an increased number of longer echoes contributing to the signal.

4-79. Approximately what TI range should be used to null fat in inversion recovery sequences?

A. 100–175 ms

B. 300 ms

C. 800 ms

D. 1,700–2,000 ms

Discussion: Fat has a short inversion time, so utilizing a short TI will help achieve fat suppression in an inversion recovery sequence.

4-80. The flip angle for a given tissue and a given T1 time that will result in maximum signal from that tissue is called the __________ angle.

A. Hahn

B. Ohm

C. Ernst

D. Damadian

Discussion: This is the definition of Ernst angle.

4-81. __________ controls the amount of T2 weighting present on the resultant imaging.

A. Flip angle

B. TR

C. TI

D. TE

Discussion: TE controls the amount of T2 weighting present. Shortening TE will decrease T2 weighting and lengthening TE will increase T2 weighting.

4-82. Parallel imaging techniques help to __________.

A. reduce artifacts in the slice direction

B. reduce scan time

C. increase T1 weighting

D. improve fat suppression

Discussion: Parallel imaging helps reduce scan time by assigning certain aspects of a coil to collect and encode imaging data.

4-83. Which of the following parameter adjustments will result in an increase in spatial resolution?

A. Decreasing FOV

B. Decreasing phase matrix size

C. Increasing slice thickness

D. Decreasing TE

Discussion: A decreased, or smaller, FOV will result in smaller voxels and, thus, increase spatial resolution.

4-84. In an FSE sequence, the effective TE echoes will be stored in __________.

A. the outer areas of k-space

B. the center areas of k-space

C. the left half of k-space

D. the top half of k-space

Discussion: The echoes from the effective TE will be stored in the center of k-space, thus contributing to the overall signal and contrast of the resultant image.

4-85. A fat suppression sequence incorporates __________ pulse prior to the excitation pulse.

A. a 90°

B. a 180°

C. a 90° pulse followed by a 180°

D. no

Discussion: Fat suppression sequences apply a 90° pulse prior to the RF excitation pulse. The initial pulse is applied at the precessional frequency of fat to null fat signal once it is moved to a full 180° after the excitation pulse.

4-86. Reducing the flip angle will have what effect on SNR?

A. Increase it

B. Decrease it

C. No change

Discussion: Smaller flip angles rotate the net magnetization less into the transverse plane, which allows less magnetization available to produce signal.

4-87. Assuming all parameters do not change, if the image matrix is reduced from 512 × 512 to 256 × 256, what happens to SNR?

A. SNR increases

B. SNR decreases

C. SNR is not affected

Discussion: Decreasing image matrices creates larger voxels. Larger voxels have more room for signal and, thus, an increased SNR.

4-88. Assuming all parameters do not change, what happens to SNR if the FOV is changed from 256 mm to 240 mm?

A. SNR increases

B. SNR decreases

C. SNR is not affected

Discussion: Decreasing FOVs create smaller voxels. Smaller voxels have less room for signal and, thus, a decreased SNR.

4-89. Lesions with prolonged T2 relaxation times are commonly hyperintense on diffusion-weighted images due to a phenomenon called__________.

A. T2-prime

B. T2*

C. T2 relaxation

D. T2 shine-through

Discussion: T2 shine-through occurs typically with pathologies with increased T2 relaxation times, including hemorrhage.

Reference: AJNR: 26, February 2005, http://www.ajnr.org/content/26/2/236.full.pdf

4-90. Why are presaturation pulses useful?

A. To improve spatial resolution

B. To reduce flow motion artifacts

C. To reduce scan time

D. To decrease flow void artifacts

Discussion: Presaturation bands can be utilized to decrease artifacts in general, and specifically to reduce flow motion artifacts.

4-91. Which of the following postcontrast techniques is optimal when imaging breast tissue?

A. T1-weighted

B. T2-weighted

C. Inversion recovery

D. T1-weighted fat saturation

Discussion: Due to the large fatty content of breast tissue, postcontrast fat saturation techniques are preferred to distinguish tumor tissue from fat tissue.

4-92. Lung tissue demonstrates as __________ on T1- and T2-weighted imaging.

A. hypointense

B. isointense

C. hyperintense

D. no signal

Discussion: Due to the lack of available signal in the lungs, a signal void is present and, thus, the lungs are black on MR images.

4-93. Which is an option to increase spatial resolution?

A. Use course matrix

B. Increase slice thickness

C. Use smaller FOV

D. Decrease TE

Discussion: Only using a smaller FOV will increase spatial resolution, as this option will create smaller voxels. All other options listed will create larger voxels or have no effect at all (decrease TE).

4-94. Which option below can help reduce Moiré pattern artifacts?

A. Reduce bandwidth

B. Use spin echo sequence

C. Increase FOV

D. Decrease TR

Discussion: Moiré pattern artifacts, or fringe artifacts, typically occur with gradient echo sequences and large FOVs. This is due to the lack of field homogeneity from one area of the FOV to another. Using spin echo sequences will help reduce magnetic field inhomogeneities due to the presence of a 180° rephasing pulse.

4-95. Which of the following is the most common sequence used in bright blood MRA imaging?

A. Fast spin echo

B. Gradient echo

C. Inversion recovery

D. Echo planar

Discussion: Only gradient echo sequences generally produce hyperintense signal on flowing nuclei. Spin echo sequences generally demonstrate hypointense signal from flowing nuclei.

4-96. To achieve thicker slices, what type of gradient is required?

A. Steep slice select gradient slope

B. Steep slice phase-encoding slope

C. Shallow slice select gradient slope

D. Shallow phase-encoding slope

Discussion: Shallow slice select gradient slopes are required to produce thicker slices. This gradient is on during the application of the 90° and 180° pulses.

4-97. What parameter change is required to decrease magic angle artifacts?

A. Increase flip angle

B. Decrease TR

C. Increase bandwidth

D. Increase TE

Discussion: Magic angle artifacts are present when molecules lie at 54.74° and, thus, cause a lengthening of T2 times. In short TE sequences, little T2 signal has decayed when the echo is read. Longer TE sequences will allow for more T2 decay and the artifact will not be as visible.

Reference: www.radiopaedia.org

4-98. When using a surface coil, SNR will __________ the farther the coil is from the region of interest.

A. increase

B. decrease

C. not be affected

Discussion: SNR is directly affected by the distance a surface coil is in relation to the anatomy to be examined. Placing the coils as close to the anatomy as possible will ensure higher SNR.

4-99. When imaging the internal auditory canal, which of the following should not be employed?

A. Smaller FOV

B. Thicker slices

C. Longer TR

D. Decreased image matrix

Discussion: Thicker slices are not optimal when imaging the internal auditory canal, since larger slices create larger voxels and cause partial volume averaging.

4-100. Which of the following is the effect of decreasing TE time?

A. Decrease in SNR

B. Increase in proton density contrast weighting

C. Decrease in image resolution

D. Increase in contrast-to-noise ratio (CNR)

Discussion: Decreasing TE will reduce T2 effects, thereby increasing proton density contrast. It also increases SNR, has no effect on resolution, and decreases CNR (due to reduced T2 effects).

4-101. One method to increase SNR is __________.

A. increasing signal averaging

B. utilizing thinner slices

C. utilizing smaller FOV

D. utilizing a shorter TR

Discussion: Only increasing signal averaging will increase the signal measured compared to noise. All other options listed will reduce SNR. Thinner slices and smaller FOVs will reduce voxel size and cause lower SNR; using a shorter TR will reduce SNR due to less transverse magnetization being available when the next application of the RF pulse is applied.

4-102. Gradient moment nulling will __________ minimum TE.

A. increase

B. decrease

C. not affect

Discussion: Gradient moment nulling uses additional gradient pulses so, therefore, will require a longer minimum TE.

4-103. In steady state gradient echo imaging, the TR is __________.

A. longer than the T1/T2 times of tissues

B. shorter than the T1/T2 times of tissues

C. equal to the T1/T2 times of tissues

D. not related to the T1/T2 times of tissues

Discussion: In order to achieve steady state, a TR that is shorter than the T1 and T2 times of tissues must be utilized. By having a TR shorter than the T1/T2 times of tissues, no transverse magnetization is allowed to decay prior to the next repetition of the TR.

4-104. A method to reduce phase mismapping, or ghosting, from respiratory motion is:

A. Increase TR

B. Gating

C. Gradient moment nulling

D. VENC

Discussion: Respiratory gating is a primary method to reduce phase mismapping caused by respiratory motion.

4-105. Increasing __________ will increase diffusion-weighting on DWI sequences.

A. b-value

B. resolution

C. slice thickness

D. concatenations

Discussion: The b-value parameter increases the amount of diffusion present on DWI sequences.

4-106. BOLD effects in functional MR imaging are short-lived; therefore, it is important to use a sequence with __________.

A. high CNR

B. high SNR

C. high spatial resolution

D. high temporal resolution

Discussion: In functional MR, high temporal resolution is crucial since BOLD effects occur very quickly and are short-lived. Using a high temporal resolution will increase the ability to detect BOLD effects.

4-107. In TOF-MRA, a TR of approximately __________ should be utilized to maximize signal.

A. 50 ms

B. 150 ms

C. 250 ms

D. 350 ms

Discussion: When used in conjunction with a flip angle of approximately 45–60, a 50 ms TR will maximize signal without suppressing signal from blood.

Reference: MRI in Practice, page 271

4-108. To achieve T1 weighting in ECG cardiac-gated imaging, a TR range of 600–900 is used and __________ R wave will trigger the pulse sequence.

A. every

B. every other

C. every third

D. every fourth

Discussion: In ECG cardiac-gated imaging, every R wave in the QRS complex will be required to trigger the pulse sequence. Triggering every second or third wave is required to achieve T2 weighting.

4-109. Which of the following is an effective method to decrease cross-talk?

A. Decrease slice gap

B. Interleaving slices

C. Increase phase-encoding steps

D. Increase number of slices

Discussion: Interleaving slices will be excited in a different order (i.e., even slices first, then odd slices), and as such will reduce cross-talk artifacts.

4-110. A __________ flip angle is typically used to achieve T2* weighting in gradient echo sequences.

A. high

B. low

C. medium

D. always 90°

Discussion: Since the flip angle helps control the amount of saturation present, a lower flip angle is required for T2* and proton density gradient echo imaging. This is used in conjunction with a longer TR and longer TE.

Reference: MRI in Practice

4-111. Approximately what inversion time should be used to null CSF in an inversion recovery sequence?

A. 150 ms

B. 800 ms

C. 1,000 ms

D. 2,000 ms

Discussion: CSF has long T1/T2 times, so a long inversion time is required to null signal from CSF.

4-112. Time-of-flight effects increase in spin echo sequences when __________ increases.

A. TR

B. TE

C. flip angle

D. slice thickness

Discussion: Time-of-flight effects will increase when TE increases due to fewer flowing nuclei being present when the 180° pulse is applied. Nuclei must receive both the 90° and 180° pulses for signal to be present.

4-113. Which is an option to increase spatial resolution?

A. Use course matrix

B. Increase slice thickness

C. Use smaller FOV

D. Decrease TE

Discussion: Only using a smaller FOV will increase spatial resolution, as this option will create smaller voxels. All other options listed will create larger voxels or have no effect at all (decrease TE).

4-114. To achieve T1 weighting on a gradient echo sequence, which flip angle listed below should be used?

A. 5°

B. 15°

C. 35°

D. 75°

Discussion: Higher flip angles in gradient echo sequences will achieve T1 weighting.

4-115. To double SNR in a sequence with 1 signal average, to what must the signal averages be increased?

A. 2

B. 4

C. 6

D. 8

Discussion: To double SNR, the signal averages must be increased by a factor of 4, or √4.

4-116. Which of the following would have the highest CNR?

A. 500 ms TR, 30 ms TE, 256 × 256 image matrix

B. 1,500 ms TR, 30 ms TE, 192 × 256 image matrix

C. 2,000 ms TR, 40 ms TE, 512 × 512 image matrix

D. 4,000 ms TR, 90 ms TE, 256 × 256 image matrix

Discussion: Increasing T2 weighting is a primary method for increasing CNR. All other options listed are either T1- or PD-weighted sequences.

4-117. Which of the following sequences will have the shortest scan time?

A. 3,500 ms TR, 256 phase encoding steps, 2 signal averages, 2 ETL

B. 2,500 ms TR, 512 phase encoding steps, 2 signal averages, 4 ETL

C. 3,000 ms TR, 256 phase encoding steps, 4 signal averages, 4 ETL

D. 2,000 ms TR, 512 phase encoding steps, 2 signal averages, 2 ETL

Discussion: To determine scan time: TR × phase encoding steps × signal averages / ETL 2.5 sec × 512 × 2 / 4 = 640 seconds, or approximately 10 minutes, 40 seconds.

4-118. Which of the following sequences would provide the most optimal image resolution?

A. 128 mm FOV, 256 × 256 matrix, 0.5 mm slice thickness

B. 256 mm FOV, 512 × 512 matrix, 1.0 mm slice thickness

C. 256 mm FOV, 256 × 256 matrix, 0.5 mm slice thickness

D. 256 mm FOV, 512 × 512 matrix, 1.0 mm slice thickness

Discussion: Option A will create an image resolution of 0.5 mm × 0.5 mm × 0.5 mm. This is an isotropic voxel as it has equal resolution on all three sides.

4-119. Applying a spatial presaturation band will __________.

A. increase the number of slices available

B. decrease the number of slices available

C. decrease RF deposition in the patient

D. have no effect on slices and RF deposition

Discussion: Applying a spatial presaturation pulse, or "sat band," will increase RF deposition as well as reduce the number of slices available, since it occurs within the allotted TR time available.

Reference: MRI in Practice, pages 210, 224

4-120. __________ controls the amount of T1 weighting present on the resultant imaging.

A. Flip angle

B. TR

C. TE

D. TI

Discussion: TR controls the amount of T1 weighting present. Shortening TR will increase T1 weighting, and lengthening TR will decrease T1 weighting.

4-121. In contrast-enhanced T1-weighted MR imaging, the TR should __________.

A. stay the same on precontrast and postcontrast imaging

B. be longer on precontrast than postcontrast imaging

C. be shorter on pre- and postcontrast imaging

D. vary from patient to patient on precontrast and postcontrast imaging

Discussion: Gadolinium shortens T1 times of surrounding water protons, so utilizing the same TR for both precontrast and postcontrast imaging is essential. If the TR is altered, signal and contrast will be affected on potential pathology.

4-122. Applying fat saturation to a pulse sequence will __________.

A. decrease the number of slices available

B. increase the number of slices available

C. decrease RF deposition

D. have no effect on the number of slices available or RF deposition

Discussion: Since fat saturation requires an additional pulse within the pulse sequence, this will decrease the number of slices available for a given TR.

Reference: MRI in Practice, page 218

4-123. To reduce image blurring on FSE imaging, the MR operator would need to __________.

A. increase echo train length (ETL)

B. decrease echo train length (ETL)

C. increase echo spacing

D. decrease effective TE

Discussion: FSE sequences with longer ETLs (echo train lengths) will have increased blurring due to late echoes with negligible signal creating a low-image resolution. Reducing ETL and/or echo spacing will reduce image blurring.

Reference: MRI in Practice, page 146

4-124. When utilizing a rectangular FOV, spatial resolution __________.

A. is decreased

B. is decreased

C. remains the same

Discussion: Rectangular FOV decreases the overall number of phase encodings but will not increase or decrease spatial resolution since the pixel dimensions remain unchanged.

Reference: MRI in Practice, pages 127, 130

4-125. Of the options listed below, which statement is true regarding decreasing phase matrix?

A. Spatial resolution will increase

B. Spatial resolution will decrease

C. SNR will decrease

D. Scan time will increase

Discussion: Decreasing phase matrix, or the number of phase-encoding steps, will decrease overall spatial resolution since pixel/voxel dimension will be larger.

4-126. Of the options listed below, which statement is true regarding decreasing slice thickness?

A. Spatial resolution will decrease

B. Scan time will increase

C. Partial volume averaging will increase

D. SNR will decrease

Discussion: Decreasing slice thickness will decrease overall SNR since pixel/voxel dimension will be smaller.

4-127. Of the options listed below, which statement is true regarding increasing FOV?

A. Spatial resolution will decrease

B. Aliasing artifact will increase

C. SNR will decrease

D. Scan time will increase

Discussion: Increasing FOV will decrease overall spatial resolution since pixel/voxel dimension will be larger.

4-128. Of the options listed below, which statement is true regarding increasing the number of signal averages?

A. Spatial resolution will increase

B. Spatial resolution will decrease

C. SNR will decrease

D. Scan time will increase

Discussion: Increasing the number of signal averages will increase overall scan time, since the signal will be collected and averaged by the number of signal averages selected. For example, if a sequence with one signal average is 2 minutes in length, increasing signal averages to "two" will double scan time, thus making the sequence 4 minutes in length.

4-129. __________ is a technique to reduce background signal in time-of-flight (TOF) MRA sequences.

A. MIP

B. VENC

C. Multi-planar reformatting

D. Magnetization transfer contrast

Discussion: Magnetization transfer contrast, or MTC, suppresses background signal from macromolecules in fat, white matter, and gray matter. MTC is considered a method to improve CNR in MRA sequences.

Reference: MRI in Practice, page 275

4-130. To reduce aliasing, which method listed below should be employed?

A. Reduce number of signal averages

B. Increase FOV in phase direction

C. Reduce TE

D. Increase receiver bandwidth

Discussion: Increasing FOV in the phase direction will reduce aliasing since the FOV in this direction will be increased. Additionally, the use of *no phase wrap*, *oversampling*, or *anti-foldover* will reduce aliasing.

Reference: MRI in Practice, page 240

4-131. Which statement below is not true concerning 3-D phase contrast MRA (PC-MRA) imaging?

A. 3-D sequences allow increased spatial resolution.

B. 3-D sequences will have decreased SNR compared to 2-D PC-MRA sequences.

C. 3-D sequences are typically used for imaging of smaller vascular structures.

D. 3-D sequences generally have longer scan times.

Discussion: 3-D PC-MRA sequences will actually have improved SNR compared to 2-D PC-MRA since the entire imaging volume will be excited at once as opposed to slice-by-slice.

Reference: MRI in Practice, pages 283–285

4-132. Which option listed would better reduce specific absorption rate (SAR)?

A. Gradient echo breath-hold on 1.5T system

B. Spin echo on 3T system

C. Fast spin echo with long echo train length on 3T system

D. Fast spin echo with a short echo train length on 3T system

Discussion: Generally, spin echo sequences, and especially fast spin echo sequences, create a higher SAR in patients since the magnitude and number of RF pulses increases. Gradient echo sequences use smaller RF pulses, so SAR is generally lower. Additionally, increasing field strength will increase SAR as well.

Reference: AJR Online (http://www.ajronline.org/doi/pdf/10.2214/AJR.14.14173); MR-Tip.com (http://www.mr-tip.com/serv1.php?type=db1&dbs=Specific%20Absorption%20Rate)

4-133. A tissue that has a higher proton density will __________.

A. appear as hypointense compared to tissues with lower proton density

B. appear as hyperintense compared to tissues with lower proton density

C. appear as isointense compared to tissues with lower proton density

D. demonstrate no signal at all compared to tissues with lower proton density

Discussion: Tissues that have higher proton density will provide more signal, thus appearing hyperintense, or brighter, on the images, compared to tissues with lower proton density.

4-134. Decreasing voxel size will __________.

A. decrease spatial resolution

B. increase spatial resolution

C. decrease temporal resolution

D. increase temporal resolution

Discussion: When voxel size decreases, spatial resolution will increase, since smaller voxel size is directly related to increased image resolution.

4-135. What method should be utilized to correct for motion artifacts?

A. Decrease phase matrix

B. Decrease number of signal averages

C. Swap phase and frequency encoding directions

D. Increase number of slices

Discussion: Swapping phase and frequency encoding directions will not reduce motion artifacts but will help correct for it, as the motion artifact will subsequently be placed into a different direction. Decreasing the phase matrix will not have any effect. Decreasing the number of signal averages may actually increase motion artifacts seen on the imaging, and increasing the number of slices will not have any effect.

MRI Questions: Data Acquisition

5-1. A spin echo pulse results from a _________ radio frequency (RF) pulse followed by a_________ RF pulse.

A. 180°; 90°

B. 90°; 180°

C. 180°; 180°

D. 90°; 90°

Discussion: A spin echo results from a 90° RF pulse followed by a 180° RF pulse.

5-2. What is the term used to describe the time between the initial 90° RF pulse and the spin echo?

A. Time-to-echo (TE)

B. Inversion recovery (IR)

C. Time-to-recovery (TR)

D. Multi-echo spin echo (MESE)

Discussion: Echo time is the time from the middle of the first pulse to the middle of the echo.

Reference: http://mri-q.com/index.html

5-3. Which of the following MRI techniques is the most commonly used to acquire the MRI image?

A. Inversion recovery (IR)

B. Spin echo (SE)

C. Turbo spin echo (TSE)

D. Gradient recall echo (GRE)

Discussion: The most commonly used MRI imaging technique is the spin echo. It was introduced by Hahn in 1950.

5-4. K-space in the spin echo sequence is filled_________.

A. Every other line

B. Top to bottom

C. All at time

D. Line by line

Discussion: The spatial frequency domain (k-space) is filled line by line sequentially from bottom to top.

5-5. In what period is the k-space of the analog spin echo sampled and converted into digital form?

A. Sample period

B. Phase-encoding period

C. Frequency-encoding period

D. Read period

Discussion: The read period is the time at which the k-space in the spin echo is sampled and converted into digital form. The frequency encoding gradient is turned on and data is recorded.

5-6. What part of the k-space contains coarse structure information of the object?

A. Central zone

B. Middle zone

C. Right zone

D. Left zone

Discussion: The signal is received and contains phase information encoded before the read period. The central zone contains coarse structure of the object.

5-7. A significant source of artifacts in MR images can result from what?

A. Changes in the patient from one echo time to the next

B. Changes in the patient from one repetition time to the next

C. Changes in frequency-encoding measurement to the next

Discussion: A significant source of artifacts from one phase-encoding measurement to the next, the Fourier transform assumes that all information in k-space comes from the same subject. If there is a change during the repetition time (TR), this assumption becomes void.

5-8. What is the purpose of the 180° refocusing RF pulse during a spin echo pulse sequence?

A. Dephase the transverse magnetization to prevent inhomogeneities

B. Relax the transverse magnetization to prevent inhomogeneities

C. Invert the phase of the spins to prevent inhomogeneities

Discussion: The 180° refocusing RF pulse inverts the phase of the spins by putting the faster components of the transverse magnetizations behind the slower to prevent inhomogeneities.

5-9. Inversion time is defined as _________.

A. the period between the beginning of a pulse sequence and the beginning of the succeeding and identical pulse sequence.

B. the time between the initial 90° RF pulse and the spin echo

C. an additional 180° RF pulse in a fast spin echo

D. the time between the 180° RF inversion pulse and the subsequent 90° RF pulse.

Discussion: The time between the 180° RF inversion pulse and the subsequent 90° RF pulse.

5-10. How does inversion recovery (IR) imaging differ from spin echo (SE) imaging?

A. The longitudinal magnetization of various tissues is larger

B. The transverse magnetization of various tissues is larger

C. The transverse magnetization of various tissues is shorter

D. The longitudinal magnetization of various tissues is shorter

Discussion: The differences among the longitudinal magnetization of various tissues can be larger in IR imaging than SE imaging; the increase in magnetization increases the T1W and improves the contrast between tissues with slightly different T1 values.

5-11. A valuable application for inversion recovery imaging includes_________.

A. The enhancement of signal from tissues having specific T1 relaxation times

B. The nulling of signal from tissues having specific T1 relaxation times

C. The enhancement of signal from tissues having specific T2 relaxation times

D. The nulling of signal from tissues having specific T2 relaxation times

Discussion: Clinical application for inversion recovery (IR) imaging is the nulling of signal from tissues having specific T1 relaxation times. The part of the spin echo (SE) sequence is started allowing the longitudinal magnetization of a relaxation time when the 90° RF pulse is applied so that there is no net magnetization flipped into the XY plane and no signal is produced for that tissue.

5-12. Fat has _________ T1 relaxation time.

A. a long

B. a short

C. no

Discussion: Fat has a short T1 relaxation time.

5-13. STIR stands for__________.

A. **Short tau inversion recovery**

B. Standard tau inversion recovery

C. Some tau inversion recovery

D. Single tau inversion recovery

Discussion: STIR stands for short tau inversion recovery.

5-14. Fluid has __________ T1 and TI times.

A. **long**

B. short

C. no

Discussion: Fluids have a relatively long T1 and TI times, 2 seconds or more, which helps to minimize signal from fluid structures.

5-15. A FLAIR sequence is used to diagnose diseases such as __________.

A. multiple sclerosis

B. infarctions

C. subarachnoid hemorrhages

D. **All the above**

Discussion: Fluids have a relatively long T1 and TI times, 2 seconds or more, which helps to minimize signal from fluid structures. This allows for better diagnosis of periventricular lesions.

5-16. What is the mathematical relationship that states k-space is symmetrical in both the x-frequency and y-phase axes?

A. **Herrmann symmetry**

B. Fourier transform

C. Half Fourier imaging

D. Hermitian symmetry

Discussion: The spatial frequency lines acquired on either side of a zero-amplitude phase-encoding gradient are symmetrical.

5-17. The technique used to increase imaging speed is called?

A. Herrmann symmetry

B. Fourier transform

C. **Half Fourier imaging**

D. Hermitian symmetry

Discussion: By using the Hermitian symmetry principle, fast imaging approaches are used so that only half the data are calculated during image reconstruction rather than by signal detection. This is called half Fourier imaging. It uses half of the filled k-space and calculates the other half to produce the MR image.

5-18. The fast spin echo (FSE) uses __________ to produce a train of spin echo (SE) within a single repetition time (TR) interval.

A. **multiple 180° refocusing RF pulses**

B. multiple 90° refocusing RF pulses

C. multiple 90° and 180° refocusing RF pulses

Discussion: Fast spin echo (FSE) uses multiple 180° refocusing pulses to produce a train of spin echoes (SE) within a single TR. This has become the preferred sequence for T2W imaging.

5-19. A fast spin echo (FSE) pulse sequence uses a TR of about __________ milliseconds.

A. 150

B. 6,000

C. **4,000**

D. 550

Discussion: A typical pulse sequence uses a TR of 4,000 ms and an effective TE of 30 ms.

5-20. When echo times are increased, the echoes become more __________ T2W.

A. slightly

B. **heavily**

C. faintly

D. consistently

Discussion: As the echo time is increased, echoes become more heavily T2W, and artifacts can be generated.

5-21. Spin echo trains usually contain __________ echoes.

A. 10–14

B. 20–24

C. 8–12

D. 4–8

Discussion: Echo trains can be as long as 64; however, as the echo time is increased, echoes become more heavily T2W, and artifacts can be generated.

5-22. High spatial frequencies influence __________ and __________ of small objects.

A. edge definition; resolution

B. blurring of edges; resolution

C. edge definition; blurring

D. resolution; loss of contrast

Discussion: High spatial frequencies influence edge definition and resolution of small objects, while low spatial frequencies influence the contrast resolution.

5-23. Using a(n) __________ measurement time in a fast spin echo sequence increases spatial and contrast resolution.

A. increased

B. decreased

C. high

D. amplified

Discussion: In fast spin echo (FSE), superior spatial resolution with better contrast resolution can be obtained with a reduced measurement time.

5-24. Simulated echoes happen during a fast spin echo sequence when a __________.

A. 90° refocusing pulse RF pulse is generated closer together than those of single- or dual-echo SE sequences

B. 180° refocusing pulse RF pulse is generated closer together than those of single- or dual-echo SE sequences

C. 90° and 180° refocusing pulse RF pulse is generated closer together than those of single- or dual-echo SE sequences

D. None of the above

Discussion: Simulated echo is another difference between fast spin echo (FSE) and spin echo (SE). The 180° refocusing RF pulse in the fast spin echo (FSE) is generated a great deal closer together in time than in single- or dual-echo SE sequences.

5-25. Simulated echoes can be produced at any time when __________ RF pulses are applied in rapid succession.

A. 1

B. 2

C. 3

Discussion: Simulated echoes can be produced any time three or more RF pulses are applied in rapid succession and if the time between the pulses is less than $T2^*$.

5-26. __________ blood is not affected by magnetization transfer saturation (MTS) phenomenon.

A. Still

B. Stagnant

C. Static

D. Moving

Discussion: Moving blood is not affected by magnetization transfer saturation. This then improves contrast for MR angiograms.

5-27. In a gradient echo sequence (GRE), simulated echoes can be eliminated through the use of __________.

A. spoiler pulses

B. refocusing pulses

C. ghost pulses

D. relocating pulses

Discussion: In gradient echo imaging, simulated pulses are eliminated through the use of gradient spoiler or RF spoiling during phase cycling.

5-28. J-coupling explains _________ fat in _________ fast spin echo (FSE) imaging.

A. dark; T1W

B. bright; T2W

C. dark; T2W

D. bright; T1W

Discussion: The term J-coupling helps to explain the bright fat in T2W imaging. For complicated molecules like fat, the coupling force spins the magnetization to more rapidly dephase despite the 180° refocusing RF pulse. The dephasing superimposed on the T2 relaxation can result in the addition of signal loss in fatty tissues in spin echo imaging (SE).

5-29. T1W images are beneficial in demonstrating anatomy because they have a _________ signal-to-noise ratio (SNR).

A. high

B. low

C. intermediate

D. T1W does not affect SNR

Discussion: T1W images are beneficial in demonstrating anatomy because they have a high SNR and, when contrast is used, they provide excellent enhancement of pathology.

5-30. By reducing _________, spatial resolution of an MRI image is reduced.

A. repetition time

B. NEX

C. scan time

D. phase encodings

Discussion: Reducing the number of phase encodings reduces the spatial resolution.

5-31. In fast spin echo (FSE), the number of 180° rephrasing pulses performed per _________ corresponds to the number of echoes produced and number of k-spaces filled.

A. TR

B. TE

C. PD

D. TI

Discussion: In fast spin echo (FSE), the number of 180° rephrasing pulses performed per TR corresponds to the number of echoes produced and number of k-spaces filled. This number is referred to as echo train length or turbo factor. The higher the turbo factor or echo train length, the shorter the scan time.

5-32. Gradient echo (GRE) spins are refocused with _________ field, rather than a 180° RF pulse.

A. spin magnetic

B. gradient magnetic

C. phase magnetic

D. frequency magnetic

Discussion: During a gradient echo sequence, spins are refocused with a gradient magnetic field, rather than a 180° RF pulse.

5-33. Which pulse sequence is depicted below?

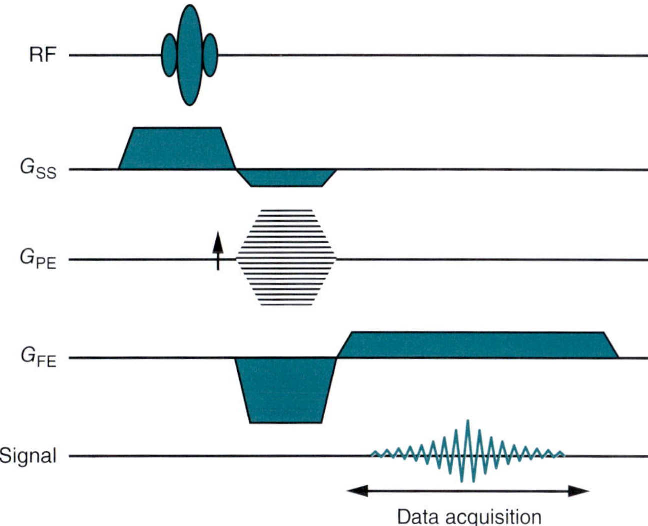

FIGURE 5-1.

Source: Reproduced with permission from Mc Robbie DW, Moore EA, Graves MJ, Prince MR. *MRI From Picture To Proton*, 2e. Cambridge University Press; 2006.

A. Spin echo (SE)

B. Inversion recovery (IR)

C. Gradient echo (GRE)

D. FLAIR

Reference: ccn.ucla.edu

5-34. A gradient echo is generated from _________ when a _________ gradient is applied early and then immediately reversed.

A. free induction decay (FID); rephasing

B. free induction decay (FID); dephasing

C. low flip angle; rephasing

D. long flip angle; dephasing

Discussion: The gradient echo signal is generated from a free induction decay (FID) when the dephasing gradient is applied early within the free induction decay (FID) and then immediately reversed.

5-35. T2* relaxation occurs as a result of _________.

A. homogeneity and dephasing

B. inhomogeneity and rephasing

C. homogeneity and rephasing

D. inhomogeneity and dephasing

Discussion: T2* relaxation occurs as a result of magnetic field inhomogeneity and dephasing. Faster relaxation will result from a gradient magnetic field that is applied to a voxel.

5-36. _________ mechanisms help contribute to the image contrast of a T2* image.

A. Dephasing

B. Rephasing

C. Long flip angle

D. Short flip angle

Discussion: In gradient echo imaging, additional dephasing mechanisms contribute to image contrast and spin-spin relaxation time in a T2* image.

5-37. _________ is the condition of a constant longitudinal magnetization after repeated alpha or partial pulses.

A. Steady state

B. Spoiled state

C. Recoiled state

D. Magnetic state

Discussion: Steady state is the condition of constant longitudinal magnetization after repeated alpha or partial pulses. This is the point at which the reduction in magnetization caused by the excitation equals the same amount of recovery during the TR.

5-38. In a steady state, a _________ excitation can occur if the longitudinal magnetization is close to equilibrium.

A. large flip angle

B. short flip angle

C. low flip angle

D. high flip angle

Discussion: When relatively long TRs and when the longitudinal magnetization is close to equilibrium and the absolute recovery is relatively low, a steady state low flip angle can occur.

5-39. The Ernst angle consists of a flip angle of _________.

A. more than 90°

B. less than 90°

C. zero

Discussion: The Ernst angle is usually less than 90°.

5-40. The Ernst angle is used to achieve _________ signal that can be produced with a _________ TR.

A. maximum; short

B. minimum; short

C. maximum; long

D. minimum; long

Discussion: Exciting an RF pulse with an Ernst angle will produce maximum signal of a tissue and can be achieved with a short TR.

5-41. RF _________ eliminates the phase coherence of the transverse magnetization by changing the phase of each successive RF pulse for each of the measured lines of k-space.

A. spoiling

B. rephrasing

C. dephasing

D. recovering

Discussion: Spoiling methods are used to make sure that only the longitudinal magnetization is recovered and involved in the next measurement.

5-42. Fast imaging with steady state precession is a pulse sequence in which a _________ establishes steady states in both the longitudinal and transverse planes.

A. refocused spin echo (SE)

B. refocused gradient echo (GRE)

C. dephased spin echo (SE)

D. dephased gradient echo (GRE)

Discussion: Fast imaging with steady state precession is a pulse sequence in which a refocused gradient echo (GRE) establishes steady states in both the longitudinal and transverse planes. This pulse sequence is similar to the crusher sequence used in spin echo to eliminate artifacts.

5-43. There is/are _________ type(s) of refocused gradient echo sequences that help to produce different tissue contrasts.

A. 1

B. 2

C. 3

D. 4

Discussion: In practice, there are three different types of refocused gradient echo sequences: fast imaging with steady state precession (FISP), precession of steady state imaging fast (PSIF), and balanced steady state free procession sequence (bSSFP).

5-44. What conditions need to be satisfied for there to be image appearance differences between a spoiled gradient echo (GRE) and refocused gradient echo (GRE)?

A. TR/T2* ratio needs to be about 10 or fewer milliseconds

B. TR/T2* ratio needs to be greater than 10 milliseconds

C. The steady state longitudinal and transverse components are the same

D. None of the above

Discussion: The conditions that need to be satisfied for there to be image appearance differences between a spoiled gradient echo (GRE) and refocused gradient echo (GRE) are a TR/T2*ratio less than 10 ms and the transverse component must be nurtured according to the projection of the longitudinal component. Manufacture sequences include GRASS, FFE, and FISP.

5-45. Refocused gradient echo (GRE) pulse sequences produce a _________ contrast and a _________ signal to noise than spoiled gradient echo (GRE) sequences.

A. better; poorer

B. poorer; better

C. enhanced; better

D. reduced; reduced

Discussion: In general, refocused gradient echo (GRE) pulse sequences produce a poorer contrast and a better signal to noise than spoiled gradient echo (GRE) sequences. At flip angles >20°, spoiled sequences have exceptional T1W, and fluids like blood appear dark, refocused images will appear with less contrast, and fluids will be bright.

5-46. _________ is a type of refocused imaging that produces an RF spin echo instead of a refocused FID.

A. Balanced steady state imaging

B. Free precession steady state imaging

C. Precession steady state imaging fast

D. None of the above

Discussion: Precession steady state imaging fast (PSIF) produces an RF SE instead of a refocused FID. It is a time-reversed fast imaging with steady state precession (FISP) sequence.

5-47. Adding an FISP echo and PSIF echo increases the _________ of a basic fast imaging with steady state precession (FISP).

A. T1W

B. T2W

C. PDW

Discussion: Adding an FISP echo and PSIF echo increases the T2W of a basic fast imaging with steady state precession (FISP). This allows for better definition of fluid, fat, and cartilage, which is helpful when imaging orthopedics.

5-48. Balanced steady state free precession (bSSFP) is a sequence used to provide a _________ signal from fluids and in cardiac imaging and MRA pulse sequences.

A. hyperintense

B. hypointense

C. uniform

Discussion: Balanced steady state free precession uses a symmetric gradient waveform to generate a net gradient magnetic moment equal to zero from one RF pulse to the next. The gradient echo signal is then both proportional to T2 and inversely proportional to T1, which provides a hyperintense signal from fluids and is used in cardiac imaging and MRA pulse sequences.

5-49. _________ is an extremely fast MRI imaging technique.

A. Conventional spin echo

B. Gradient echo planar

C. Echo-planar imaging

D. Fast spin echo

Discussion: Echo-planar imaging (EPI) is a method used to acquire extremely fast MRI images.

5-50. Echo-planar (EPI) sequences can acquire images in _________ milliseconds.

A. 5

B. 10

C. 30

D. 50

Discussion: EPI imaging sequences allow an operator to acquire images at imaging times of as little as 50 milliseconds.

5-51. K-space filling for echo-planar imaging (EPI) can be accomplished during _________ radiofrequency (RF) excitation(s).

A. 0

B. 1

C. 2

D. 3

Discussion: A unique feature of echo-planar imaging is that k-space for the sequence can be filled in a single radio frequency excitation, enabling extremely fast imaging.

5-52. To accomplish echo-planar imaging (EPI), a system must have what components?

A. Low-amplitude gradient switching and rapid data-acquisition capabilities

B. High-amplitude gradient switching and rapid data-acquisition capabilities

C. Shallow-amplitude gradient switching and rapid data-acquisition capabilities

D. High-amplitude gradient switching and slow data-acquisition capabilities

Discussion: All raw data measurements for k-space during echo-planar imaging (EPI) must be acquired before the transverse magnetization is altered in magnitude by $T2^*$ relaxation; therefore, scanners must be equipped with high-amplitude gradient switching and rapid data-acquisition capabilities.

5-53. Acquisition times for echo-planar imaging (EPI) are about _________ times greater than those of gradient echo (GRE) imaging.

A. 10

B. 20

C. 40

D. 50

Discussion: Each echo has different k-space encoding and can be used to fill k-space, allowing for acquisition times for echo-planar imaging (EPI) that are about 10 times greater than those of gradient echo (GRE) imaging.

5-54. A hardware requirement for echo-planar imaging includes a _________.

A. frequency-encoding gradient that receives MR signals continuously and rapidly

B. phase-encoding gradient that receives MR signals continuously and rapidly

C. frequency-encoding gradient that receives MR signals consistently and slowly

D. phase-encoding gradient that receives MR signals consistently and slowly

Discussion: Hardware requirements of EPI include switching the frequency-encoding gradients and receiving MR signals rapidly and continuously. There is a need for fast, high-intensity gradient magnetic fields.

5-55. A more recent version of echo-planar imaging developed is called __________.

A. rapid echo-planar imaging

B. instant echo-planar imaging

C. blipped echo-planar imaging

D. gradient echo-planar imaging

Discussion: In blipped echo-planar imaging, there is only one RF pulse, the phase-encoding gradient waveform that consists of a string of short, weak "blips." Signals are acquired between blips.

5-56. During a blipped echo-planar imaging series, k-space __________ lines indicate the signal is decaying from left to right, while __________ lines indicate the signal decays from right to left.

A. even; odd

B. odd; even

C. top; bottom

D. bottom; top

Discussion: Alternate lines are scanned in the reverse direction in the k_x direction during blipped echo-planar imaging. Odd lines indicate the signal is decaying from left to right, while even lines indicate the signal decays from right to left. To minimize artifacts created, the raw data matrix must be reversed before the Fourier transform is applied.

5-57. Gradient magnetic fields for echo-planar imaging (EPI) usually exceeding __________ are common.

A. 10 mT/m

B. 15 mT/m

C. 20 mT/m

D. 25 mT/m

Discussion: Gradient magnetic fields exceeding 25 mT/m are common.

5-58. The rise and fall time required for gradients used in echo-planar imaging (EPI) is __________.

A. 25 μs

B. 50 μs

C. 75 μs

D. 100 μs

Discussion: Extremely fast, high-intensity gradient magnetic fields are required for echo-planar imaging (EPI).

5-59. K-space of echo-planar (EPI) sequences can be done in which of the following ways?

A. Spirals

B. Square spirals

C. Rosettes

D. All of the above

Discussion: K-space in echo-planar imaging (EPI) can be filled in many ways including spirals, square spirals, and rosettes. These acquisition methods map the entire k-space with the magnetization from a single RF pulse.

5-60. K-space filling in echo-planar imaging (EPI) is restricted due to __________ in the center and __________ in the peripheral regions.

A. undersampling; oversampling

B. oversampling; undersampling

C. oversampling; oversampling

D. undersampling; undersampling

Discussion: K-space filling in echo-planar imaging (EPI) is restricted due to oversampling in the center and undersampling in the peripheral regions. This leads to poor spatial resolution. The data also need to be manipulated so the proper positions of k-space are filled before the Fourier transform can be performed.

5-61. The biggest advantage to echo-planar imaging (EPI) is __________ motion.

A. create

B. visualize

C. freeze

D. produce

Discussion: The biggest advantage to echo-planar imaging (EPI) is freeze motion. With imaging times from 50–100 milliseconds, cardiac motion (10 cm/s) can be reduced.

5-62. The biggest concern of echo-planar imaging (EPI) is __________ stimulation.

A. nerve

B. cartilage

C. bone

D. organ

Discussion: The biggest concern of echo-planar imaging (EPI) is nerve stimulation. A rapidly changing magnetic field (dB/dt) can result in nerve stimulation through magnetic induction and lead to muscle contraction.

5-63. __________ is a ghost artifact that is displayed in exactly ½ of the field of view (FOV).

A. Nyquist ghost

B. Mansfield ghost

C. Tesla ghost

D. Feinberg ghost

Discussion: Nyquist ghost is a ghost artifact that is displayed in exactly ½ of the field of view (FOV). This can happen because of imperfections of the rephrasing-dephasing cycle of the rapidly switching frequency-encoding gradients, including gradient instabilities, eddy currents, and poor B_0 magnetic field uniformity.

5-64. __________ spatial frequencies are more important to image contrast than __________ frequencies.

A. High; low

B. Low; high

C. Low; low

D. High; high

Discussion: Low spatial frequencies are more important to image contrast than high frequencies. High frequencies contribute to edge enhancement and spatial resolution.

5-65. Low spatial frequencies contain a patient's __________ structure, while high spatial frequencies contain the patient's __________ structure.

A. coarse; coarse

B. fine; fine

C. coarse; fine

D. fine; coarse

Discussion: Low spatial frequencies contain a patient's coarse structure, while high spatial frequencies contain the patient's fine structure. Low spatial frequencies follow weak phase-encoding gradients. High spatial frequency follows strong phase-encoding gradients.

5-66. Turbo imaging contains:

A. 90° spin echo pulse at the beginning of the sequence to generate T1W contrast

B. 90° inversion pulse at the beginning of the sequence to generate T1W contrast

C. 180° spin echo pulse at the beginning of the sequence to generate T1W contrast

D. 180° inversion pulse at the beginning of the sequence to generate T1W contrast

Discussion: A common approach to turbo imaging contains a 180° inversion pulse at the beginning of the sequence to generate T1W contrast.

5-67. For a turbo sequence to generate T2W contrast, which of the following happens?

A. Data are collected while the tissue relaxes

B. Data are collected while the tissue is excited

C. Data are collected during both relaxation and excitation cycles of tissue

D. None of the above

Discussion: Another spin preparation method for turbo sequences that generate T2W contrast collects data while the tissue relaxes.

5-68. Motion artifacts are greatly reduced during turbo imaging sequences because they:

A. Result in multiple images at one time

B. Result in one image at a time

C. Result in decreased image contrast

D. Result from a long TR

Discussion: Turbo imaging acquires one image at a time, thus allowing for short breath-hold times and a reduction in motion artifacts.

5-69. Use of turbo imaging can dramatically increase diagnostic capabilities for MR imaging in an area such as:

A. Skeletal

B. Spines

C. Arterial studies using gadolinium

D. Musculoskeletal

Discussion: Use of turbo imaging can dramatically increase diagnostic capabilities for MR imaging in an area such as imaging of first-pass contrast agents or when imaging the temporal lobe, liver, or breast. These scans result in better temporal resolution and may increase signal-to-noise ratio (SNR) over a gradient echo image (GRE).

5-70. Which pulse sequence is depicted below?

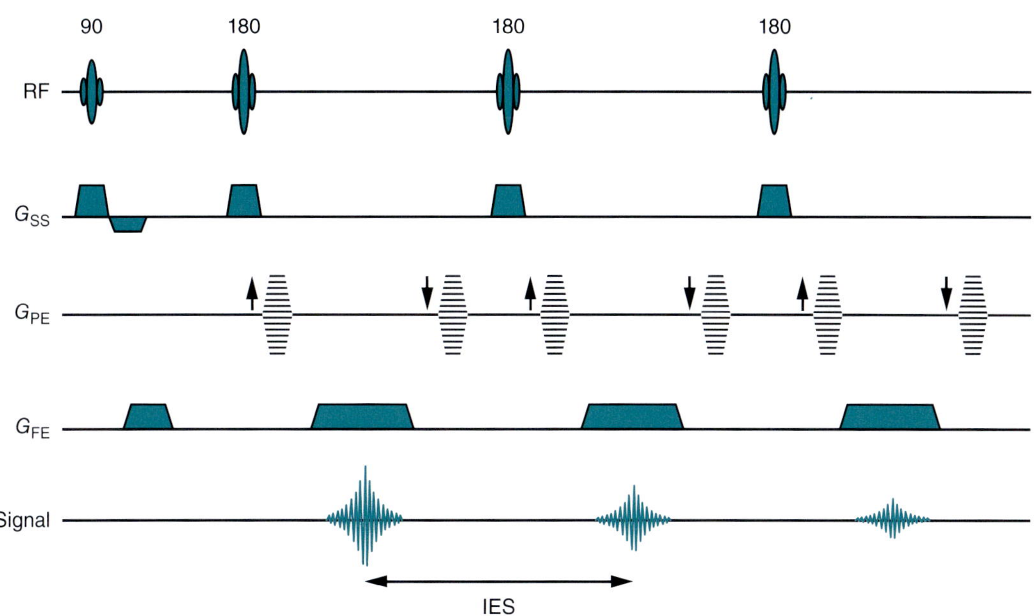

FIGURE 5-2.

Source: Reproduced with permission from Mc Robbie DW, Moore EA, Graves MJ, Prince MR. *MRI From Picture To Proton,* 2e. Cambridge University Press; 2006.

A. Gradient echo

B. Spin echo

C. Inversion recovery

D. Turbo imaging

5-71. During a turbo gradient echo (GRE), the _________ is different from gradient echo to gradient echo.

A. TE

B. TI

C. TR

D. Nothing changes from gradient echo to gradient echo

Discussion: Turbo gradient echo (GRE) is similar to fast spin echo (FSE) where the TE is different from spin echo to spin echo; however, during the turbo gradient echo (GRE), the TI is different from gradient echo to gradient echo.

5-72. Desired contrast for turbo imaging is determined by _________.

A. TR

B. TE

C. TI

D. k-space filling

Discussion: The k-space ordering scheme becomes an adjustable parameter to achieve the desired contrast. It can be filled sequentially from the smallest phase-encoding gradient to the largest or by selecting the amplitude of the phase-encoding gradient.

5-73. A combination of fast spin echo and gradient echo imaging is referred to as GRASE. An advantage to this type of turbo imaging includes:

A. Longer echo train and fewer slices per TR

B. Shorter echo train and more slices per TR

C. Shorter echo train and fewer slices per TR

D. Longer echo train and more slices per TR

Discussion: A gradient echo and fast spin echo image, referred to as a GRASE, only samples one echo between refocusing pulses, and three gradient echoes (GRE) are acquired. The advantage to this type of turbo imaging sequence is the shorter echo train and more slices per TR with a lower power disposition.

5-74. What is the term used to describe a discrete Fourier transform (FT) that is optimized specifically for the binary architecture of computers?

A. Continuous Fourier transform

B. Sampled Fourier transform

C. Fast Fourier transform

D. Signaling Fourier transform

Discussion: Fast Fourier transform (FFT) is the term used to describe a discrete Fourier transform (FT) that is optimized specifically for the binary architecture of computers.

5-75. A fast Fourier transform (FFT) requires __________ complex multiplications to reconstruct images and to compute a 256 × 256 image.

A. 512

B. 1,024

C. 2,048

D. 4,048

Discussion: A fast Fourier transform (FFT) requires 2,048 complex multiplications to reconstruct images and to compute a 256 × 256 image.

5-76. The most accurate preservation of resolution for the fast Fourier transform (FFT) needs to be computed using __________.

A. floating-point numbers

B. flop numbers

C. four numbers

D. fix-point numbers

Discussion: The most accurate preservation of resolution for the fast Fourier transform (FFT) needs to be computed using floating-point numbers. Floating-point numbers are referred to as a flop, or reconstruction speed of the image.

5-77. K-space filled using multiple energizations of phase and frequency-encoding gradients immediately after the RF excitation pulse is called __________.

A. sequential filling

B. segmental filling

C. spiral filling

D. centric filling

Discussion: Spiral filling of k-space uses multiple energizations of phase and frequency-encoding gradients immediately after the RF excitation pulse. Filling begins at the center of k-space and spirals outward.

5-78. Contrast resolution is improved when k-space is filled using spiral filling because:

A. Data is filled line by line during acquisition

B. Data is filled in the center during acquisition of the image

C. Data is filled per segment during acquisition of the image

D. Data is filled from the edges to the center during acquisition of the image

Discussion: During spiral imaging, the center of k-space is filled in more than the periphery of the image, improving contrast resolution.

5-79. What is the most common algorithm manipulated from projection data into an angiographic view that has been created from a 3-D dataset?

A. Multiplanar projections (MPR)

B. Minimum intensity projections (minP)

C. Maximum intensity projections (MIP)

D. Subtracted projections (SP)

Discussion: Maximum intensity projections are the most common algorithm manipulated from projection data into an angiographic view that has been created from a 3-D dataset.

5-80. Maximum intensity projection (MIP) advantages include all of the following except:

A. They can be created from arbitrary points of view.

B. Carotid arteries cannot be separated so that they can be viewed individually.

C. Maximum intensity projections can be produced from using a partial volume data set.

D. Maximum intensity projections look natural.

Discussion: Maximum intensity projection (MIP) advantages do include the ability to individually separate and view the right and left carotid arteries.

5-81. A maximum intensity projection image (MIP) is created from which of the following:

A. A ray line perpendicular to each pixel of the maximum intensity projection (MIP) image projected through a 3-D dataset and assigned the brightest pixel of the ray image for the MIP image

B. A ray line parallel to each pixel of the maximum intensity projection (MIP) image projected through a 3-D dataset and assigned the brightest pixel of the ray image for the MIP image

C. A ray line parallel to each pixel of the maximum intensity projection (MIP) image projected through a 3-D dataset and assigned the dullest pixel of the ray image for the MIP image

D. A ray line parallel to each pixel of the maximum intensity projection image (MIP) image projected through a 2-D dataset and assigned the brightest pixel of the ray image for the MIP image

Discussion: A maximum intensity projection (MIP) image is created when a ray line perpendicular to each pixel of the MIP image is projected through a 3-D dataset and assigned the brightest pixel of the ray image for the MIP image.

5-82. A disadvantage to a maximum intensity projection (MIP) image is:

A. Overwhelming depth information

B. Misleading depth information

C. Misrepresented depth information

D. Underrepresented depth information

Discussion: A disadvantage to a maximum intensity projection (MIP) image is misleading depth information. This occurs as a result of small, low-intensity structures overshadowed by larger, brighter structures.

5-83. A maximum intensity projection (MIP) image can be used to visualize:

A. Multiple sclerosis

B. Lesions

C. Herniated disks

D. Brain lesions

Discussion: A maximum intensity projection (MIP) image can be used to visualize lesions of blood vessels.

5-84. __________ is the random motion of molecules from a region of high concentration to one of low concentration.

A. Diffusion imaging

B. Perfusion imaging

C. Phase contrast imaging

D. Gradient echo imaging

Discussion: Diffusion imaging is the random motion of molecules from a region of high concentration to one of low concentration. Diffusion is a step closer to the cell than capillary perfusion.

5-85. Diffusion coefficient (D) refers to:

A. The time required for atoms to diffuse from one medium to another

B. The time required for atoms to perfuse from one medium to another

C. The time required for molecules to diffuse from one medium to another

D. The time required for molecules to perfuse from one medium to another

Discussion: Diffusion coefficient (D) refers to the time required for molecules to diffuse from one medium to another.

5-86. The diffusion coefficient (D) is measured by:

A. cm^2/s

B. cm/s

C. mm/s

D. $\mathbf{mm^2/s}$

Discussion: Units used to express the diffusion coefficient (D) are mm^2/s.

5-87. __________ values for the diffusion coefficient (D) represent __________ rates of molecular diffusion.

A. Higher; higher

B. Slower; slower

C. Higher; slower

D. Slower; higher

Discussion: Higher values for the diffusion coefficient (D) represent higher rates of molecular diffusion.

5-88. Which pulse sequence is depicted below?

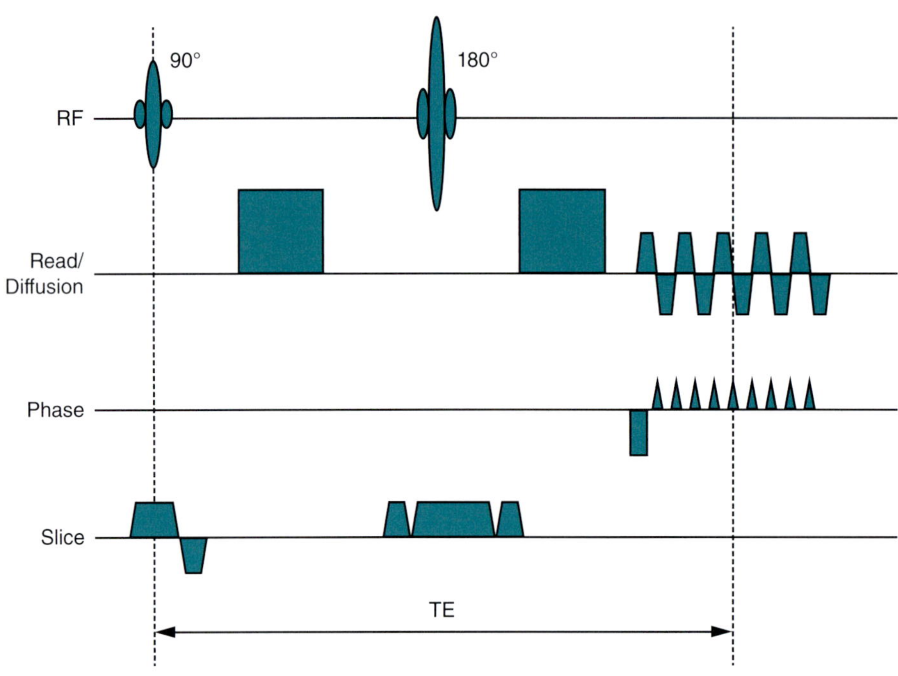

FIGURE 5-3.

Source: H. Douglas Morris, PhD. Uniform Services University Bethesda, Department of Radiology & Radiological Sciences, Bethesda, MD USA.

A. Gradient echo imaging

B. Diffusion imaging

C. Perfusion imaging

D. Phase contrast imaging

Reference: www.mritutor.org

5-89. Which of the following ratios represents signal attenuation of a diffusion sequence?

A. M/M_0

B. M_0/M

C. S_0/S

D. S/S_0

Discussion: S/S_0 ratio represents signal attenuation of a diffusion sequence.

5-90. Which pulse sequences can be used during the acquisition of diffusion imaging?

A. Steady-state free precession (SSFP)

B. Gradient echo (GRE)

C. Spin echo (SE)

D. All of the above

Discussion: To acquire a diffusion image, two of more pulse sequences are necessary. Applicable pulse sequences can include steady-state free precession (SSFP), gradient echo (GRE), spin echo (SE), or echo-planar imaging (EPI).

5-91. What gradient field strength is necessary to make diffusion imaging possible?

A. 10 mT/m

B. 20 mT/m

C. 30 mT/m

D. 40 mT/m

Discussion: The gradient field strength necessary for diffusion imaging to be possible is 40 mT/m. This allows for more intense gradient magnetic fields to produce higher gradient value.

5-92. Slew rate refers to:

A. The time required to switch on or off a gradient magnetic field

B. The time required to switch off a gradient magnetic field

C. The time required to switch on a gradient magnetic field

D. The time the gradient magnetic field is active

Discussion: The slew rate is the time required to switch on or off a gradient magnetic field.

5-93. Diffusion is sometimes also referred to as:

A. Bowanian motion

B. Brownian motion

C. Boeing motion

D. Brawnian motion

Discussion: Diffusion is sometimes also referred to as Brownian motion, named for the English scientist Robert Brown, who first identified this process as thermal, or heat-induced.

5-94. Magnetic resonance angiography (MRA) is a sequence that is acquired to:

A. Visualize bony trabeculae

B. Visualize spinal abnormalities

C. Visualize flowing blood

D. Visualize brain lesions

Discussion: Magnetic resonance angiography (MRA) is a sequence that is acquired to visualize flowing blood.

5-95. A term that describes the movement of fluid at the same speed is:

A. Turbulent flow

B. Laminar flow

C. Pulsatile flow

D. Plug flow

Discussion: Plug flow describes the movement of fluid at the same speed.

5-96. Laminar flow describes flow that:

A. Varies in speed

B. Moves at the same speed

C. Moves very fast

D. Moves very slowly

5-97. A term that describes random motion of blood in regions of discontinuity is:

A. Pulsatile

B. Turbulence

C. Laminar flow

D. Plug flow

Discussion: Turbulence describes the random motion of blood flow through regions of discontinuity, such as stenosis and bifurcation.

5-98. Pulsatile describes the __________ and __________ of blood through an artery.

A. acceleration; acceleration

B. deceleration; deceleration

C. acceleration; deceleration

D. consistent; inconsistent

Discussion: Pulsatile describes the acceleration and deceleration of blood through an artery. The velocity may accelerate (plug-like) or to a more consistent speed (parabolic).

5-99. Time of flight (TOF) and phase contrast (PC) are two ways to:

A. Display stagnant blood and produce MRA

B. Display flowing blood and produce MRA

C. Display flowing blood and produce MRI

D. Display stagnant blood and produce MRI

Discussion: The two basic ways in which flowing blood and MRA can be produced are through time of flight (TOF) and phase contrast (PC) acquisitions.

5-100. _________ blood flow results in dark blood; while _________ flow results in bright blood.

A. Rapid; slow

B. Slow; rapid

C. Stagnant; rapid

D. Slow; stationary

Discussion: The appearance of blood on an MRA sequence depends on the velocity of flow. Rapid blood flow results in dark blood, while slow flow results in bright blood.

5-101. During the radio frequency (RF) excitation, the _________ of the proton spin results in the time of flight (TOF) effects.

A. inflow/outflow

B. signal sampling

C. laminar flow

D. plug flow

Discussion: During the radio frequency (RF) excitation, the outflow/inflow of the proton spin results in the time of flight (TOF) effects.

5-102. Gradient magnetic field intensity, pulse sequence, and slew rate are three contributing factors to:

A. Flow void

B. Flow rate

C. Appearance of blood

D. Phase contrast

Discussion: Gradient magnetic field intensity, pulse sequence, and slew rate are three contributing factors to the appearance of blood. The other contributing factor for blood visualization is flow-compensating gradients.

5-103. What three factors impact flow-void and signal loss during rapid blood flow?

A. Low velocity, turbulence, dephasing

B. High velocity, turbulence, rephrasing

C. Low velocity, turbulence, rephrasing

D. High velocity, turbulence, dephasing

Discussion: High velocity, turbulence, and dephasing are the three factors that impact flow-void and signal loss during rapid blood flow. Flow-related enhancement, even-echo rephrasing, and gating impact signal gain.

5-104. _________ flow occurs in a vessel that has a stenosis or bifurcation, which causes intravoxel dephasing and leads to a loss of signal within the vessel.

A. Pulsatile

B. Turbulent

C. Laminar

D. Plug

Discussion: The lumen of the vessel contains different spins during the acquisition of an MRI image, so if flow is disturbed due to turbulent flow in the vessel due to stenosis or bifurcation, intravoxel dephasing will occur leading to a loss of signal within the vessel.

5-105. Flow-related enhancement (FRE) happens as a result of:

A. Fast-moving blood

B. Stationary blood

C. Slow-moving blood

D. Is not a result of blood flow

Discussion: Flow-related enhancement is a result of slow-moving blood when multislice imaging of slow-moving blood entering the first slice has a different spin property as the tissue slice. Flow-related enhancement is most visible on T1W imaging. Unsaturated blood emits a higher-intensity signal.

5-106. Motion artifact suppression technique (MAST) and gradient moment nulling (GMN) are types of:

A. Flow

B. Flow artifacts

C. Flow suppression

D. Flow compensation

Discussion: Motion artifact suppression technique (MAST) and gradient moment nulling (GMN) are types of flow compensation.

5-107. The term moment refers to:

A. The order of blood flow

B. The order of blood flow artifacts

C. Blood-flow equilibrium

D. Is not related to blood flow

Discussion: The term moment refers to zero order (stationary), first order (velocity), second order (acceleration), and third order (pulsatility motion). The gradient magnetic fields are set up to null each other to avoid flow artifacts.

5-108. Which of the following produce phase shifts during MRA image acquisition?

A. Chemical shift differences

B. Magnetic susceptibility differences

C. Velocity of blood

D. All of the above

Discussion: Multiple effects produce phase shifts during the MRA, including chemical shift differences, magnetic susceptibility differences, velocity, and motion.

5-109. What are the two categories of motion artifacts related to blood flow?

A. Frequency-shift errors; intensity errors

B. Intensity errors; phase-shift errors

C. Phase-shift errors; misregistration errors

D. Frequency-shift errors; misregistration errors

Discussion: The two categories of motion artifacts related to blood flow are intensity errors and phase-shift errors, which present as streaks that arise from the arteries.

5-110. One of the most common magnetic resonance angiography (MRA) procedures is done to evaluate which of the following structures?

A. Circulation of the neck

B. Function of the urinary system

C. Lesions of the breast

D. Cirrhosis of the liver

Discussion: Magnetic resonance angiography (MRA) is done to evaluate circulation of the neck to include both carotid and vertebral arteries, arteriovenous malformations, and aneurysms.

5-111. During which sequence are the thickness of the excited region, the flip angle of the RF pulses, and the TR optimized for speed and direction of blood flood?

A. Phase contrast

B. Spin echo

C. Inversion recovery

D. Time of flight

Discussion: To acquire a time of flight (TOF) magnetic resonance angiograph (MRA) sequence, the thickness of the excited region, the flip angle of the RF pulses, and the TR must be optimized for speed and direction of blood flood. This helps to maximize the contrast between blood and surrounding tissues.

5-112. The time of flight (TOF) magnetic resonance angiograph (MRA) sequence is best accomplished with which of the following sequences?

A. Phase contrast

B. Spin echo

C. Inversion recovery

D. Gradient echo

Discussion: The time of flight (TOF) magnetic resonance angiography (MRA) sequence is best accomplished with fast gradient echoes. The short TR tissue is partially saturated and exhibits a low signal intensity, the flow-related enhancement (FRE) is optimized, and vessels appear bright.

5-113. Problems acquiring images of tortuous blood vessels, the carotid bulb, some aneurysms, bifurcations, or stenosis occur during which sequence?

A. Phase contrast

B. Spin echo

C. Inversion recovery

D. Time of flight

Discussion: Problems acquiring images of tortuous blood vessels, the carotid bulb, some aneurysms, bifurcations, or stenosis occur during a time of flight (TOF) magnetic resonance angiography (MRA) sequence due to the struggle of completely replenishing the saturated blood with fresh blood.

5-114. Phase contrast (PC) MRA takes two measurements with different __________ sensitivities to acquire an image.

A. velocity

B. frequency

C. blood

D. contrast

Discussion: Phase contrast (PC) MRA takes two measurements with different velocity sensitivities to acquire an image. There must be nonzero velocities within the blood vessels to be visualized as blood vessels.

5-115. Which type of MRA sequence allows for the visualization of structural and functional measurements?

A. Time of flight

B. Phase contrast

C. Maximum intensity projection

D. Flow-related enhancement

Discussion: Phase contrast MRA has the potential for allowing both visualization of structural and functional measurements.

5-116. What type of image is produced utilizing a 2-D MRA technique that is acquired through the use of a thick slice, which allows for differentiation of vessels and the surrounding tissues?

A. Time of flight

B. Phase contrast

C. Maximum intensity projection

D. Flow-related enhancement

Discussion: The 2-D approach is a sequence that is acquired using a thick slice; therefore, it produces a high contrast between the vessels and surrounding tissue, allowing for better differentiation of the two structures, also referred to as a maximum intensity projection (MIP).

5-117. 3-D MRA provides for better__________ and __________.

A. spatial resolution; noise

B. noise; contrast resolution

C. spatial resolution; contrast resolution

D. spatial resolution; signal-to-noise ratio

Discussion: 3-D MRA can be used to acquire both phase contrast and time of flight images with increased spatial resolution and signal to noise; however, 2-D acquisition of these images is faster.

5-118. __________ is an approach that helps the human visual system with misleading perception of different intensities.

A. Depth-weighted MIP

B. Volume MIP

C. Intensity MIP

D. Spatial MIP

Discussion: Depth-weighted MIP is an approach that helps the human visual system with misleading perception of different intensities. Depth-weighted MIP attenuates the intensity of the brightest pixel along the ray line to provide improved depth perception.

5-119. Imaging of the blood flow within the capillaries is called:

A. Diffusion

B. Magnetic resonance angiography

C. Perfusion

D. Maximum intensity projection

Discussion: As the blood flows through the vessels, the diameter of the vessels gets smaller and smaller. Capillaries are the smallest of those vessels that provide the tissue with nutrients and oxygen. The imaging of these capillaries is called perfusion.

5-120. Perfusion and diffusion imaging are two types of:

A. Structural magnetic resonance imaging

B. Magnetic resonance angiography

C. Cardiac magnetic resonance imaging

D. Functional magnetic resonance imaging

Discussion: Perfusion and diffusion imaging are two types of functional magnetic resonance imaging.

5-121. What are the two approaches to perfusion imaging?

A. Extrinsic/intrinsic

B. Exogenous/endogenous

C. Esoteric/inherent

D. External/internal

Discussion: The two approaches to perfusion imaging are exogenous and endogenous. Exogenous is the use of a contrast material outside the tissue, whereas endogenous refers to a contrast agent produced by the spins of hydrogens within the tissue.

5-122. What is the challenge associated with perfusion imaging and use of the contrast media gadolinium?

A. Perfusion requires a drip injection and specific imaging timing.

B. Perfusion requires a bolus injection and specific imaging timing.

C. Perfusion requires a hand injection and specific imaging timing.

D. Contrast injections are not a requirement for perfusion imaging.

Discussion: When utilizing the contrast media gadolinium when performing perfusion imaging, the timing of the injection must be such that the sequence is acquired during the first pass of contrast media.

5-123. An extremely effective method of acquiring perfusion images is a combination of which of the following:

A. Single photon computed tomography (SPECT), positron emission tomography (PET), x-ray computed tomography (CT)

B. Single photon computed tomography (SPECT), positron emission tomography (PET), ultrasound (U/S)

C. Single photon computed tomography (SPECT), conventional radiography (x-ray), ultrasound (U/S)

D. Single photon computed tomography (SPECT), conventional radiography (x-ray), x-ray computed tomography (CT)

Discussion: An extremely effective method of acquiring perfusion images is a combination of single photon computed tomography (SPECT), positron emission tomography (PET), and x-ray computed tomography (CT)

5-124. Perfused tissue acquired utilizing _________ weighted pulse sequences will show an increased signal.

A. T2

B. PD

C. T1

D. $T2^*$

Discussion: T1 weighted pulse sequences will show perfused tissue better than other pulse sequences. $T2^*$ weighted pulse sequences result in reduced signal intensity.

5-125. The pulse sequence used most commonly to acquire a perfusion protocol is _________.

A. T1 FID-EPI (free induction decay echo-planar imaging)

B. T2* FID-EPI (free induction decay echo-planar imaging)

C. T2 FID-EPI (free induction decay echo-planar imaging)

D. PD (free induction decay echo-planar imaging)

Discussion: The pulse sequence used most commonly to acquire a perfusion protocol is T2* FIR-EPI (free induction decay echo-planar imaging). It is used for tumor characterization, tumor recurrence, and stroke.

5-126. Added time, added expense, and delay for repeated scans are disadvantages of _________ contrast agents.

A. endogenous

B. exogenous

C. inherent

D. intrinsic

Discussion: Several disadvantages accompany exogenous contrast agents including added time, added expense, possible side effects of an invasive procedure, and delay for repeated scans.

5-127. Oxyhemoglobin is _________.

A. diamagnetic

B. paramagnetic

C. hemomagnetic

D. unaffected by the magnetic

Discussion: Oxyhemoglobin is diamagnetic. Arterial capillary blood carries oxygen fixed to the hemoglobin molecule.

5-128. Cerebral blood flow _________ in response to brain activity.

A. decreases

B. increases

C. declines

D. stays the same

Discussion: Neuroscientists have determined that cerebral blood flow increases as a response to brain activity. The activity can include mechanisms such as tapping a finger, viewing pictures, or speaking.

5-129. Functional magnetic resonance imaging is done using echo-planar imaging techniques with TRs of _________ to prevent effects of patient motion.

A. less than 100 ms

B. less than 200 ms

C. less than 300 ms

D. less than 400 ms

Discussion: Functional magnetic resonance imaging is done using echo-planar imaging techniques with TRs of less than 100 ms to prevent effects of patient motion.

5-130. What is the effective TE?

A. The TE used on the initial echo produced in an FSE sequence

B. The TE used on the last echo produced in an FSE sequence

C. The TE used on the middle echo produced in an FSE sequence

D. The TE used in an FSE sequence to produce the desired contrast

Discussion: The effective TE is the TE that will produce the desired contrast on an image. For example, if the desired contrast is T2 weighting and the TEs used in a 4-ETL are 20 ms, 40 ms, 60 ms, and 80 ms, the effective TE should be 80 ms. All other options will not produce significant T2 weighting.

5-131. A STIR sequence uses an inversion time (TI) of approximately _________.

A. 150 ms

B. 450 ms

C. 850 ms

D. 1,150 ms

Discussion: The TI for a STIR sequence should be a short to null signal from fat since fat has a short T1 relaxation time. This is to prevent a longitudinal component of fat and, thus, no magnetization to relax back through the transverse plane.

Reference: MRI in Practice, pages 157–158

5-132. How many lines of k-space are filled per TR in a conventional spin echo sequence?

A. 1

B. 2

C. 4

D. 8

Discussion: Only one line of k-space data is filled per TR as there is only one echo produced per TR in a conventional spin echo sequence.

5-133. The number of lines of k-space to be filled directly corresponds to the _________.

A. number of slices

B. frequency matrix

C. phase matrix

D. slice thickness

Discussion: The phase matrix determines how many lines of data are filled in k-space. For example, if the phase matrix selected is 224, then 224 lines of data will be required to fill k-space.

Reference: MRI in Practice, page 81

5-134. To visualize signal in MR spectroscopy, what must be suppressed?

A. Background signal

B. Water signal

C. Flowing nuclei signal

D. White matter signal

Discussion: The chemical content of tissue is measured in MR spectroscopy, and these signals are typically very small compared to a water (hydrogen) signal, so the signal from water must be suppressed to visualize these signals.

5-135. A primary result of using 180° refocusing pulses in spin echo sequences is the _________.

A. rephasing of spins

B. dephasing of spins

C. increased T1 weighting

D. decreased T1 weighting

Discussion: 180° refocusing pulses will rephase spins that have been dephased and allow them to move back together in the transverse plane. When all spins are aligned, they are "in phase."

5-136. A pulse sequence that utilizes two TEs and creates two separate echoes is called a _________.

A. multiecho

B. fast spin echo

C. modified spin echo

D. inversion recovery spin echo

Discussion: Spin echo sequences that produce two echoes are called multiecho or dual-echo pulse sequences. They will produce one echo with proton-density weighting and one with T2 weighting.

5-137. What is a primary disadvantage of using gradient echo pulse sequences?

A. They take longer to scan

B. They cannot use variable flip angles

C. They have increased magnetic susceptibility

D. They cannot produce T1 weighting

Discussion: There is no compensation for magnetic susceptibility in gradient echoes primarily due to the lack of a 180° refocusing pulse. In gradient echo imaging, gradients perform rephasing rather than the 180° refocusing pulse in spin echo imaging.

5-138. The duration of the frequency-encoding gradient is called the _________.

A. sampling frequency

B. sampling bandwidth

C. acquisition window

D. frequency matrix

Discussion: This is also called sampling time and refers to how long the frequency-encoding gradient is on during the time of readout of the signal.

Reference: MRI in Practice, page 75

5-139. Lines in k-space are typically numbered with the lowest number near the _________.

A. highest portion of k-space

B. lowest portion of k-space

C. left or right portion of k-space

D. central portion of k-space

Discussion: K-space numbering typically starts in the center of k-space and with the lowest line numbers. For example, if there are 256 lines of k-space, lines +1 and −1 will typically start at the two central lines then move up/down from there.

Reference: MRI in Practice, page 81

5-140. When does the FID occur during spin echo pulse sequence?

A. After the 180° refocusing pulse

B. After the 90° excitation pulse and before the 180° refocusing pulse

C. Immediately before the 180° refocusing pulse

D. Before the 90° excitation pulse

Discussion: The FID signal is created immediately after the 90° excitation pulse is removed and before the 180° refocusing pulse is applied.

5-141. _________ is the series of mathematical calculations that convert raw MR data to image data.

A. Integral transformation

B. Fourier technology

C. Fourier transform

D. Integral technology

Discussion: Fourier transform is the process used to convert raw, analog k-space data into digital image data.

5-142. The transmit bandwidth is related to the _________.

A. slice select gradient

B. phase-encoding gradient

C. frequency-encoding gradient

D. all three gradients

Reference: MRI in Practice, pages 65–66

Discussion: The transmit bandwidth is applied at the same time as the RF excitation and RF refocusing pulses in order for resonance to occur with an individual slice.

5-143. The spatial encoding process that usually follows the initial RF pulse application is _________.

A. slice selection

B. phase encoding

C. frequency encoding

D. FID

Reference: MRI in Practice, pages 69–71

5-144. The technique that fills only half the area of the k-space along the frequency axis is called _________.

A. zero fill

B. partial echo

C. partial acquisition

D. fractional averaging

Reference: MRI in Practice, pages 99–100

5-145. Where are the effective TE echoes placed in k-space?

A. Center lines of k-space

B. Outer lines of k-space

C. Throughout k-space

D. It is dependent upon the effective TE

Reference: MRI in Practice, pages 144–145

5-146. To achieve thick slices, what type of transmit bandwidth is applied?

A. Narrow

B. Broad

C. Deep

D. Shallow

Reference: MRI in Practice, pages 65–66

5-147. How is k-space filled if the polarity of the frequency-encoding gradient is negative?

A. Top to bottom

B. Bottom to top

C. Left to right

D. Right to left

Reference: MRI in Practice, pages 96–97

5-148. The receiver bandwidth is related to the __________.

A. slice select gradient

B. phase-encoding gradient

C. **frequency-encoding gradient**

D. all three gradients

Reference: MRI in Practice, page 115

5-149. The method of filling one line of k-space for one slice, then filling the same line in k-space in adjacent lines is called __________.

A. **2-D volumetric**

B. 3-D volumetric

C. sampling

D. sequential

Reference: MRI in Practice, pages 101–102

5-150. The outer portion of k-space contains data that have both _____ signal amplitude and ____ resolution.

A. **low, high**

B. low, low

C. high, low

D. high, high

Reference: MRI in Practice, pages 81–82

5-151. Gradient magnetic field strength is measured in ________ or ________.

A. **mT/m, G/cm**

B. mT/cm, G/cm

C. cm/T, m/G

D. cm/kg, m/lb

Reference: MRI in Practice, page 326

5-152. The slice-select gradient must be turned on during which of the following events of an SE pulse sequence?

A. 90° RF excitation pulse only

B. **90° and 180° pulses**

C. 180° RF refocusing pulse only

D. Readout of the MR signal

Reference: MRI in Practice, page 67

5-153. To collect scan data using thin slices, applying a __________ is required.

A. **steep slice select gradient slope**

B. shallow slice select gradient slope

C. shallow frequency-encoding gradient slope

D. high amount of steep phase-encoding gradient slopes

Reference: MRI in Practice, page 65

5-154. To collect scan data using a small FOV, applying a __________ is required.

A. steep slice select gradient slope

B. shallow slice select gradient slope

C. **steep frequency-encoding gradient slope**

D. shallow frequency-encoding gradient slope

Reference: MRI in Practice, page 133

5-155. To collect scan data using a fine matrix, applying a __________ is required.

A. steep frequency-encoding gradient slope

B. shallow frequency-encoding gradient slope

C. high amount of shallow phase-encoding gradient slopes

D. **high amount of steep phase-encoding gradient slopes**

Reference: MRI in Practice, page 133

5-156. The number of lines of k-space to be filled is directly related to the __________.

A. number of slices

B. **phase matrix**

C. frequency matrix

D. combination of all the above

Reference: MRI in Practice, pages 94–96

5-157. In volume imaging, optimal reformatting will occur if the voxel size is:

A. Anisotropic

B. **Isotropic**

C. Oblique

D. Spherical

Reference: MRI in Practice, pages 138–139

5-158. What aspect of k-space is filled if the polarity of the phase-encoding gradient is positive?

A. Top

B. Bottom

C. Left

D. Right

Reference: MRI in Practice, pages 96–97

5-159. Which of the following is directly related to the time to fill k-space?

A. Phase-encoding steps

B. Frequency-encoding data points

C. Slice select gradient slope

D. Echo time

Reference: MRI in Practice, pages 94–96

5-160. What is the effect on sampling time if receiver bandwidth is reduced?

A. Sampling time is decreased

B. Sampling time is increased

C. It is directly proportional to sampling time

D. It has no effect on sampling time

Reference: MRI in Practice, pages 76–79

5-161. The time-reducing technique that fills less than 100% of the area of k-space along the phase axis is called _________.

A. zero fill

B. partial echo

C. partial acquisition

D. fractional averaging

Reference: MRI in Practice, pages 99–191

5-162. The method of filling all lines of k-space for one slice before filling k-space in adjacent lines is called _________.

A. 2-D volumetric

B. 3-D volumetric

C. sampling

D. sequential

Reference: MRI in Practice, page 101

5-163. The center portion of k-space contains data that have both ____ signal amplitude and ___ resolution.

A. low, high

B. low, low

C. high, low

D. high, high

Reference: MRI in Practice, page 82

5-164. The sampling rate is _________ receiver bandwidth.

A. inversely proportional to

B. proportional to

C. not related to

D. half of the

Reference: MRI in Practice, pages 76–79

Procedures: Brain-Spine-Body-MSK

6-1. What is the most likely type of tissue being pointed to in the noncontrast images (Figure 6.1) by arrows #1 and #2?

A. **Fluid like mass**

B. Solid homogenous mass

C. Metastatic tumor mass

D. Hyper-enhancing mass

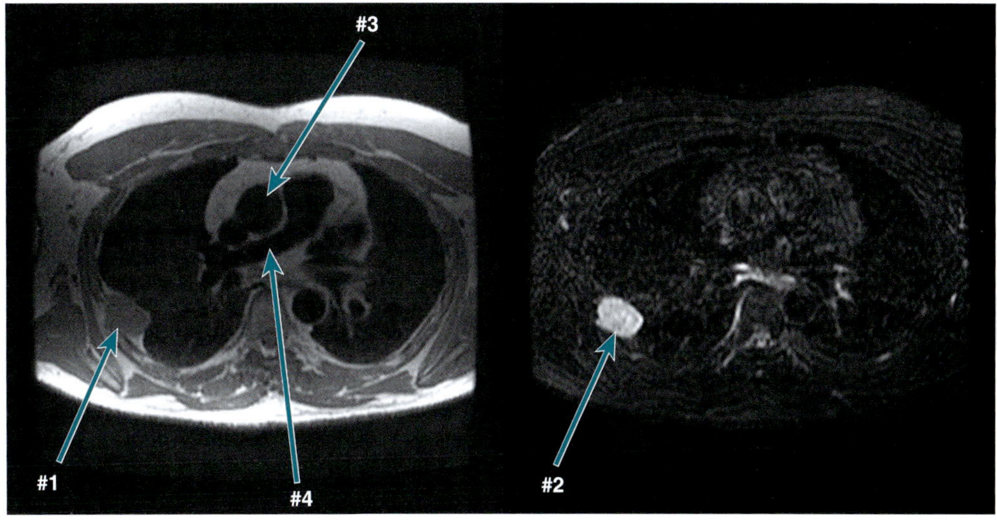

FIGURE 6-1.
(Walter Reed National Military Medical Center)

6-2. What is the structure in Figure 6.1 being pointed to by #3?

A. Pulmonary artery

B. Pulmonary vein

C. **Ascending aorta**

D. Descending aorta

6-3. What is the structure in Figure 6.1 being pointed to by #4?

A. Right pulmonary artery

B. Pulmonary vein

C. Ascending aorta

D. Left pulmonary artery

Additional reading:

McRobbie DW, Moore EA, Graves MJ, Prince MR. MRI from Picture to Proton, Third Edition. Cambridge University Press; 2017.

Norton PT, Nacey NC, Caovan DB, Gay SB, Krmaer CM, Jeun BS. Cardaic MRI: The Bascis. https://introductiontoradiology.net/courses/rad/CardiacMR/Anatomy/Normal.html

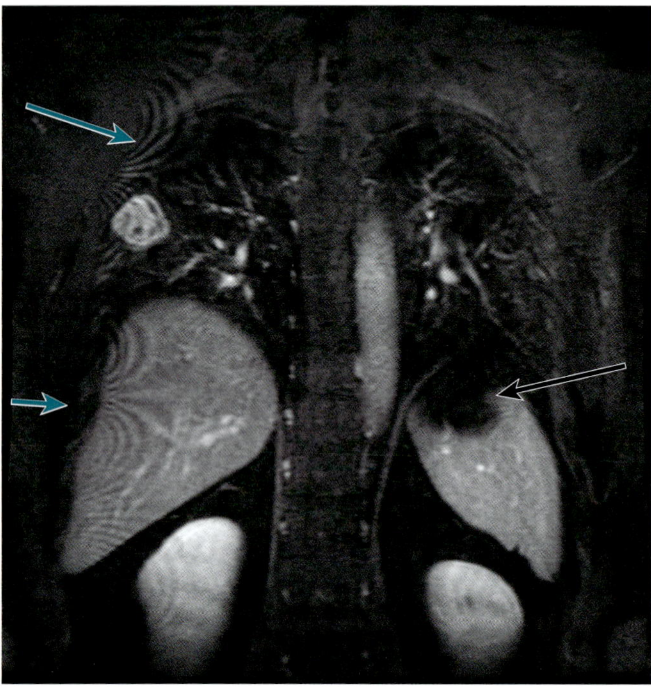

FIGURE 6-2.
(Walter Reed National Military Medical Center)

6-4. What artifact is being pointed to by the two blue arrows on the left side of Figure 6-2?

A. Susceptibility artifact

B. Eddy currents

C. Non-uniform banding artifact

D. Edge artifact

6-5. What artifact is being pointed to by the black arrow on the right side of Figure 6-2?

A. Susceptibility artifact

B. Eddy currents

C. Banding artifact

D. Edge artifact

Additional reading:

Huang SY, Seethamraju RT, Patel P, Hahn PF, Kirsch JE, Guimaraes AR. Body MR Imaging: Artifacts, k-Space, and Solutions. Radiographics. 2015 Sep-Oct;35(5):1439-60.

6-6. What pathology is depicted in Figure 6.3?

A. Mediastinal mass

B. Abdominal mass

C. Anatomy within normal limits

D. Cardiomegaly

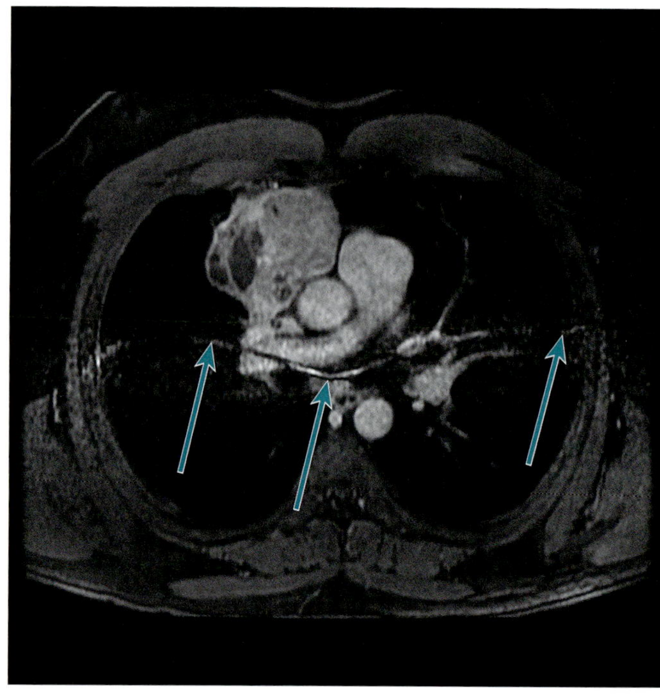

FIGURE 6-3.
(Walter Reed National Military Medical Center)

6-7. What is the artifact being pointed to by the arrows in Figure 6.3?

A. Breathing Motion

B. Breathing Motion with accelerated parallel imaging

C. Wrap around artifact

D. Gibbs artifact

Additional reading:

Ferreira PF, Gatehouse PD, Mohiaddin RH, Firmin DN. Cardiovascular magnetic resonance artefacts. J Cardiovasc Magn Reson. 2013 May 22;15:41.

6-8. What imaging sequence is shown by the images in Figure 6.4?

A. Magnitude and speed images

B. Phase contrast

C. T1- and T2-weighted double echo

D. Both a and b

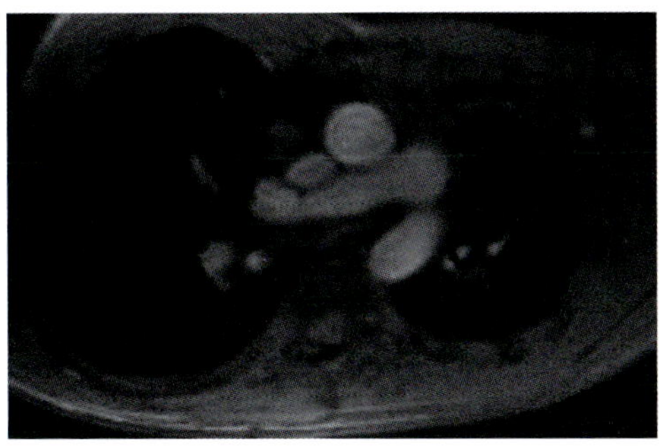

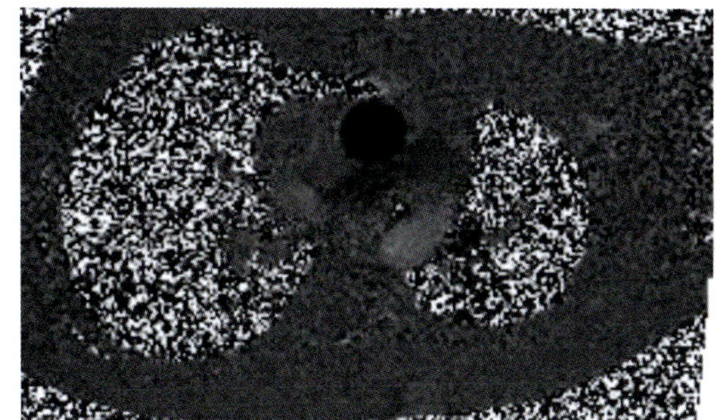

FIGURE 6-4.
(Walter Reed National Military Medical Center)

6-9. What is the best use of phase contrast imaging in the great vessels of the chest?

A. Quantifying cerebral flow

B. Quantifying flow velocities

C. Quantifying ejection fractions

D. Quantifying cardiac output

6-10. What key parameter do you adjust in phase contrast imaging for different rates of flow?

A. Flip angle

B. Gradient direction

C. Velocity encoding

D. Field of view

Additional reading:

Schneider G, Prince MR, Meaney JFM, Ho VB (Eds). Magnetic Resonance Angiography: Techniques, Indications and Practical Applications. 2005. Spinger-Verlag Italia, Milan, Italy.

6-11. What is the difference between slices #1 and #2 in the axial slices shown in Figure 6.5?

A. Gadolinium contrast

B. T1 versus T2 weighting

C. Fat suppression

D. Flip angle

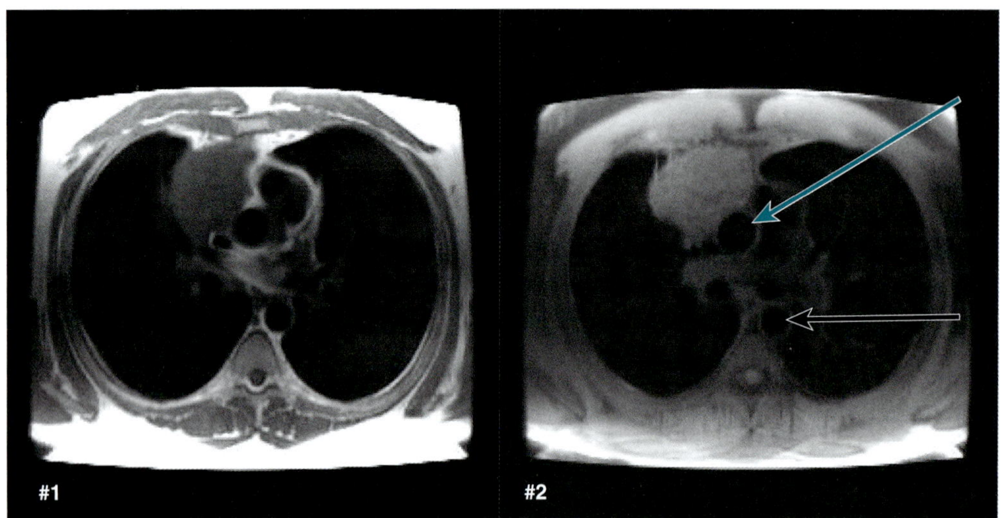

FIGURE 6-5.
(Walter Reed National Military Medical Center)

6-12. What main motion reducing technique being used in the image of the mediastinum?

A. Respiratory gating

B. Cardiac gating

C. Multiple acquisition averaging

D. K-space spiral filling

6-13. What is the blue arrow pointing to in Figure 6.5?

A. Ascending aorta

B. Descending aorta

C. Pulmonary artery

D. Inferior vena cava

6-14. What is the black arrow pointing to in Figure 6.5?

A. Ascending aorta

B. Descending aorta

C. Pulmonary artery

D. Inferior vena cava

Additional reading:

Hochhegger B, de Souza VV, Marchiori E, Irion KL, Souza AS Jr, Elias Junior J, Rodrigues RS, Barreto MM, Escuissato DL, Mançano AD, Araujo Neto CA, Guimarães MD, Nin CS, Santos MK, Silva JL. Chest magnetic resonance imaging: a protocol suggestion. Radiol Bras. 2015 Nov-Dec;48(6):373-80.

6-15. What is the major congenital abnormality in Figure 6.6?

A. Marfan syndrome

B. Dextrocardia

C. Triple chamber syndrome

D. Bicuspid valve

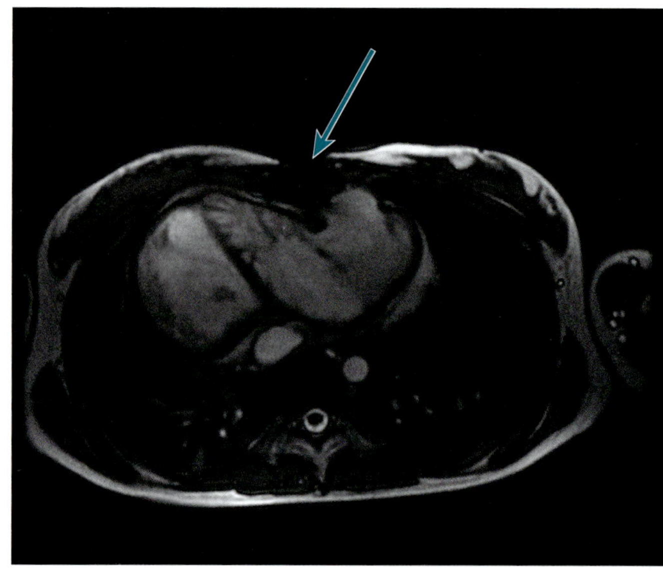

FIGURE 6-6.
(Walter Reed National Military Medical Center)

6-16. What is most likely causing the susceptibility artifact pointed to by the arrow in Figure 6.6?

- **A. Sternal wires**
- **B.** Cardiac gating leads
- **C.** Surgical plate
- **D.** Pacemaker

6-17. What is the pulse sequence being used in Figure 6.6?

- **A.** T1 fast/turbo spin echo
- **B.** T2 fast/turbo spin echo
- **C. Steady-state free precession**
- **D.** Double echo steady state

Additional reading:

Maldjian PD, Saric M. Approach to dextrocardia in adults: review. AJR Am J Roentgenol. 2007 Jun;188(6 Suppl):S39-49.

6-18. In Figure 6.7 #1, what weighting is this image?

- **A.** T1
- **B.** T2
- **C. T2 with fat suppression**
- **D.** T1 with fat suppression

6-19. In Figure 6.7, the white arrow is pointing to what type of artifact?

- **A.** Eddy current
- **B.** Coil drop off
- **C. Inhomogeneous fat saturation and shimming**
- **D.** Metallic artifact

6-20. In breast MRI, what is the optimal patient positioning?

- **A.** Patient's breast should be centered one at a time since they are scanned separately
- **B. Patient should be centered over the bilateral breast coil symmetrically with the sternum overlying the center bar**
- **C.** Patient place themselves in the bilateral breast coil for comfort
- **D.** Patient should be centered over the bilateral breast coil, but allowed to adjust themselves for comfort for maximum stillness during exam

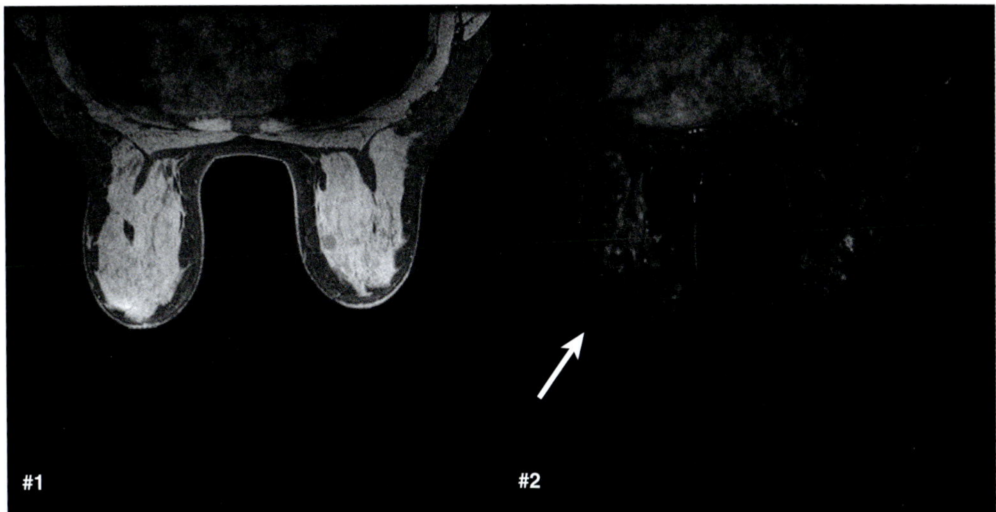

FIGURE 6-7.
(Walter Reed National Military Medical Center)

6-21. In breast MRI, what is the coil prep to reduce artifacts?

A. Use fresh linens for each patient that do not have printed designs

B. Simply clean the coil between uses

C. Use disposable coil covers

D. Fold linen to provide for more padding in the coil

6-22. What artifact is NOT a direct result of poor patient positioning?

A. Poor fat suppression

B. Uneven fat-air interface with inhomogeneous fat suppression

C. Inhomogeneous tissue with nonuniform contrast media enhancement

D. Decoupling

6-23. What is depicted in the breast MRI images in Figure 6.8?

A. Incomplete fat suppression

B. Saline implants

C. Solid silicone implants

D. Large cysts

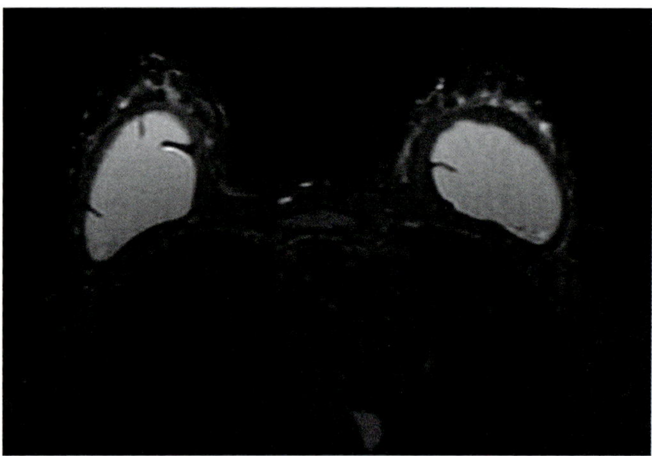

FIGURE 6-8.
(Walter Reed National Military Medical Center)

6-24. When scanning breast implants, what combination of sequences is most helpful?

A. T1-weighted unsuppressed, T1-weighted water suppressed, (optional: T1-weighted silicone suppressed)

B. T2-weighted unsuppressed, T1-weighted water suppressed, (optional: T1-weighted silicone suppressed)

C. T2-weighted unsuppressed, T2-weighted water suppressed, (optional: T2- weighted silicone suppressed)

D. T1-weighted unsuppressed, T1-weighted water suppressed, (optional: T2-weighted silicone suppressed)

Discussion:

Coils must be protected and the patient needs comfort. Therefore, it is recommended to use disposable linen or pads to protect the coil and on which the patient lies. Cloth towels and sheets can cause artifacts from many sources: starch in laundering process, skin folds due to cloth lines placing pressure on the skin, other artifacts if the cloth is printed.

Surgical scars and therapy can result in scar tissue making the skin surface uneven, resulting in an artifact unrelated to patient positioning.

Additional reading:

Yeh ED, Georgian-Smith D, Raza S, Bussolari L, Pawlisz-Hoff J, Birdwell RL. Positioning in breast MR imaging to optimize image quality. Radiographics. 2014 Jan-Feb;34(1):E1-17. doi: 10.1148/rg.341125193.

Harvey JA, Hendrick RE, Coll JM, Nicholson BT, Burkholder BT, Cohen MA. Breast MR imaging artifacts: how to recognize and fix them. Radiographics. 2007 Oct;27 Suppl 1:S131-45. doi: 10.1148/rg.27si075514.

6-25. What structure is the red arrow (a) pointing to in Figure 6.9?

A. Descending thoracic aorta

B. Ascending thoracic aorta

C. Pulmonary artery

D. Superior vena cava

6-26. What structure is the yellow arrow (b) pointing to in Figure 6.9?

A. Descending thoracic aorta

B. Ascending thoracic aorta

C. Pulmonary artery

D. Superior vena cava

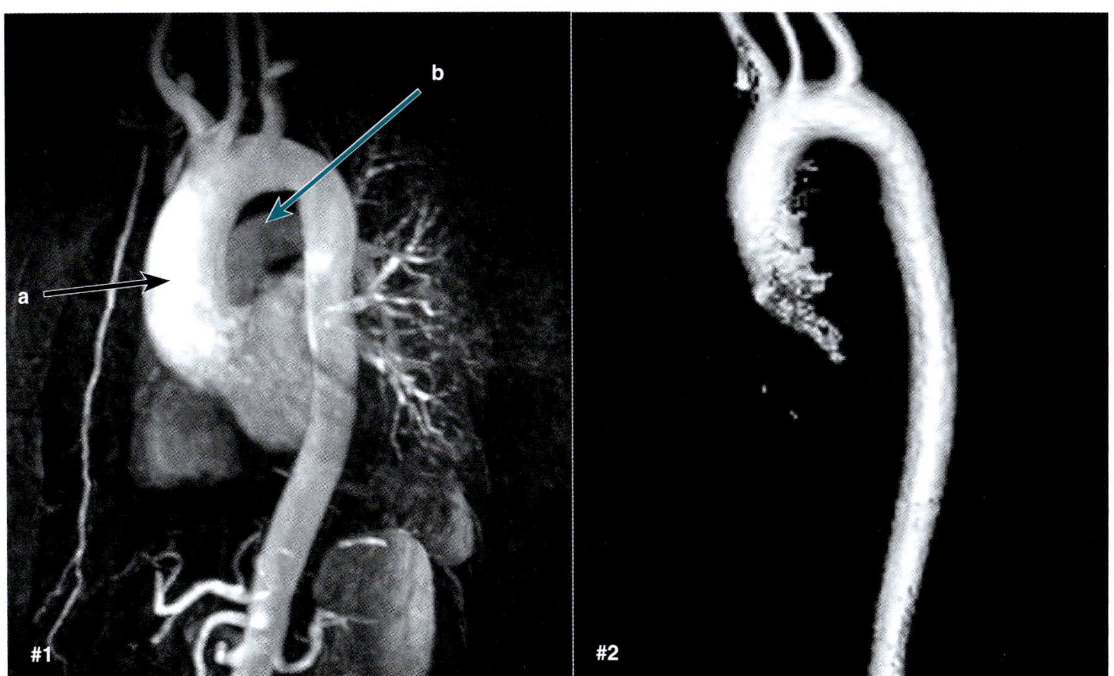

FIGURE 6-9.
(Walter Reed National Military Medical Center)

6-27. What post processing technique is shown in Figure 6.9, #2?

A. 2-D Maximum intensity pixel (MIP)

B. 2-D Multiplanar reconstruction (MPR)

C. Noncontrast MRA

D. 3-D volume rendering (VR)

Additional reading:

Garg I, Grist TM, Nagpal P. MR Angiography for Aortic Diseases. Magn Reson Imaging Clin N Am. 2023 Aug;31(3):373-394. doi: 10.1016/j.mric.2023.05.002. Epub 2023 Jun 7. PMID: 37414467.

Lichtenberger JP 3rd, Franco DF, Kim JS, Carter BW. MR Imaging of Thoracic Aortic Disease. Top Magn Reson Imaging. 2018 Apr;27(2):95-102. doi: 10.1097/RMR.0000000000000165.

6-28. In Figure 6.10, what is pathology is the arrow pointing to?

- **A. Coarctation of the aorta**
- B. Aneurism of the aorta
- C. Fistula of the pulmonary artery
- D. Partial anomalous venous return

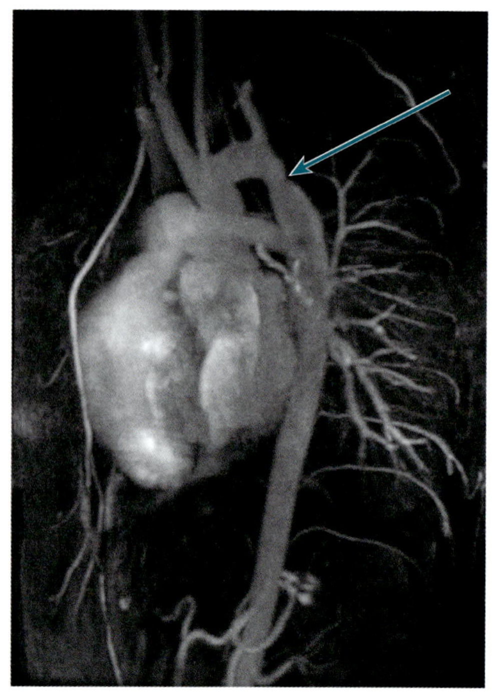

FIGURE 6-10.
(Walter Reed National Military Medical Center)

Additional reading:

Dijkema EJ, Leiner T, Grotenhuis HB. Diagnosis, imaging and clinical management of aortic coarctation. Heart. 2017 Aug;103(15):1148-1155. doi: 10.1136/heartjnl-2017-311173. Epub 2017 Apr 4. Erratum in: Heart. 2019 Jul;105(14):e6. PMID: 28377475.

Ho VB, Bakalov VK, Cooley M, Van PL, Hood MN, Burklow TR, Bondy CA. Major vascular anomalies in Turner syndrome: prevalence and magnetic resonance angiographic features. Circulation. 2004 Sep 21;110(12):1694-700. doi: 10.1161/01.CIR.0000142290.35842.B0. Epub 2004 Sep 7. PMID: 15353492.

6-29. In Figure 6.11, what MRA technique is being depicted?

- A. Traditional contrast enhanced 3-D MRA in the coronal view
- B. Traditional contrast enhanced 2-D MRA in the coronal view
- C. Fluoro-triggered contrast enhanced 3-D MRA in the axial view
- **D. Time resolved contrast enhanced 3-D MRA in the coronal view**

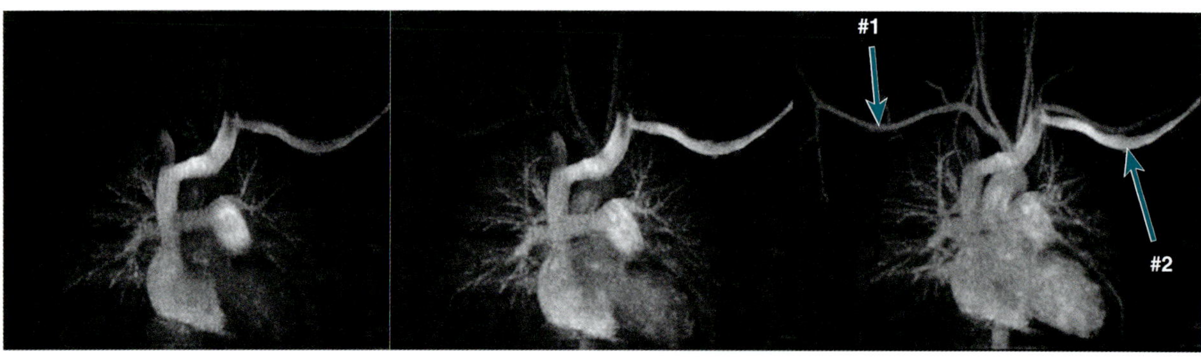

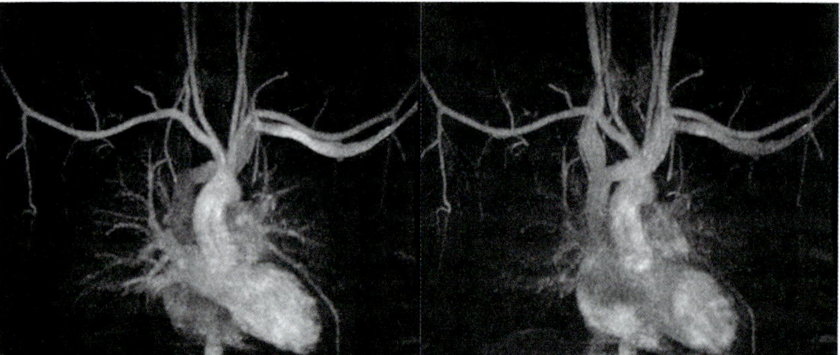

FIGURE 6-11.
(Walter Reed National Military Medical Center)

6-30. For provocative thoracic outlet syndrome MRA, how does the technologist position the patient?

A. Coil is over the upper chest with the patients arms down by their sides

B. Coil is over the upper chest with the patients arms down by their sides and patient coached on when to take a deep breath and bear down

C. Coil is over the upper chest with the patients arms up over their head

D. Coil is over the upper chest with the patients arms crossed over the chest

6-31. In Figure 6.11, what is arrow #1 pointing to?

A. Right subclavian artery

B. Brachiocephalic artery

C. Right subclavian vein

D. Left subclavian artery

6-32. In Figure 6.11, what is arrow #2 pointing to?

A. Right subclavian artery

B. Left subclavian vein

C. Right subclavian vein

D. Brachiocephalic vein

Additional reading:

Raptis CA, Sridhar S, Thompson RW, Fowler KJ, Bhalla S. Imaging of the Patient with Thoracic Outlet Syndrome. Radiographics. 2016 Jul-Aug;36(4):984-1000. doi: 10.1148/rg.2016150221.

6-33. What liver specific contrast agent was used in the liver study pictured in Figure 6.12?

A. ProHAnce

B. MultiHance

C. Eovist

D. Gadovist

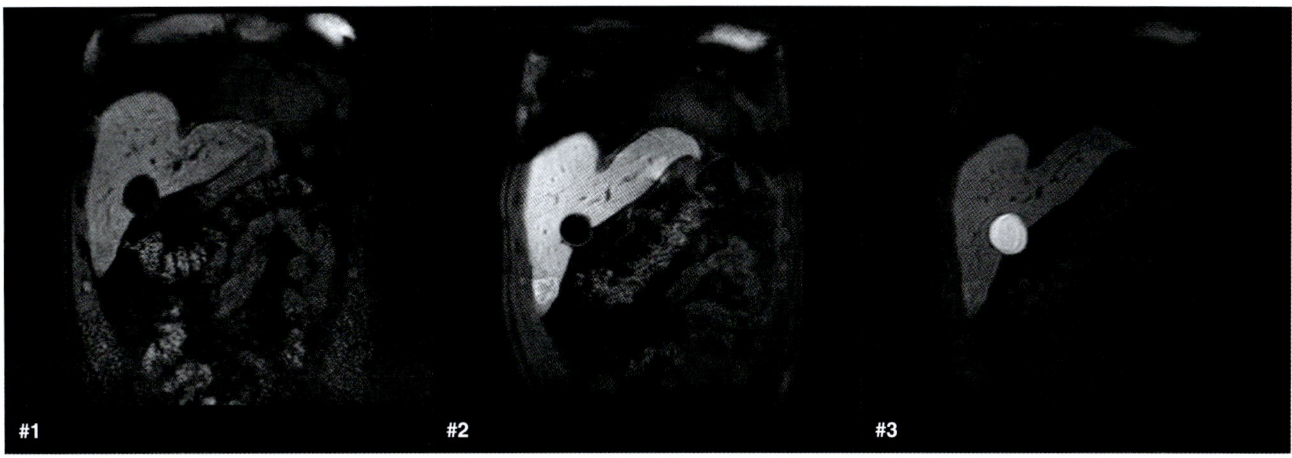

FIGURE 6-12.
(Walter Reed National Military Medical Center)

6-34. The images in Figure 6.12 are all post contrast. How are the three images in this figure defined?

A. Pre phase, early phase, and late phase

B. Arterial phase, venous phase, and hepatocellular phase

C. TE short, TE medium, and TE Long

D. TE early, TE optimal, and TE late

Additional reading:

Jhaveri K, Cleary S, Audet P, Balaa F, Bhayana D, Burak K, Chang S, Dixon E, Haider M, Molinari M, Reinhold C, Sherman M. Consensus statements from a multidisciplinary expert panel on the utilization and application of a liver-specific MRI contrast agent (gadoxetic acid). AJR Am J Roentgenol. 2015 Mar;204(3):498-509. doi: 10.2214/AJR.13.12399.

6-35. What pathology is demonstrated in Figure 6.13?

A. **Cirrhosis**

B. Splenic rupture

C. Gall stones

D. Aortic dissection

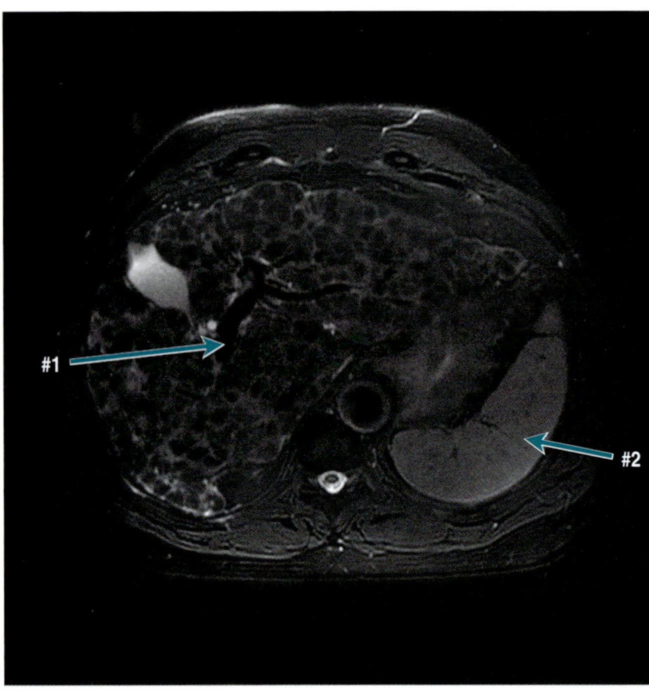

FIGURE 6-13.
(Walter Reed National Military Medical Center)

6-36. What is the structure labeled #1 in Figure 6.13?

A. Left portal vein

B. Left portal artery

C. **Right portal vein**

D. Right portal artery

6-37. Identify the sequence weighting demonstrated in Figure 6.13.

A. T1

B. Perfusion

C. Diffusion

D. **T2 with fat suppression**

6-38. What is the structure labeled #2 in Figure 6.13?

A. Left lobe of the liver

B. **Spleen**

C. Pancreas

D. Left kidney

6-39. Eovist is a contrast agent for liver imaging. What unique aspect does it have for liver imaging?

A. A 20-minute postinjection set of images at peak enhancement should be acquired

B. 50% of the contrast is taken up and eliminated via the biliary system

C. 5% of the contrast is taken up and eliminated via the biliary system

D. **Both a and b**

Additional reading:

Cruite I, Schroeder M, Merkle EM, Sirlin CB. Gadoxetate disodium-enhanced MRI of the liver: part 2, protocol optimization and lesion appearance in the cirrhotic liver. AJR Am J Roentgenol. 2010 Jul;195(1):29-41. doi: 10.2214/AJR.10.4538. PMID: 20566795.

Van Beers BE, Pastor CM, Hussain HK. Primovist, Eovist: what to expect? J Hepatol. 2012 Aug;57(2):421-9. doi: 10.1016/j.jhep.2012.01.031. Epub 2012 Apr 12. PMID: 22504332.

https://www.radiologysolutions.bayer.com/products/contrast-agents/eovist-injection

6-40. What sequence is used in the liver to detect lipid either in the hepatic parenchyma or within hepatocellular tumors?

A. Dual echo T2 fast spin echo with fat suppression

B. Steady-state free precession

C. **Gradient recalled echo in-phase and out-of-phase**

D. Volume interpolated gradient recalled echo

Additional reading:

Lebert P, Adens-Fauquembergue M, Azahaf M, Gnemmi V, Behal H, Luciani A, Ernst O. MRI for characterization of benign hepatocellular tumors on hepatobiliary phase: the added value of in-phase imaging and lesion-to-liver visual signal intensity ratio. Eur Radiol. 2019 Nov;29(11):5742-5751. doi: 10.1007/s00330-019-06210-y. Epub 2019 Apr 16. PMID: 30993437.

6-41. Iron overload is measured through a quantitative method using what type of sequence?

A. T1 mapping

B. **T2***

C. T1*

D. T2 mapping

Additional reading:

Meloni A, Pistoia L, Restaino G, Missere M, Positano V, Spasiano A, Casini T, Cossu A, Cuccia L, Massa A, Massei F, Cademartiri F. Quantitative T2* MRI for bone marrow iron overload: normal reference values and assessment in thalassemia major patients. Radiol Med. 2022 Nov;127(11):1199-1208. doi: 10.1007/s11547-022-01554-w. Epub 2022 Sep 10. PMID: 36087241.

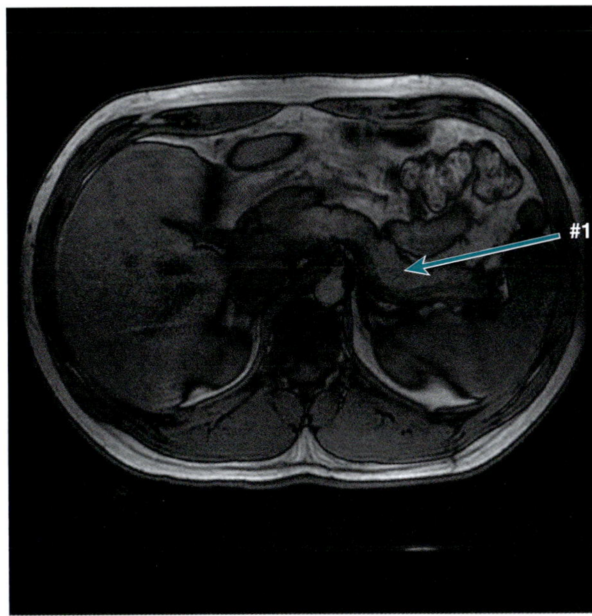

FIGURE 6-14.
(Walter Reed National Military Medical Center)

6-42. What are the dark bands around the organs and structures in Figure 6.14 caused by?

A. Optimal TE

B. In-phase TE

C. **Out-of-phase TE**

D. Out-of-phase TR

6-43. What is #1 pointing to in Figure 6.14?

A. Spleen

B. **Pancreas**

C. Jejunum

D. Duodenum

6-44. The kidneys are "capped" by what glands?

A. Pineal bodies

B. Thymus

C. **Adrenal glands**

D. Hypothalamus

Additional reading:

Netter FH. Netter's Anatomy, 1989, CIBA-Geigy Corporation: Summit, NJ.

d'Amuri FV, Maestroni U, Pagnini F, Russo U, Melani E, Ziglioli F, Negrini G, Cella S, Cappabianca S, Reginelli A, Barile A, De Filippo M. Magnetic resonance imaging of adrenal gland: state of the art. Gland Surg. 2019 Sep;8(Suppl 3):S223-S232. doi: 10.21037/gs.2019.06.02. PMID: 31559189; PMCID: PMC6755942.

6-45. In Figure 6.15, what is #1 pointing to?

A. **Left adrenal gland**

B. Right adrenal gland

C. Left parotid gland

D. Right parotid gland

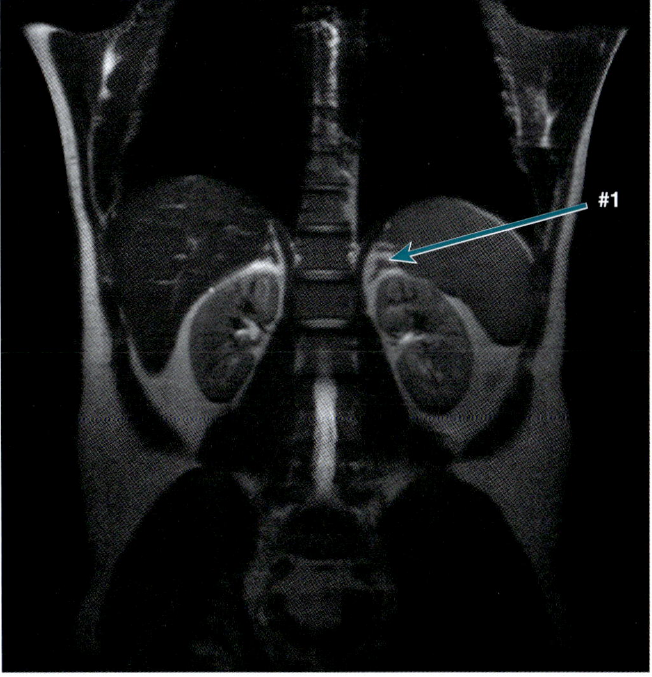

FIGURE 6-15.
(Walter Reed National Military Medical Center)

6-46. Imaging of the kidneys should include all EXCEPT?

- **A. Inclusion of innominate artery**
- **B.** Pay attention as to whether the kidney of clinical concern is a renal transplant in the pelvis
- **C.** Should include entire abdominal aorta through iliac artery bifurcation
- **D.** Must cover kidneys through aortic bifurcation on the non-MRA sequences and MRA images

6-47. In Figure 6.15, why are the lungs dark?

- **A.** Inversion time has turned the lungs dark
- **B.** The fluid in the lungs has caused a paradoxical effect
- **C. The air in lungs has no signal**
- **D.** This sequence makes the lungs dark

Additional reading:

d'Amuri FV, Maestroni U, Pagnini F, Russo U, Melani E, Ziglioli F, Negrini G, Cella S, Cappabianca S, Reginelli A, Barile A, De Filippo M. Magnetic resonance imaging of adrenal gland: state of the art. Gland Surg. 2019 Sep;8(Suppl 3):S223-S232. doi: 10.21037/gs.2019.06.02. PMID: 31559189; PMCID: PMC6755942.

6-48. What pathology is demonstrated in Figure 6.16, #1?

- **A.** AVM
- **B.** Cyst
- **C.** Lipoma
- **D. Angiomyolipoma**

6-49. Identify the sequence demonstrated in Figure 6.16.

- **A.** T1
- **B. T1 post contrast**
- **C.** STIR
- **D.** T2

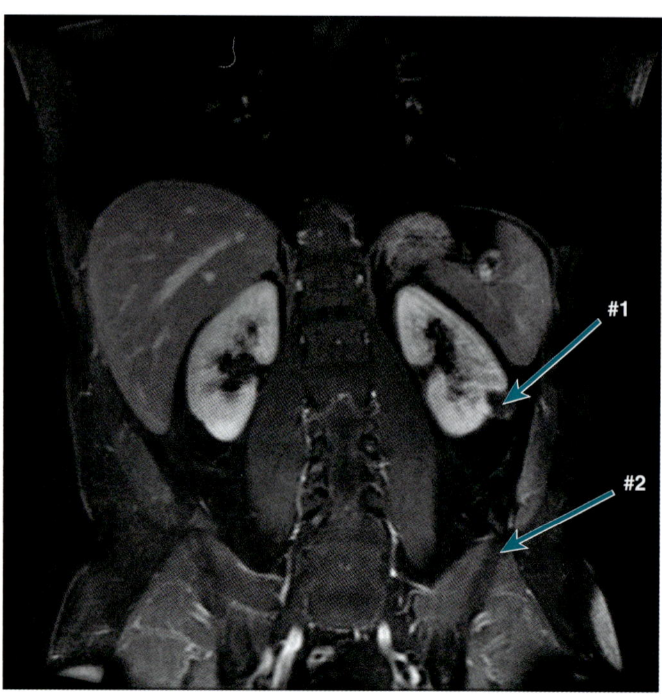

FIGURE 6-16.
(Walter Reed National Military Medical Center)

6-50. What is the structure labeled #2 in Figure 6.16?

- **A. Left iliac crest**
- **B.** Left anterior superior iliac crest
- **C.** Right anterior superior iliac crest
- **D.** Right iliac crest

6-51. On SSFSE images of the abdomen, certain pathologies can be obscured due to the presence of abdominal ______ ?

- **A.** Fluid
- **B. Fat**
- **C.** Free air
- **D.** Stool in the bowel

Additional reading:

Renzulli M, Brocchi S, Pettinari I, Biselli M, Clemente A, Corcioni B, Cappabianca S, Gaudiano C, Golfieri R. New MRI series for kidney evaluation: Saving time and money. Br J Radiol. 2019 Jul;92(1099):20190260. doi: 10.1259/bjr.20190260. Epub 2019 Jun 12. PMID: 31046410; PMCID: PMC6636269.

Flum AS, Hamoui N, Said MA, Yang XJ, Casalino DD, McGuire BB, Perry KT, Nadler RB. Update on the Diagnosis and Management of Renal Angiomyolipoma. J Urol. 2016 Apr;195(4 Pt 1):834-46. doi: 10.1016/j.juro.2015.07.126. Epub 2015 Nov 21. PMID: 26612197.

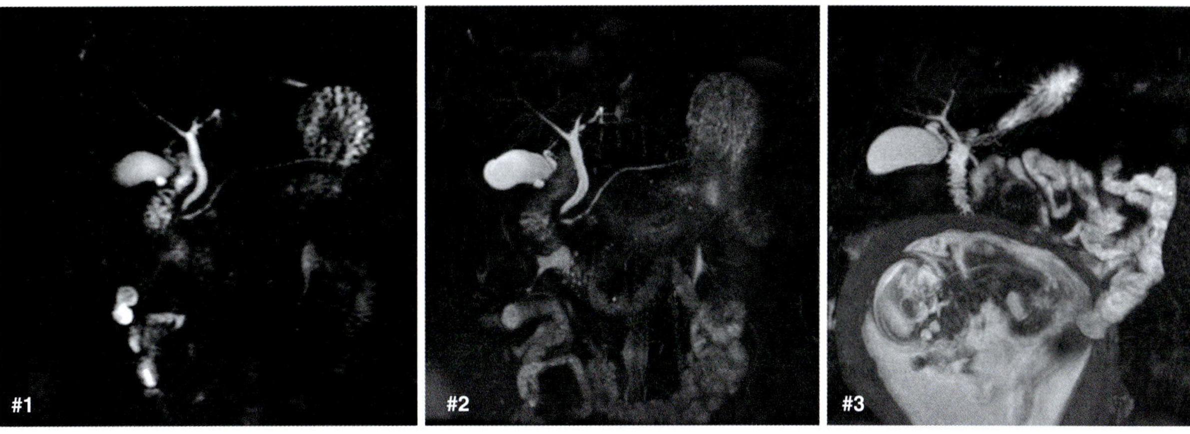

FIGURE 6-17.
(Walter Reed National Military Medical Center)

6-52. The pictures in Figure 6.17 are from what type of sequence?

A. Heavily weighted T1

B. Heavily weighted PD

C. Heavily weighted IR

D. Heavily weighted T2

6-53. Figure 6.17, #3 is also showing what unexpected finding?

A. A large dermoid

B. A large fibroid

C. A fetus

D. A large malignant tumor

6-54. Magnetic resonance cholangiopancreatography (MRCP) includes images of the hepatobiliary and pancreatic systems, including:

A. The liver, pancreas, pancreatic duct, interlobar artery, and bile ducts

B. The liver, gallbladder, bile ducts, pancreas, and pancreatic duct

C. The liver, pancreas, pancreatic duct, haustra, and bile ducts

D. The liver, gallbladder, bile ducts, pancreas, cisterna chyli, and pancreatic duct

Additional reading:

Griffin N, Charles-Edwards G, Grant LA. Magnetic resonance cholangiopancreatography: the ABC of MRCP. Insights Imaging. 2012 Feb;3(1):11-21. doi: 10.1007/s13244-011-0129-9.

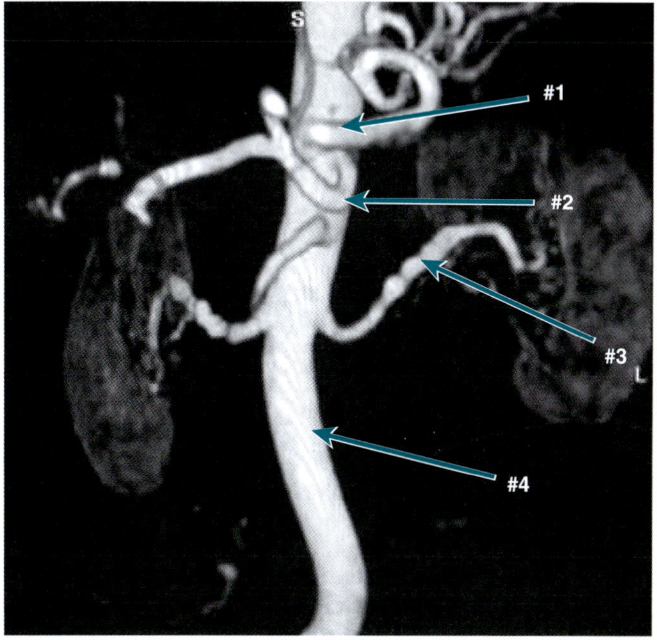

FIGURE 6-18.
(Walter Reed National Military Medical Center)

6-55. What is #1 pointing to in Figure 6.18?

A. Abdominal aorta

B. Superior mesenteric artery

C. Renal artery

D. Celiac artery

6-56. What is #2 pointing to in Figure 6.18?

A. Abdominal aorta

B. Superior mesenteric artery

C. Renal artery

D. Celiac artery

6-57. What is #3 pointing to in Figure 6.18?

- **A.** Abdominal aorta
- **B.** Thoracic aorta
- **C.** **Renal artery**
- **D.** Celiac artery

6-58. What is #4 pointing to in Figure 6.18?

- **A.** **Abdominal aorta**
- **B.** Thoracic aorta
- **C.** Renal artery
- **D.** Celiac artery

6-59. What type of image is Figure 6.18?

- **A.** Noncontrast MRA
- **B.** **Gadolinium contrast MRA**
- **C.** Iodinated contrast MRA
- **D.** Renografin contrast MRA

Discussion:

One of the keys to the arteries coming off the abdominal aorta is to remember that the superior mesenteric artery (SMA) generally arises about 1 cm below the celiac artery. The renal arteries generally arise below the SMA. Variations in arterial anatomy do occur, including duplex renal arteries to a single kidney.

Additional reading:

Leiner T, Michaely H. Advances in contrast-enhanced MR angiography of the renal arteries. Magn Reson Imaging Clin N Am. 2008 Nov;16(4):561-72, vii. doi: 10.1016/j.mric.2008.07.013. PMID: 18926422.

Braidy C, Daou I, Diop AD, Helweh O, Gageanu C, Boyer L, Chabrot P. Unenhanced MR angiography of renal arteries: 51 patients. AJR Am J Roentgenol. 2012 Nov;199(5):W629-37. doi: 10.2214/AJR.12.8513. PMID: 23096208.

Hagspiel KD, Leung DA, Angle JF, Spinosa DJ, Pao DG, de Lange EE, Butty S, Matsumoto AH. MR angiography of the mesenteric vasculature. Radiol Clin North Am. 2002 Jul;40(4):867-86. doi: 10.1016/s0033-8389(02)00027-1. PMID: 12171189.

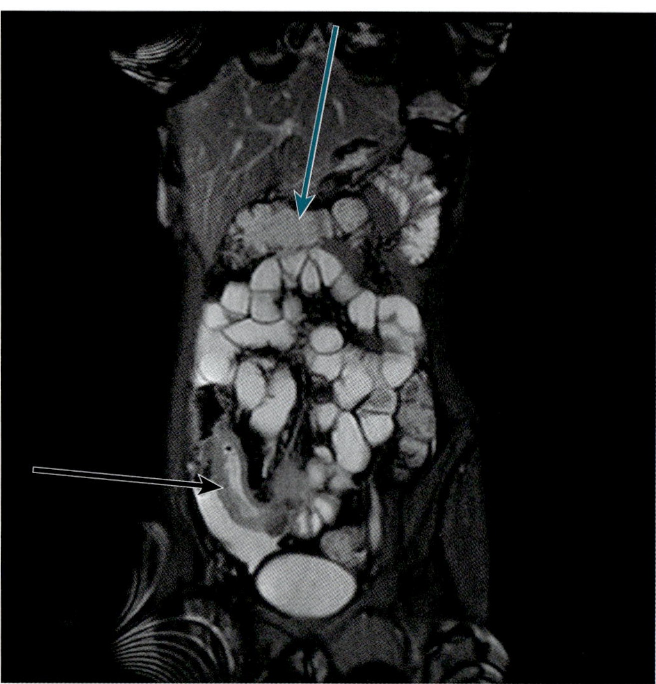

FIGURE 6-19.
(Walter Reed National Military Medical Center)

6-60. The black arrow in Figure 6.19 is pointing to an area of diseased bowel. What type of imaging is this depicted in this figure?

- **A.** Bowel MR with gadolinium-based contrast
- **B.** Bowel MR with iodine-based contrast
- **C.** **MR enterography**
- **D.** MR angiography

6-61. The blue arrow is pointing to what anatomy in Figure 6.19?

- **A.** Jejunum
- **B.** Ascending colon
- **C.** **Transverse colon**
- **D.** Left colic flexure

6-62. For an MR Enterography exam, what aspect of patient prep is essential once the patient has arrived to the MRI suite?

- **A.** Drink 3 bottles of water, 1 every 15 minutes prior to MRI
- **B.** **Drink 3 bottles of oral barium sulfate, 1 every 15 minutes prior to MRI**
- **C.** Drink 3 bottles of water, 1 every 20 minutes prior to MRI
- **D.** Drink 3 bottles of oral gadolinium, 1 every 15 minutes prior to MRI

6-63. Bowel preparation is generally regarded as helpful for improving diagnostic performance of MR Enterography exam (MRE) and improve compliance with the enteric contrast. Which of the following is NOT considered a goal of bowel prep?

A. Achieve maximal distension of bowel loops to improve visibility of luminal disease

B. Reduce bowel peristaltic activity to improve diagnostic quality of motion-sensitive MR sequences

C. **Reducing fluid in the ureters improves visualization of the bowel**

D. Displace air within bowel loops that can cause susceptibility artifact on gradient-echo sequences

6-64. For abdominal and pelvic imaging, what non-medication technique helps reduce artifacts from peristalsis?

A. Drinking 500 mL of cold water 30 minutes prior to the MRI

B. Drinking 500 mL of warm water 30 minutes prior to the MRI

C. **Fasting for 4–6 hours prior to the MRI**

D. Fasting for 2 hours prior to the MRI

Additional reading:

ACR–SAR–SPR Practice Parameter for the Performance of Magnetic Resonance (MR) Enterography. https://www.acr.org/-/media/ACR/Files/Practice-Parameters/MR-Enterog.pdf

Guglielmo FF, Anupindi SA, Fletcher JG, Al-Hawary MM, Dillman JR, Grand DJ, Bruining DH, Chatterji M, Darge K, Fidler JL, Gandhi NS, Gee MS, Grajo JR, Huang C, Jaffe TA, Park SH, Rimola J, Soto JA, Taouli B, Taylor SA, Baker ME. Small Bowel Crohn Disease at CT and MR Enterography: Imaging Atlas and Glossary of Terms. Radiographics. 2020 Mar-Apr;40(2):354-375. doi: 10.1148/rg.2020190091. Epub 2020 Jan 17. PMID: 31951512.

Zand KR, Reinhold C, Haider MA, Nakai A, Rohoman L, Maheshwari S. Artifacts and pitfalls in MR imaging of the pelvis. J Magn Reson Imaging. 2007 Sep;26(3):480-97. doi: 10.1002/jmri.20996. PMID: 17623875.

6-65. You know you have captured the late arterial phase properly when you can see:

A. Hepatic artery and branches are dark, Portal vein is enhanced, and the Hepatic veins are fully enhanced

B. Hepatic artery and branches are dark, bile duct is enhanced, and the Hepatic veins are not yet enhanced by antegrade flow

C. Hepatic artery and branches, bile duct, and the gall bladder are fully enhanced

D. **Hepatic artery and branches are fully enhanced, Portal vein is enhanced, and the Hepatic veins are not yet enhanced by antegrade flow**

Additional reading:

ACR–SAR–SPR Practice Parameter for the Performance of Magnetic Resonance Imaging (MRI) of the Liver. https://www.acr.org/-/media/ACR/Files/Practice-Parameters/MR-Liver.pdf

6-66. What anatomy is depicted by the bright structures in Figure 6.20?

A. Lungs

B. Seminole vesicles

C. Ovaries

D. **Kidneys**

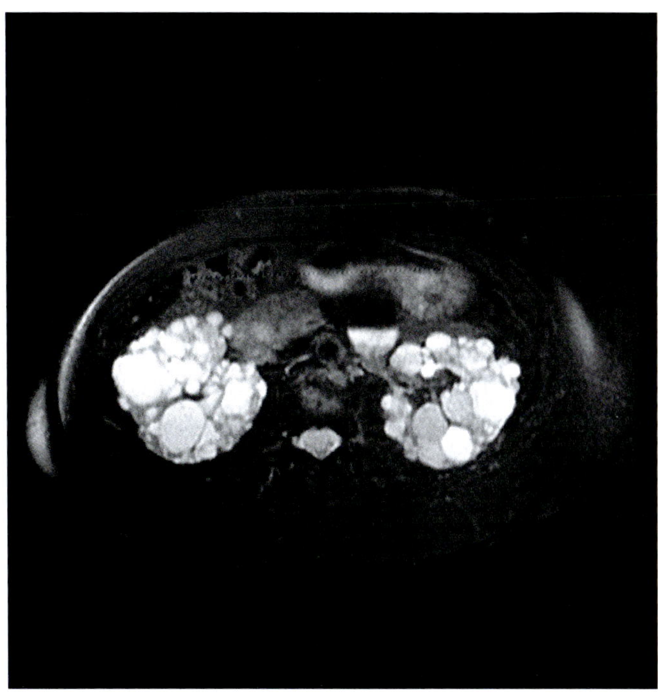

FIGURE 6-20.
(Walter Reed National Military Medical Center)

6-67. What pathology is depicted by the bright structures in Figure 6.20?

A. Metastasis

B. Primary cancer

C. Polycystic disease

D. Crohn's disease

6-68. Abnormal accumulation of serous fluid in the abdominopelvic anatomy is called what?

A. Ascites

B. Pus

C. Abscess

D. Purulent fluid

6-69. What key change is required when imaging the abdomen for a transplanted kidney?

A. Ensure no contrast is ever given

B. Place the patient prone

C. Extend field of view as transplanted kidney is usually in the pelvis

D. Make the slice thickness as small as possible

6-70. For excretory MR urography, what is given to the patient in addition to IV contrast material that improves uniformity in contrast distribution?

A. RF blanket over the abdomen

B. Oral barium sulfate suspension

C. IV administration of saline solution and a diuretic

D. SQ administration of glucagon

Additional reading:

Leyendecker JR, Barnes CE, Zagoria RJ. MR urography: techniques and clinical applications. Radiographics. 2008 Jan-Feb;28(1):23-46; discussion 46-7. doi: 10.1148/rg.281075077. PMID: 18203929.

6-71. Figure 6.21 shows two pictures from a dynamic pelvis exam. What problem is this exam best for?

A. Bladder cancer

B. Prolapsed rectum

C. Peptic ulcer

D. Hiatal hernia

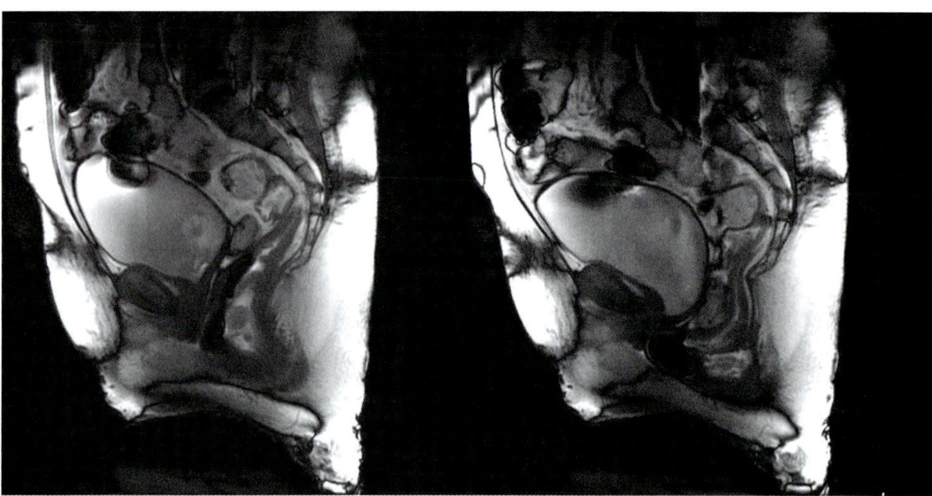

FIGURE 6-21.
(Walter Reed National Military Medical Center)

6-72. In dynamic pelvic defecography, what additional prep is the technologist to prepare for?

A. Have a bag of normal saline ready

B. Keep a crash cart nearby

C. Prepare for rectal contrast

D. Have an emesis basin ready

6-73. In dynamic pelvis exam for any kind of pelvic floor dysfunction, the technologist must instruct the patient to do what for the dynamic imaging?

A. Drink a cold beverage

B. Squeeze their pelvis to hold in any fluids

C. Breath very regularly

D. Bare down with maximal strain, trying to defecate

6-74. In dynamic pelvis exam for any kind of pelvic floor dysfunction, which preparation step is optional?

A. Completely cover table in absorbent, disposable padding

B. Instruct patient to defecate while on the MR scanner table

C. Patient wears adult size absorbent underwear

D. Clear instruction on straining with holding versus straining and completely defecating

Additional reading:

Maccioni F, Alt CD. MRI of the Pelvic Floor and MR Defecography. In: Hodler J, Kubik-Huch RA, von Schulthess GK, eds. Diseases of the Abdomen and Pelvis 2018-2021: Diagnostic Imaging - IDKD Book. Cham (CH): Springer; March 21, 2018.13-20.

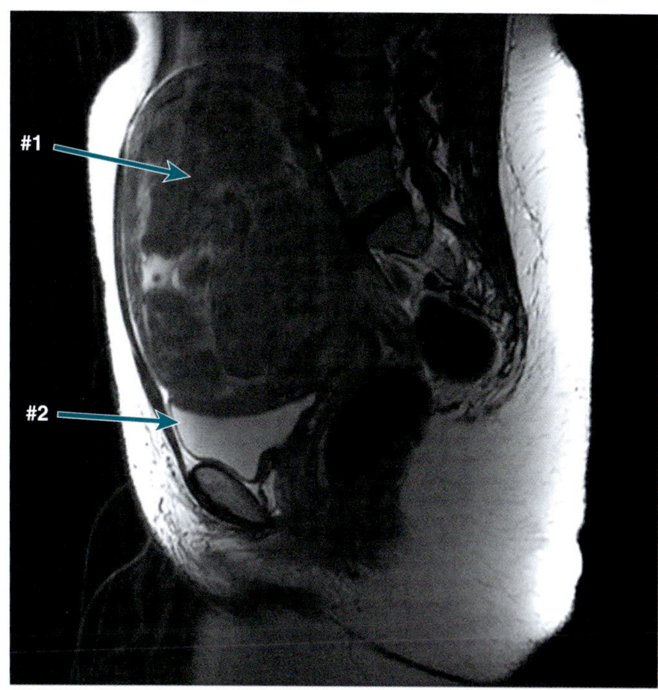

FIGURE 6-22.
(Walter Reed National Military Medical Center)

6-75. What structure is being pointed to by Arrow #1 in Figure 6.22?

A. Transplanted kidney

B. Urinary bladder

C. Uterine fibroid

D. Enlarged prostate gland

6-76. What structure is being pointed to by Arrow #2 in Figure 6.22?

A. Transplanted kidney

B. Urinary bladder

C. Uterine fibroid

D. Enlarged prostate gland

6-77. What area of the body is being shown in Figure 6.23?

A. Female pelvis

B. Abdomen

C. Male pelvis

D. Thorax

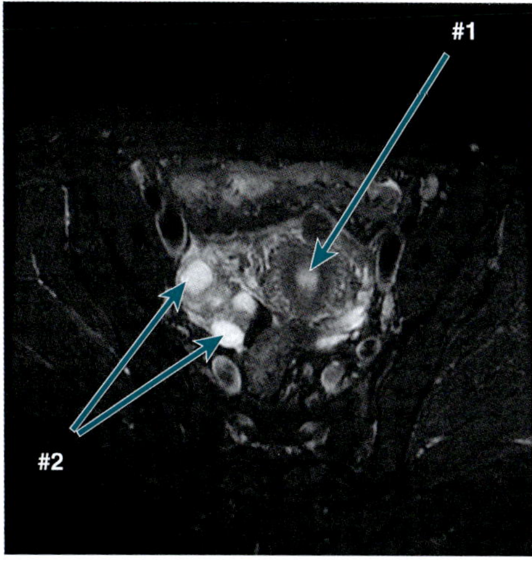

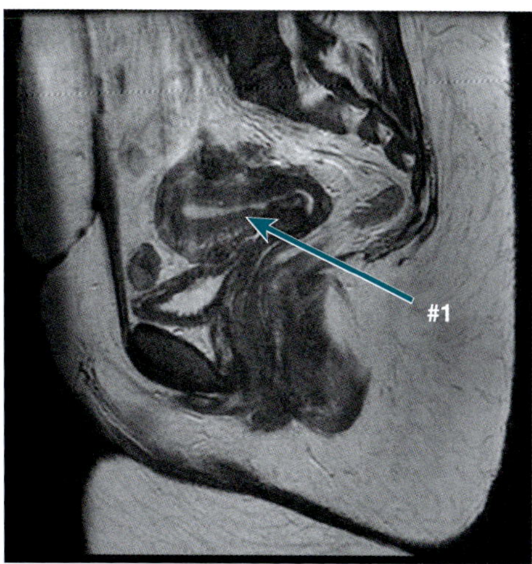

FIGURE 6-23.
(Walter Reed National Military Medical Center)

6-78. What structure is being pointed to by the arrows labeled #1 in Figure 6.23?

A. Large loop of the colon

B. Cecum

C. Uterus

D. Sigmoid colon

6-79. What structure is being pointed to by the arrow labeled #2 in Figure 6.23?

A. Ovaries

B. Right paraovarian cysts

C. Cecum

D. Loops of bowel

Discussion:

It is recommended that patients fast approximately 4 hours prior to MRI of the female pelvis. Protocols should be optimized for the specific indication.

Additional reading:

https://www.appliedradiology.com/articles/part-i-mr-of-the-female-pelvis

6-80. What is the arrow labeled #1 pointing to in Figure 6.24?

A. Prostate

B. Rectal tumor

C. Uterine fibroid

D. Fistula

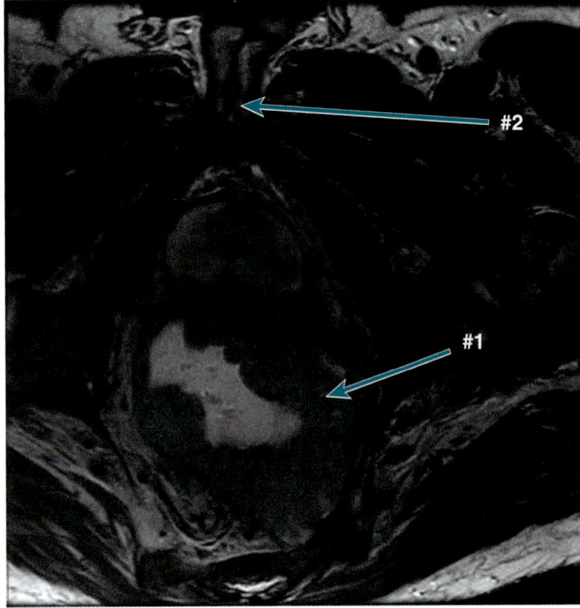

FIGURE 6-24.
(Walter Reed National Military Medical Center)

6-81. What is the arrow labeled #2 pointing to in Figure 6.24?

A. Penile urethra

B. Seminal vesicle

C. Umbilicus

D. Fistula

Discussion:

For detailed male anatomy, visit https://mrimaster.com/anatomy%20pelvis%20male%20axial.html

Additional reading:

For detailed male anatomy https://mrimaster.com/anatomy%20pelvis%20male%20axial.html

Horvat N, Carlos Tavares Rocha C, Clemente Oliveira B, Petkovska I, Gollub MJ. MRI of Rectal Cancer: Tumor Staging, Imaging Techniques, and Management. Radiographics. 2019 Mar-Apr;39(2):367-387. doi: 10.1148/rg.2019180114. Epub 2019 Feb 15. PMID: 30768361; PMCID: PMC6438362.

6-82. What is the main finding in this coronal image of the male pelvis in Figure 6-25?

A. Penile urethra

B. Seminal vesicle

C. Undescended testes

D. Fistula

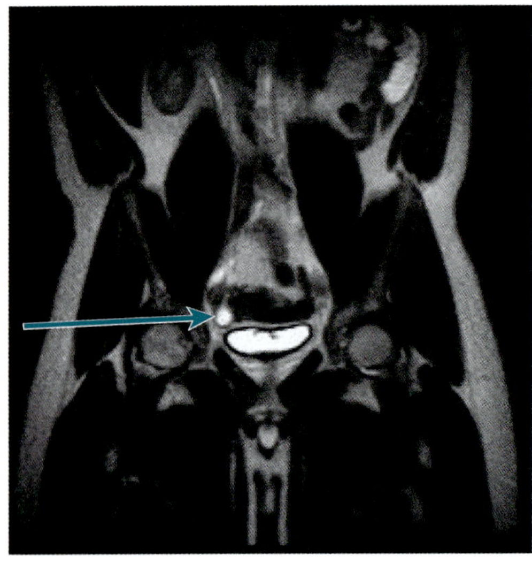

FIGURE 6-25.
(Walter Reed National Military Medical Center)

6-83. The images in Figure 6.26 depict what anatomy?

A. A/C joints

B. S/I joints

C. Prostate

D. Bladder

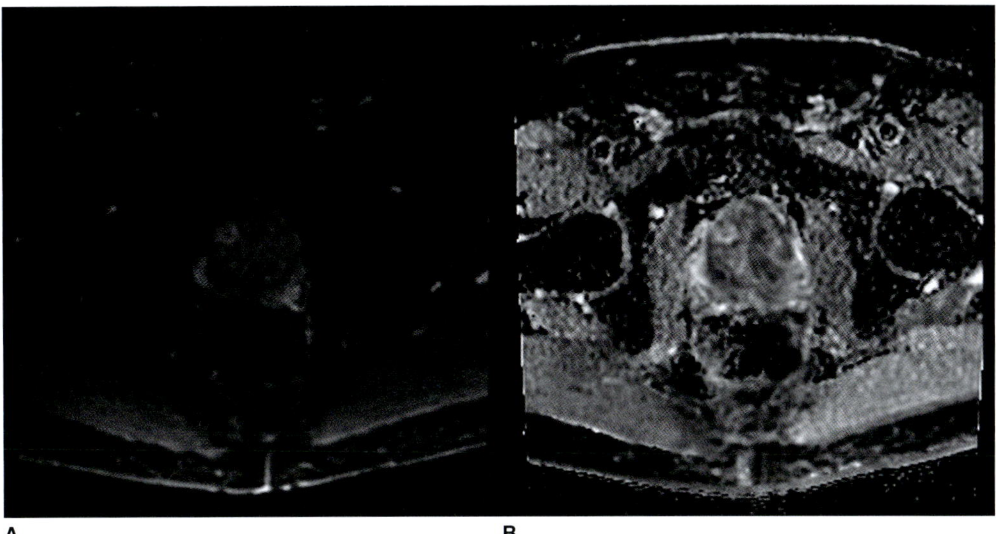

FIGURE 6-26.
(Walter Reed National Military Medical Center)

6-84. The image labeled B in Figure 6.26 is what type of technique?

A. T2 weighted

B. Diffusion weighted

C. Perfusion weighted

D. Susceptibility weighted

Additional reading:

Although the use of ADC maps have long been a mainstay of prostate imaging, more recent work is moving toward multiparametric imaging.

Lo WC, Panda A, Jiang Y, Ahad J, Gulani V, Seiberlich N. MR fingerprinting of the prostate. MAGMA. 2022 Aug;35(4):557-571. doi: 10.1007/s10334-022-01012-8. Epub 2022 Apr 13. PMID: 35419668; PMCID: PMC10288492.

Raczeck P, Frenzel F, Woerner T, Graeber S, Bohle RM, Ziegler G, Buecker A, Schneider GK. Noninferiority of Monoparametric MRI Versus Multiparametric MRI for the Detection of Prostate Cancer: Diagnostic Accuracy of ADC Ratios Based on Advanced "Zoomed" Diffusion-Weighted Imaging. Invest Radiol. 2022 Apr 1;57(4):233-241. doi: 10.1097/RLI.0000000000000830. PMID: 34743133.

6-85. The yellow arrow in Figure 6.27 is pointing to what?

A. Gas in the rectum

B. Prostate coil probe in the rectum

C. Surgical scar

D. Bladder

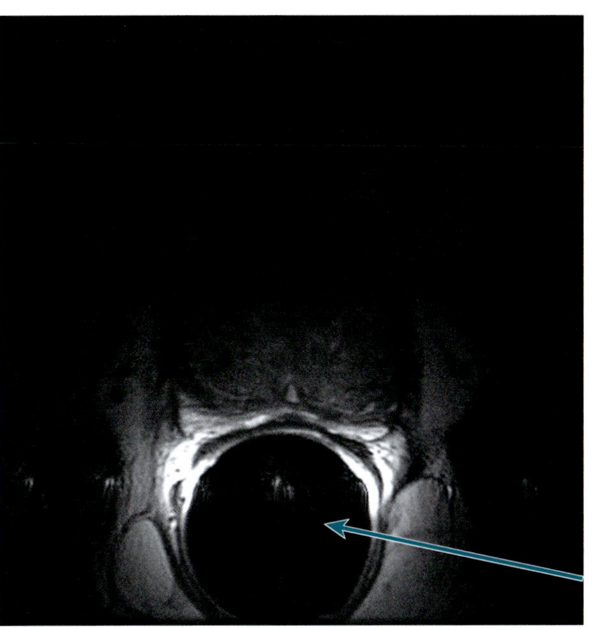

FIGURE 6-27.
(Walter Reed National Military Medical Center)

6-86. Prostate imaging prep for the patient consists of

A. Light meals or liquids the day before, enema the night before, NPO except for medications with clear liquids

B. Normal meals and liquids the day before, enema the night before, NPO after midnight except for medications with clear liquids

C. Light meals or liquids the day before, no other prep

D. Light meals or liquids the day before, NPO 1 hour prior

Discussion:

Prostate imaging recommends that the patient be prepped a day in advance of the exam in order to obtain optimal results whether they are having an exam with an endorectal coil or not.

Additional reading:

Barrett T, Haider MA. The Emerging Role of MRI in Prostate Cancer Active Surveillance and Ongoing Challenges. AJR Am J Roentgenol. 2017 Jan;208(1):131-139. doi: 10.2214/AJR.16.16355.

Purysko AS, Rosenkrantz AB. Technique of Multiparametric MR Imaging of the Prostate. Radiol Clin North Am. 2018 Mar;56(2):211-222. doi: 10.1016/j.rcl.2017.10.004. Epub 2017 Dec 6. PMID: 29420977

6-87. What is Figure 6.28 showing?

A. Mass in the pelvis

B. Aneurism off the iliac artery

C. Loop of colon with inflammation

D. Transplanted kidney

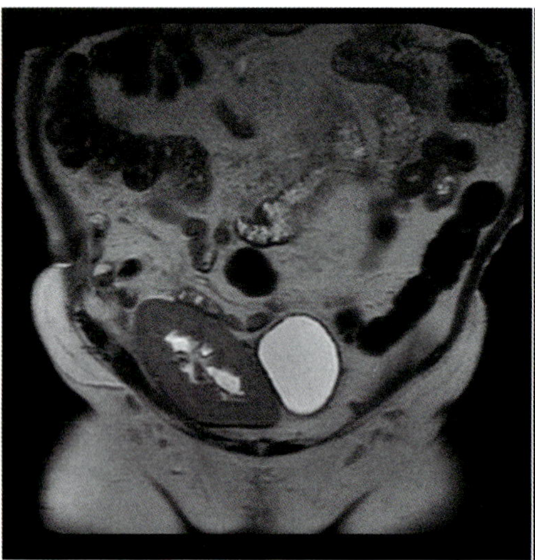

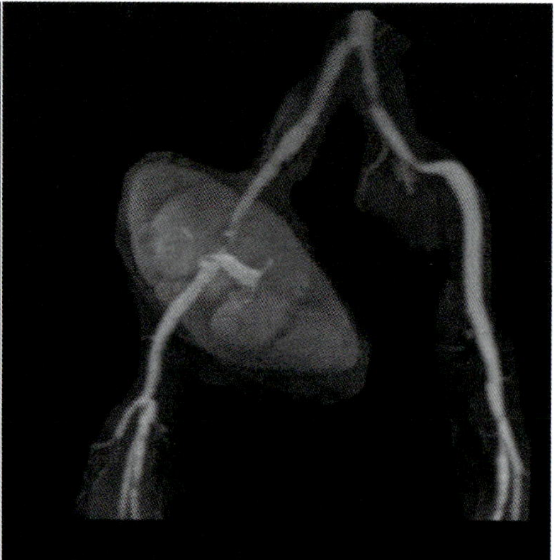

FIGURE 6-28.
(Walter Reed National Military Medical Center)

6-88. When setting up for a request to image a transplanted kidney, what must the technologist due when setting up the patient?

A. Carefully center the bottom of the surface coil at the top of the iliac crest

B. Select the smallest surface coil for the abdomen to ensure best image quality

C. Select a surface coil to cover the area of interest, making sure the coil covers down below the symphysis pubis

D. Set up multiple surface coils to cover the entire chest, abdomen, and pelvis as the transplanted kidney could be anywhere.

Discussion:

The location of the transplanted kidney can vary with the right iliac fossa being a common location.

Additional reading: Sugi MD, Joshi G, Maddu KK, Dahiya N, Menias CO. Imaging of Renal Transplant Complications throughout the Life of the Allograft: Comprehensive Multimodality Review. Radiographics. 2019 Sep-Oct;39(5):1327-1355. doi: 10.1148/rg.2019190096. PMID: 31498742

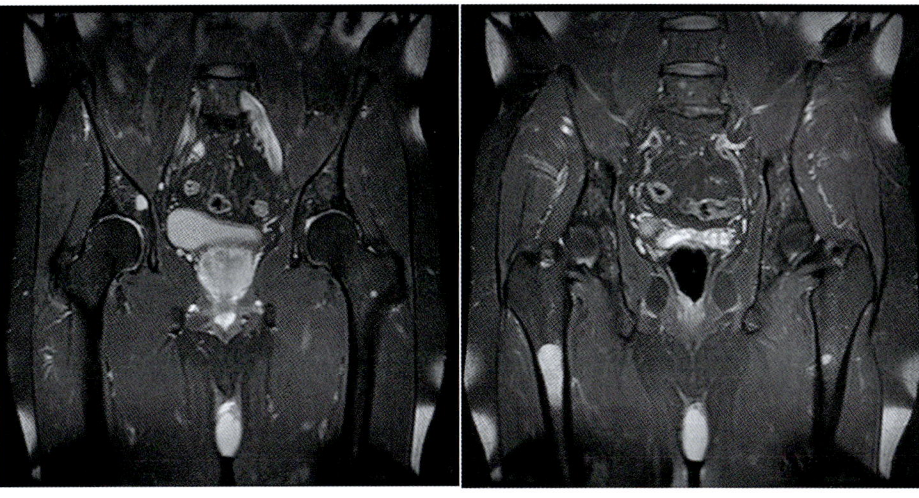

FIGURE 6-29.
(Walter Reed National Military Medical Center)

6-89. Figure 6.29 shows two images of a post contrast T1-weighted image with fat suppression technique. What is the pathology in the bony pelvis?

A. No pathology, just B1 inhomogeneity artifacts
B. Multiple foci of mass-like marrow replacement
C. Incomplete fat suppression
D. Multiple fractures

6-90. For fetal imaging, what MR sequences are generally best to show anatomy well?

A. A variety MRI sequences in 2-D and 3-D to obtain T1-, PD- and T2-weighted images
B. A variety of fast MRI sequences to obtain T1- and T2-weighted images
C. A variety of 3-D MRI sequences are used to obtain T1- and T2-weighted images
D. A variety of 2-D MRI sequences are used to obtain T1- and T2-weighted images, plus a 3-D volume to show total anatomy

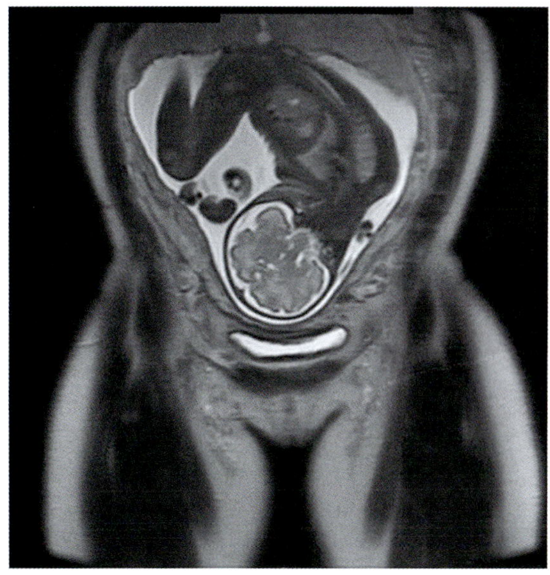

FIGURE 6-30.
(Walter Reed National Military Medical Center)

6-91. In Figure 6.30, what MR sequences is this?

A. Steady-state free precession
B. Fast/turbo spin echo with T1 weighting
C. Gradient echo with T1 weighting
D. Susceptibility weighted imaging

Additional reading:

Saleem SN. Fetal MRI: An approach to practice: A review. J Adv Res. 2014 Sep;5(5):507-23. doi: 10.1016/j.jare.2013.06.001.

6-92. In Figure 6.31, what is the structure pointing to on #1?

A. Undescended testes

B. Ovaries

C. Seminal vesicles

D. Lower bowel loop

6-93. In Figure 6.31, what is the structure pointing to on #2?

A. Rectum

B. Uterus

C. Bladder

D. Prostate

Additional reading:

Langer JE, Oliver ER, Lev-Toaff AS, Coleman BG. Imaging of the female pelvis through the life cycle. Radiographics. 2012 Oct;32(6):1575-97. doi: 10.1148/rg.326125513. PMID: 23065159.

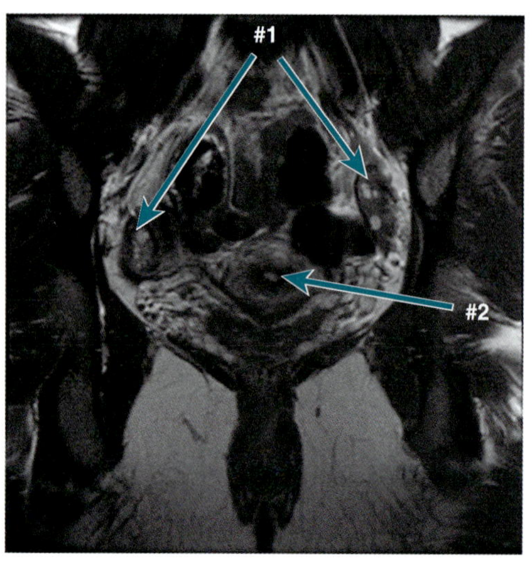

FIGURE 6-31.
(Walter Reed National Military Medical Center)

Additional reading:

Wasnik AP, Mazza MB, Liu PS. Normal and variant pelvic anatomy on MRI. Magn Reson Imaging Clin N Am. 2011 Aug;19(3):547-66; viii. doi: 10.1016/j.mric.2011.05.001.

Paramasivam S, Proietto A, Puvaneswary M. Pelvic anatomy and MRI. Best Pract Res Clin Obstet Gynaecol. 2006 Feb;20(1):3-22. Epub 2005 Nov 7.

6-94. Label the pelvic anatomy in Figure 6.32

A. Rectus abdominus muscle_____2_____

B. Iliac artery/vein_____3_____

C. Psoas muscle_____1_____

D. Descending colon_____5_____

E. Ilium_____4_____

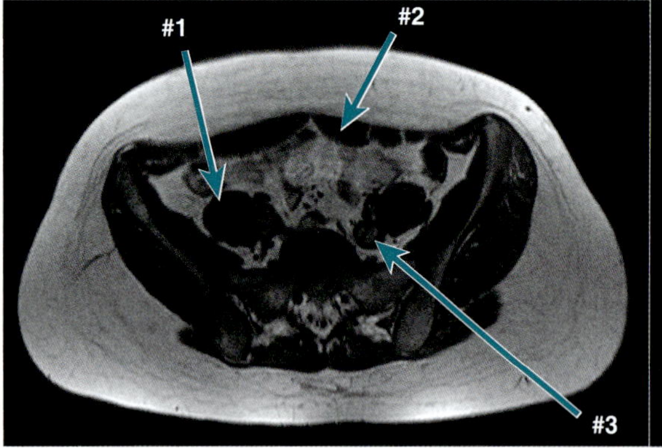

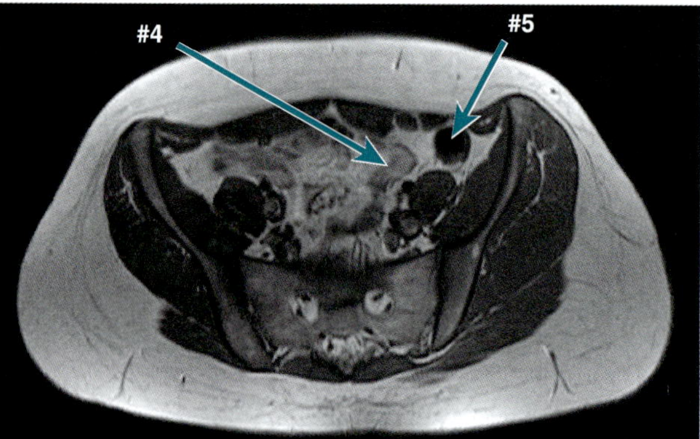

FIGURE 6-32.
(Walter Reed National Military Medical Center)

6-95. In Figure 6.33, where is arrow #1 is pointing to?

A. **Right iliac artery**

B. Right iliac vein

C. Fem-Fem graft

D. Left iliac artery

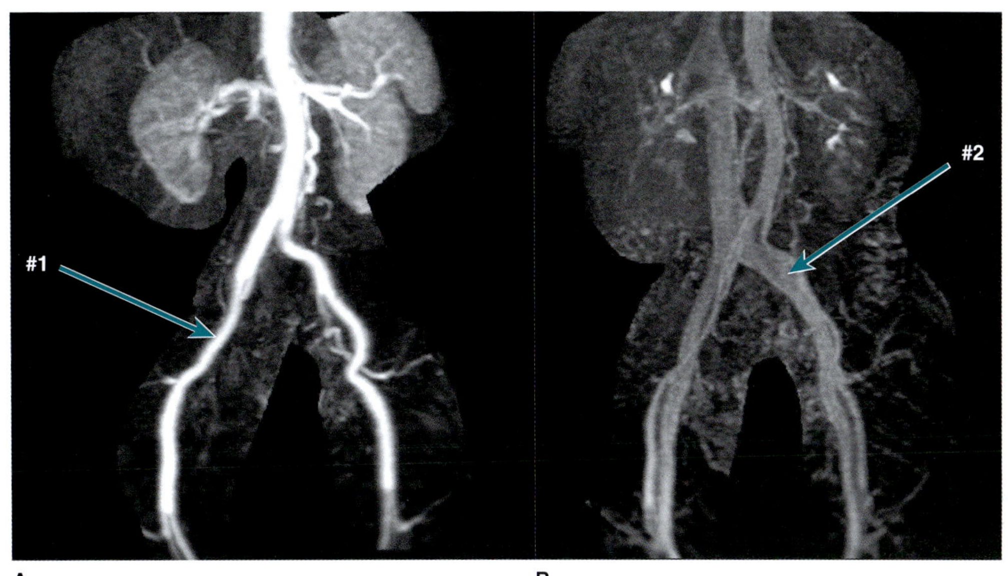

FIGURE 6-33.
(Walter Reed National Military Medical Center)

6-96. In Figure 6.33, where is arrow #2 is pointing to?

A. Right iliac artery

B. **Left iliac vein**

C. Fem-Fem graft

D. Left iliac artery

6-97. In Figure 6.33, the image labeled B is considered what kind of image?

A. Optimal phase arterial MRA

B. Early phase arterial MRA

C. **Delayed arteriovenous phase MRA**

D. Optimal phase venogram

Additional reading:

Ho VB, Corse WR. MR angiography of the abdominal aorta and peripheral vessels. Radiol Clin North Am. 2003 Jan;41(1):115-44.

Kuo AH, Nagpal P, Ghoshhajra BB, Hedgire SS. Vascular magnetic resonance angiography techniques. Cardiovasc Diagn Ther. 2019 Aug;9(Suppl 1):S28-S36. doi: 10.21037/cdt.2019.06.07. PMID: 31559152; PMCID: PMC6732109.

6-98. What structure is the yellow arrow pointing to in Figure 6.34?

A. Left testicle

B. Right testicle

C. Prostate gland

D. Ishial tuberosity

Additional reading:

Marko J, Wolfman DJ, Aubin AL, Sesterhenn IA. Testicular Seminoma and Its Mimics: From the Radiologic Pathology Archives. Radiographics. 2017 Jul-Aug;37(4):1085-1098. doi: 10.1148/rg.2017160164.

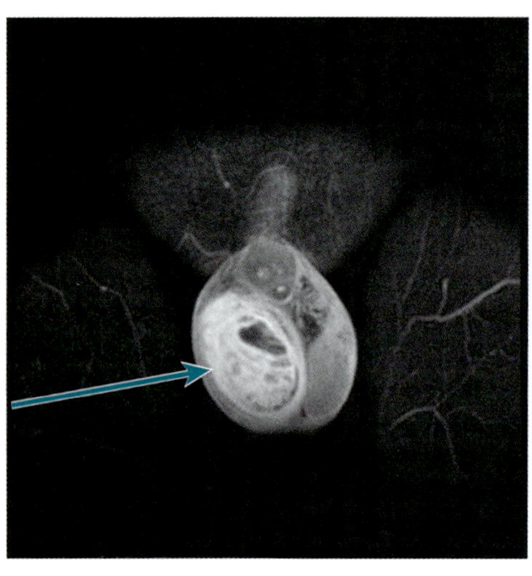

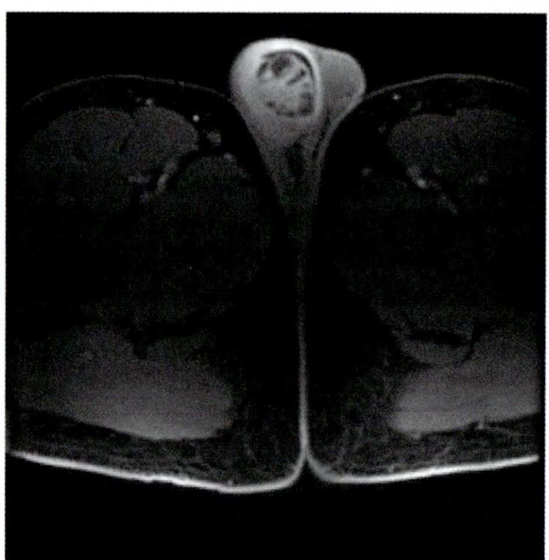

FIGURE 6-34.
(Walter Reed National Military Medical Center)

6-99. What structure is the yellow arrow pointing to in Figure 6.35?

A. Rectum

B. Anal canal

C. Ureter

D. Urethra

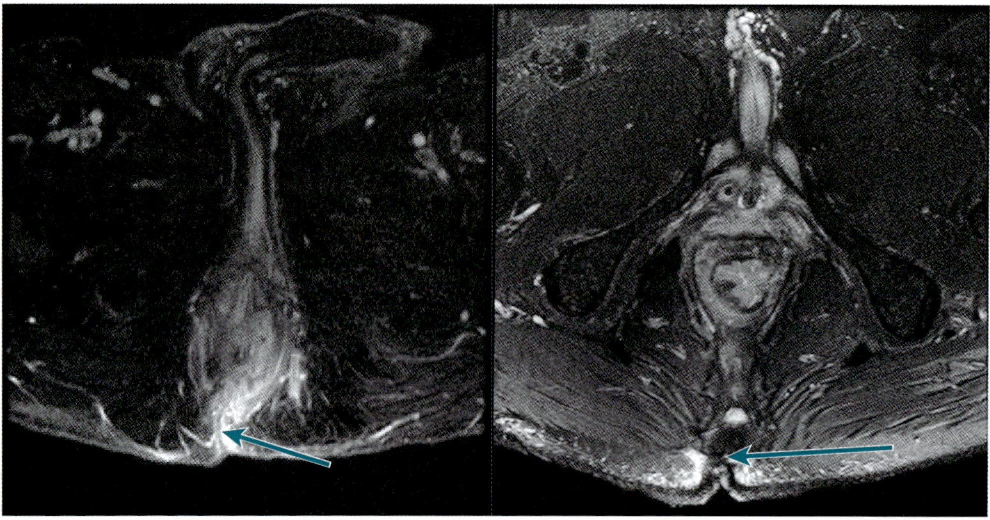

FIGURE 6-35.
(Walter Reed National Military Medical Center)

6-100. What is demonstrated by the two images in Figure 6.35?

A. Malignant bladder cancer

B. MRI gel contrast in the rectum

C. Extensive perianal disease with edema

D. Meningocele with complex connection

Additional reading:

Sneider EB, Maykel JA. Anal abscess and fistula. Gastroenterol Clin North Am. 2013 Dec;42(4):773-84. doi: 10.1016/j.gtc.2013.08.003.

6-101. What imaging plane is pictured in Figure 6.36?

A. Coronal

B. Oblique

C. Transverse

D. Sagittal

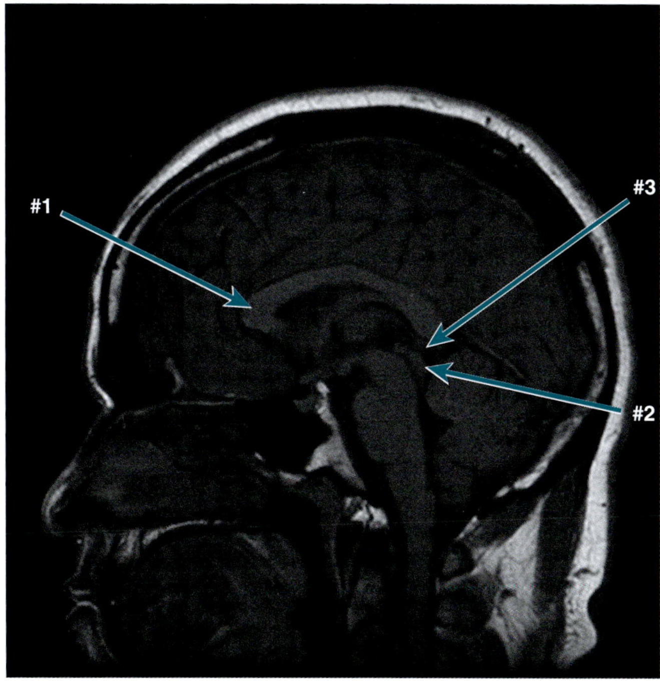

FIGURE 6-36.

(Walter Reed National Military Medical Center)

6-102. What is the structure labeled #1 in Figure 6.36?

A. Genu of the corpus callosum

B. Body of the corpus callosum

C. Thalamus

D. Splenium of the corpus callosum

6-103. Identify the structure labeled #2 in Figure 6.36?

A. Thalamus

B. Pineal body

C. Corpora quadrigemina

D. Cerebral aqueduct

6-104. Identify the structure labeled #3 in Figure 6.36?

A. Thalamus

B. Pineal body

C. Corpora quadrigemina

D. Cerebral aqueduct

Discussion:

The Corpora Quadrigemina, also known as the Quadrigeminal plate, tectal plate or tectum, is part of the midbrain that consists of four parts, two superior colliculi and two inferior colliculi that contain visual and auditory centers. The Pineal Body sits superior and posterior to the Corpora Quadrigemina and is a small endocrine gland involved circadian rhythm and produces melatonin.

Additional Reading:

Patton KT, Thibodeau GA. *Anatomy & Physiology, 9th Edition.* Mosby, 2016.

6-105. The inner membrane covering the brain is the:

A. Pia mater

B. Dura mater

C. Arachnoid

D. Endosteum

Discussion:

The brain in enclosed with three membranes or meninges. The pia mater covers the brain matter followed by the arachnoid and then the outer dura mater. The pia mater is vascular and directly covers the entire surface of the brain. The arachnoid is a very delicate avascular membrane, but just inside this layer is cerebral spinal fluid in the space referred to as the subarachnoid space. The tough outer layer is the dura mater, which actually consist of two layers, the endosteal layer lines the inner surface of the skull and the meningeal layer lines the cranial cavity.

Additional Reading:

Bo WJ, Carr JJ, Krueger WA, Wolfman NT, Bowden RL. Basic Atlas of Sectional Anatomy: With Correlated Imaging, 4th Edition. WB Saunders, 2006.

6-106. What aspect of extracellular gadolinium-based contrast agents is desirable in neuroradiology?

A. They are freely distributed in the extravascular space and easily cross the blood brain barrier.

B. They are freely distributed in the extravascular space, but do not cross the blood brain barrier.

C. They are only distributed in the intravascular space, but do not cross the blood brain barrier.

D. They are only distributed in the intravascular space, and do cross the blood brain barrier.

Additional reading:

Wahsner J, Gale EM, Rodríguez-Rodríguez A, Caravan P. Chemistry of MRI Contrast Agents: Current Challenges and New Frontiers. *Chem Rev.* 2019;119(2):957-1057.

Roberts TP, Mikulis D. Neuro MR: principles. J Magn Reson Imaging. 2007 Oct;26(4):823-37.

6-107. Multiple Sclerosis (MS) is an autoimmune inflammatory condition that primarily affects the:

A. Afferent fibers

B. Basal ganglia

C. Myelin sheath of CNS axons

D. Neuron cell bodies

Additional reading:

Multiple sclerosis (MS) is a neuroinflammatory disease that primarily affects the myelin sheath that wraps around nerve fibers (axons) in the white matter of the brain and spinal cord. MS can also damage the nerve cell bodies, of the gray matter, as well as the axons themselves in the brain, spinal cord, and optic nerve.

http://www.ninds.nih.gov/disorders/multiple_sclerosis/detail_multiple_sclerosis.htm#3215_2

6-108. Match Structures on axial slice in Figure 6.37

A. Pituitary stalk_____a_____

B. Aqueduct of Sylvius_____b_____

C. Cerebral peduncle_____c_____

D. Straight sinus_____d_____

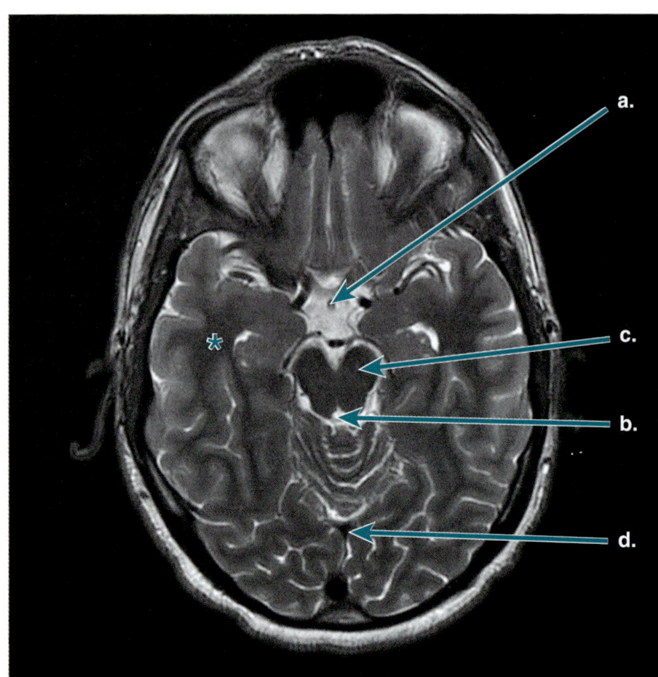

FIGURE 6-37.
(Walter Reed National Military Medical Center)

6-109. The dark areas throughout the brain tissue (marked with*), adjacent to lighter grey tissue are what?

A. White matter

B. Grey matter

C. Arachnoid layers

D. Moderate matter

Discussion:

Grey and white matter differ in composition. Grey matter contains more neurons, glial cells and other cell bodies whereas white matter is primarily composed of long nerve fibers with myelinated axons and other supporting cells. Thus, on T2 weighted imaging, white matter appears darker than grey matter.

6-110. What pathology is demonstrated in Figure 6.38?

A. Stroke

B. Multiple sclerosis

C. Tuberculosis

D. Brain metastasis

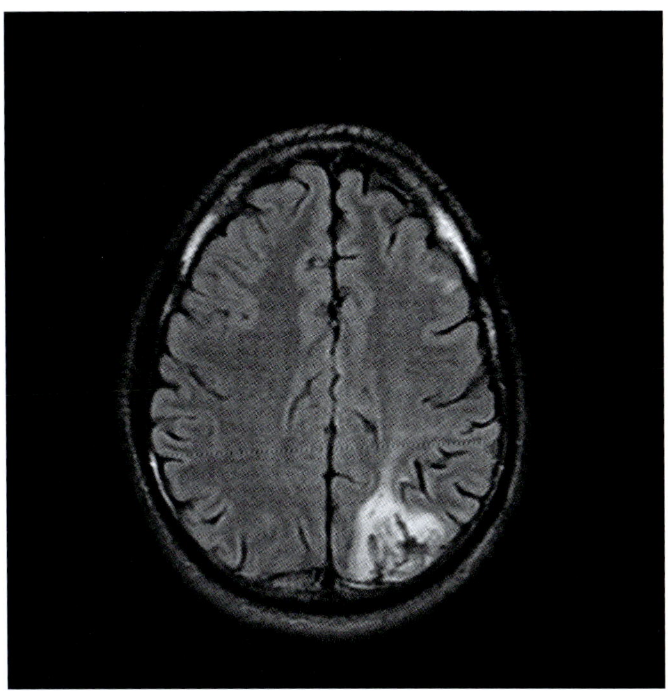

FIGURE 6-38.
(Walter Reed National Military Medical Center)

6-111. Figure 6.38 uses a fluid attenuated inversion recovery. Why is this such a desirable sequence for finding pathology in the brain?

A. Short TR and TE times make the anatomy more clear

B. Long TR and TE times, combined with the proper inversion time, show pathology while suppressing brightness from CSF

C. Long TR and TE times, combined with the proper flip angle, show Brownian motion of fluid

D. Long TR and TE times, combined with the proper flip angle, show pathology while suppressing brightness from CSF

6-112. What would be an appropriate fast MR brain protocol for an emergent acute stroke patient?

A. Sag T1 FSE, Ax T2 FSE, Ax DWI/ADC, Ax T2 FLAIR, Ax GRE, PWI

B. Ax DWI/ADC, Ax T2 FLAIR, Ax GRE, COR SPGR, 3-D TOF COW

C. Ax DWI/ADC, Ax T2 FLAIR, Ax GRE, spectroscopy

D. Ax DWI/ADC, Ax T2 FLAIR, Ax GRE

Discussion:

The key word here is fast. Time is of the essence to determine the appropriate therapy for the patient. Three quick sequences to include DWI will be sufficient to determine whether an ischemic stroke is happening. SWI imaging may also be of use but may be reserved for follow-up imaging.

Additional Reading:

Greer DM, Koroshetz WJ, Cullen S, Gonzalez RG, Lev MH. Magnetic resonance imaging improves detection of intracerebral hemorover computed tomography after intra-arterial thrombolysis. *Stroke.* 2004;35(2):491-495.

6-113. Why is a gradient recalled echo a desirable type of pulse sequence for stroke imaging?

- **A. It is sensitive to T2* shortening associated with iron**
- **B.** It is sensitive to T2 shortening associated with iron
- **C.** High resolution with few artifacts
- **D.** Insensitive to susceptibly artifacts

Discussion:

Because gradients do not refocus field inhomogeneities, GRE sequences with long TEs are T2*-weighted rather than T2-weighted like SE sequences.

Additional Reading:

Roberts TP, Mikulis D. Neuro MR: principles. *J Magn Reson Imaging.* 2007;26(4):823-837.

6-114. Figure 6.39 shows a coronal T2-weighted with fat suppression. Why is the left eye conal/extraconal space (#1) bright?

- **A.** Patient has inflammation of the orbit
- **B.** Coil element is out
- **C.** Patient has an eye infection
- **D. Uneven fat suppression caused by metallic dental work**

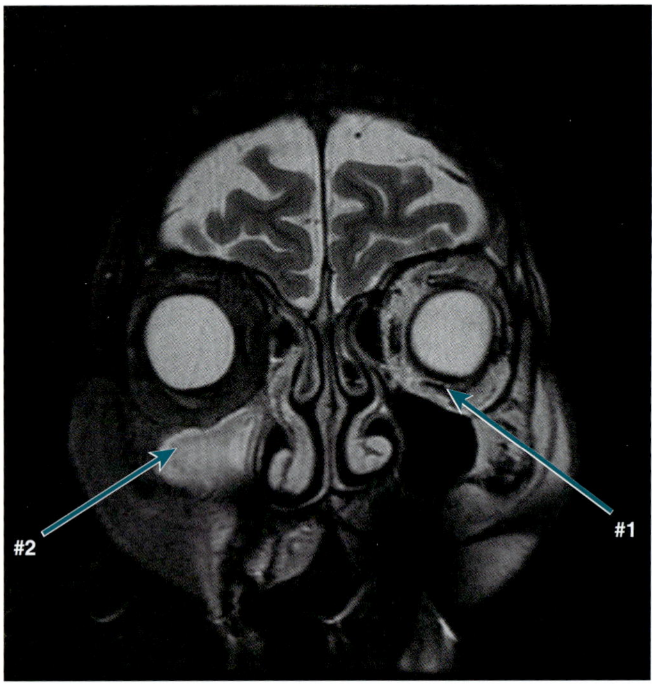

FIGURE 6-39.
(Walter Reed National Military Medical Center)

6-115. What is #2 pointing to in Figure 6.39?

- **A.** Ethmoid sinus tumor
- **B. Maxillary sinus with fluid/mucosal thickening**
- **C.** Uneven fat suppression
- **D.** Mandibular tumor

Additional reading:

Varma DR, Ponnaganti S, Dandu RV. Beware of artifacts in orbital magnetic resonance imaging. Indian J Ophthalmol. 2020 Nov;68(11):2516-2518. doi: 10.4103/ijo.IJO_640_20. PMID: 33120664; PMCID: PMC7774208.

Mossa-Basha M, Ilica AT, Maluf F, Karakoç Ö, Izbudak I, Aygün N. The many faces of fungal disease of the paranasal sinuses: CT and MRI findings. Diagn Interv Radiol. 2013 May-Jun;19(3):195-200. doi: 10.5152/dir.2012.003. PMID: 23271503.

6-116. Figure 6.40 is probably what type of sequence?

- **A.** T1 Spin Echo
- **B.** Inversion recovery T1
- **C. Gradient recalled echo/susceptibility weighted image**
- **D.** Diffusion weighted

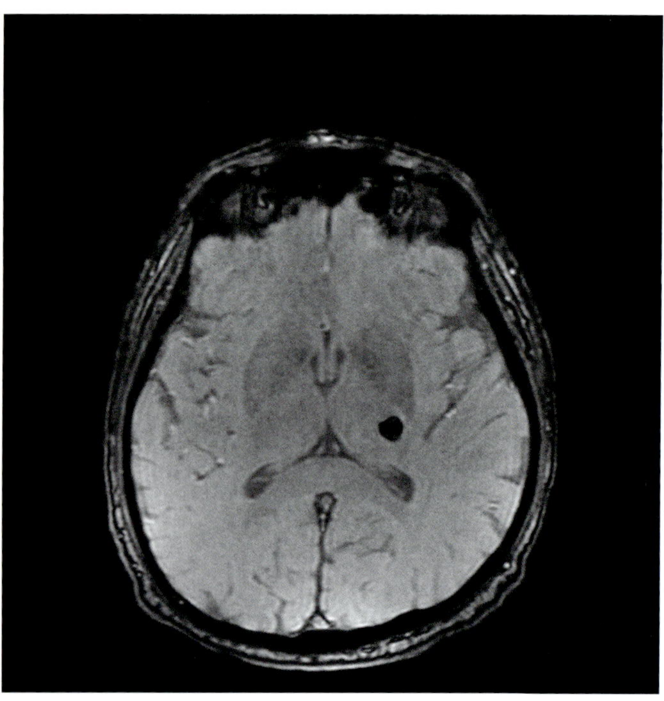

FIGURE 6-40.
(Walter Reed National Military Medical Center)

6-117. Figure 6.40 is demonstrating what type of pathology?

A. Astrocytoma

B. Hemorrhage

C. Meningioma

D. Multiple sclerosis

Additional reading:

Rubin A, Waszczuk Ł, Trybek G, Kapetanakis S, Bladowska J. Application of susceptibility weighted imaging (SWI) in diagnostic imaging of brain pathologies - a practical approach. *Clin Neurol Neurosurg.* 2022;221:107368.

Roberts TP, Mikulis D. Neuro MR: principles. J Magn Reson Imaging. 2007 Oct;26(4):823-37. doi: 10.1002/jmri.21029. PMID: 17685415.

6-118. What pathology is demonstrated on the images in Figure 6.41?

A. Bleed

B. Multiple sclerosis

C. Tuberculosis

D. Primary brain tumor

6-119. Identify the sequence demonstrated in Figure 6.41.

A. T1

B. FLAIR

C. Diffusion

D. T2

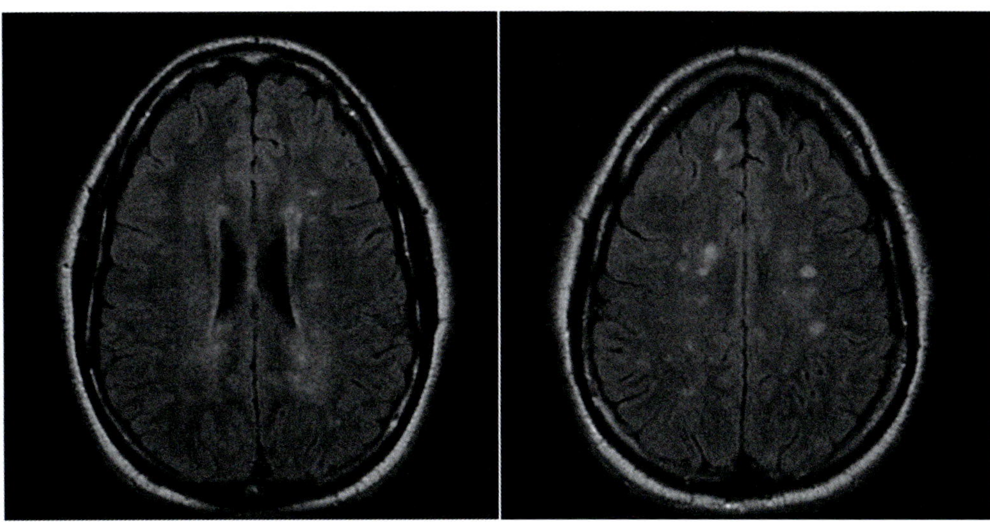

FIGURE 6-41.
(Walter Reed National Military Medical Center)

6-120. Why is this sequence depicted in Figure 6.41, most desirable for imaging pathology near the ventricles?

A. It is highly sensitive to pathology

B. Shows white and gray matter best

C. Helps differentiate pathology from CSF

D. Obviates the use of contrast media

Additional reading:

Cappelle S, Pareto D, Sunaert S, Smets I, Laenen A, Dubois B, Demaerel P. T1w/FLAIR ratio standardization as a myelin marker in MS patients. Neuroimage Clin. 2022;36:103248. doi: 10.1016/j.nicl.2022.103248. Epub 2022 Oct 25. PMID: 36451354; PMCID: PMC9668645.

6-121. Why are thin slices of coronal images important for a seizure work up?

A. Coronal allows for side to side comparison of size and shape of the hippocampus

B. Coronal is the only sequence that can see anomalies related to seizures

C. Seizure lesions are always extremely small and hard to see on axial images

D. The hippocampus is extremely small

6-122. Which section of the brain is the hippocampus located in Figure 6.42?

A. A

B. B

C. **C**

D. D

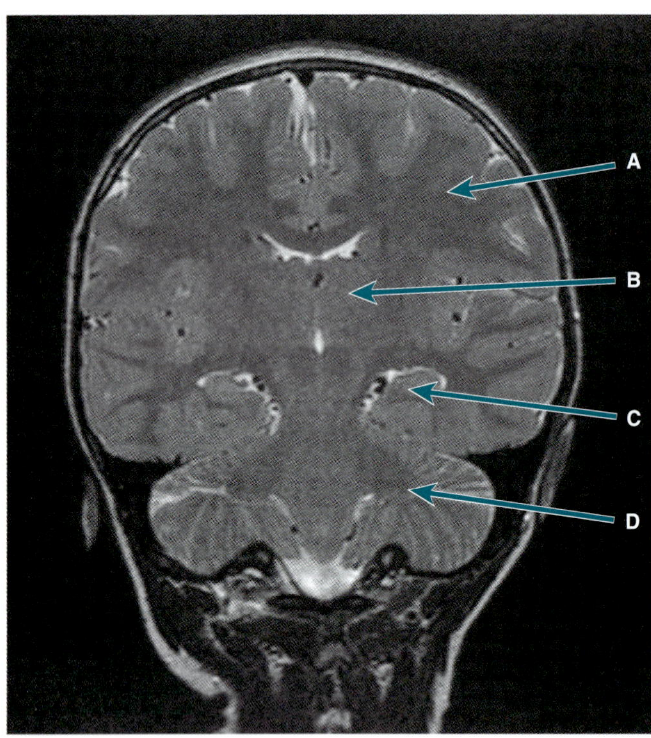

FIGURE 6-42.
(Walter Reed National Military Medical Center)

6-123. Besides coronal imaging, what other type of MR images are desired for a seizure work up?

A. 2-D whole brain axial T2 with thick slices for speed

B. **3-D high-resolution imaging**

C. Contrast MRA of the C.O.W.

D. Gradient recalled imaging looking for hemosiderin

Discussion:

Many lesions that cause seizures or epileptic symptoms can be detected using routine MRI protocols. However, smaller or subtle lesions can be missed with standard brain sequences. Therefore, an optimized seizure protocol with adequate spatial resolution, including 3-D imaging and multiplanar reformatting, is essential.

Additional reading:

Gaillard WD, Cross JH, Duncan JS, et al. Epilepsy imaging study guideline criteria: commentary on diagnostic testing study guidelines and practice parameters. Epilepsia. 2011;52(9):1750–1756.

6-124. MRI using CSF Flow is performed for what?

A. Evaluate the flow of cerebral spinal fluid

B. Hydrocephalus

C. Aqueductal stenosis

D. **All of the above**

6-125. What type of sequence is depicted in the CSF flow image in Figure 6.43?

A. 2-D time of flight

B. **2-D phase contrast**

C. 2-D susceptibility weighted imaging

D. 2-D diffusion weighted imaging

Additional reading:

Lucic MA, Koprivsek K, Kozic D, Spero M, Spirovski M, Lucic S. Dynamic magnetic resonance imaging of endoscopic third ventriculostomy patency with differently acquired fast imaging with steady-state precession sequences. Bosn J Basic Med Sci. 2014 Aug 16;14(3):165-70. doi: 10.17305/bjbms.2014.3.37. PMID: 25172977; PMCID: PMC4333999.

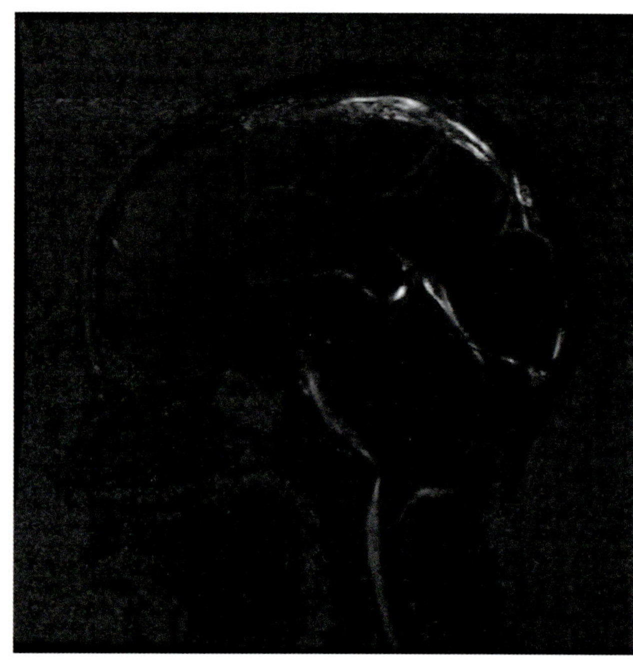

FIGURE 6-43.
(Walter Reed National Military Medical Center)

6-126. What is the age of the patient pictured in Figure 6.44?

A. Geriatric

B. Middle age

C. Pediatric

D. Bariatric

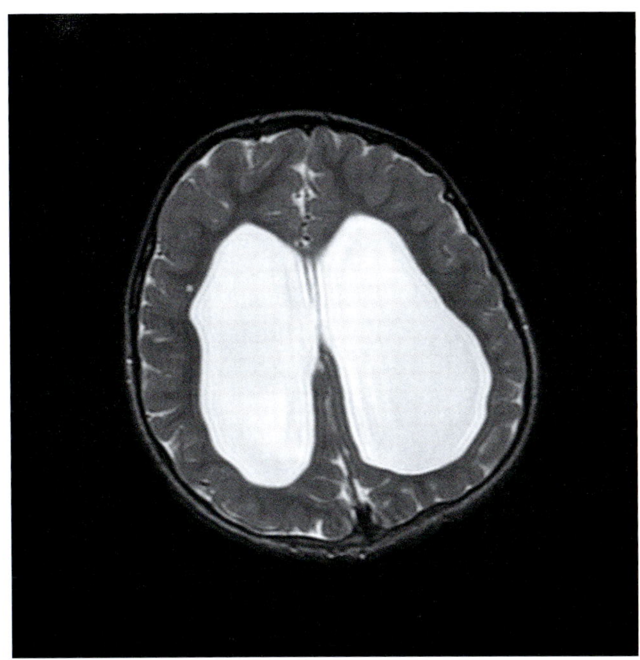

FIGURE 6-44.
(Walter Reed National Military Medical Center)

6-127. What pathology is demonstrated in Figure 6.44?

A. Bleed

B. Hydrocephalus

C. Tuberculosis

D. Brain metastasis

6-128. Identify the sequence demonstrated in Figure 6.44.

A. T1

B. FLAIR

C. Diffusion

D. T2

Additional reading:

El-Sayed Sakr, G.A., Hamisa, M.F., El Sawaf, Y.F. et al. Phase-contrast magnetic resonance imaging in evaluation of hydrocephalus in pediatric patients. *Egypt J Radiol Nucl Med* 54, 25 (2023). https://doi.org/10.1186/s43055-023-00970-w

6-129. What is the structure labeled #1 in Figure 6.45?

A. Cranial nerve IV

B. Cranial nerve V

C. Cranial nerve VI

D. Cranial nerve VII

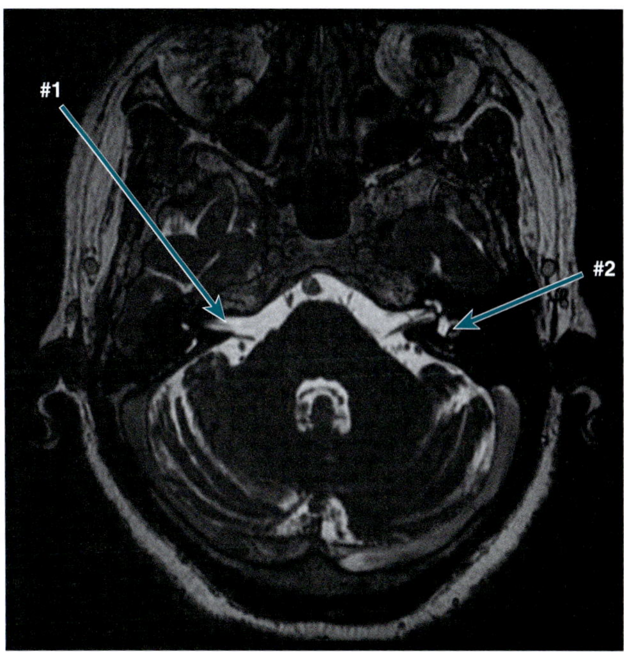

FIGURE 6-45.
(Walter Reed National Military Medical Center)

6-130. What is the structure labeled #2 in Figure 6.45?

A. Cochlea

B. Vestibule

C. Semicircular canal

D. Cranial nerve VII

6-131. The sequence in Figure 6.45 was most likely done using what slice thickness?

A. **1–2 mm**

B. 4–6 mm

C. 6–8 mm

D. 8–10 mm

Additional reading:

Benson JC, Carlson ML, Lane JI. MRI of the Internal Auditory Canal, Labyrinth, and Middle Ear: How We Do It. Radiology. 2020 Nov;297(2):252-265. doi: 10.1148/radiol.2020201767. Epub 2020 Sep 22. PMID: 32960730.

Bailey, K. Imaging the Internal Auditory Canals. https://www.youtube.com/watch?v=HbEOhqxjtiE

6-132. What is the structure labeled #1 in Figure 6.46?

A. **Pituitary gland**

B. Infundibulum

C. Cranial nerve VI

D. Optic chiasm

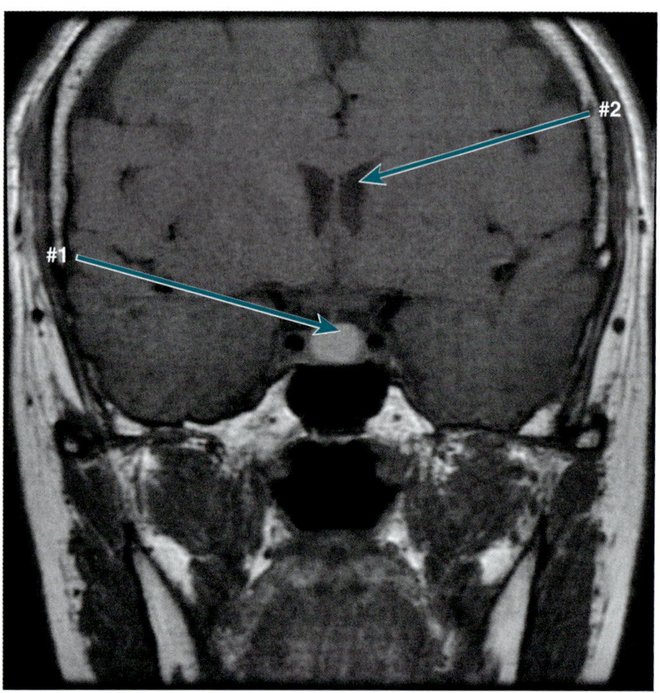

FIGURE 6-46.
(Walter Reed National Military Medical Center)

6-133. Identify the artifact present on Figure 6.46?

A. Metal artifact

B. Magnetic susceptibility artifact

C. **Motion**

D. Aliasing

6-134. What is the structure labeled #2 in Figure 6.46?

A. Central sinus

B. **Lateral ventricle**

C. 3rd ventricle

D. Left lateral recess

Additional reading:

Chapman PR, Singhal A, Gaddamanugu S, Prattipati V. Neuroimaging of the Pituitary Gland: Practical Anatomy and Pathology. Radiol Clin North Am. 2020 Nov;58(6):1115-1133. doi: 10.1016/j.rcl.2020.07.009. Epub 2020 Sep 17. PMID: 33040852.

6-135. What is the structure labeled #1 in Figure 6.47?

A. Optic chiasm

B. Pituitary gland

C. Pons

D. **Clivus**

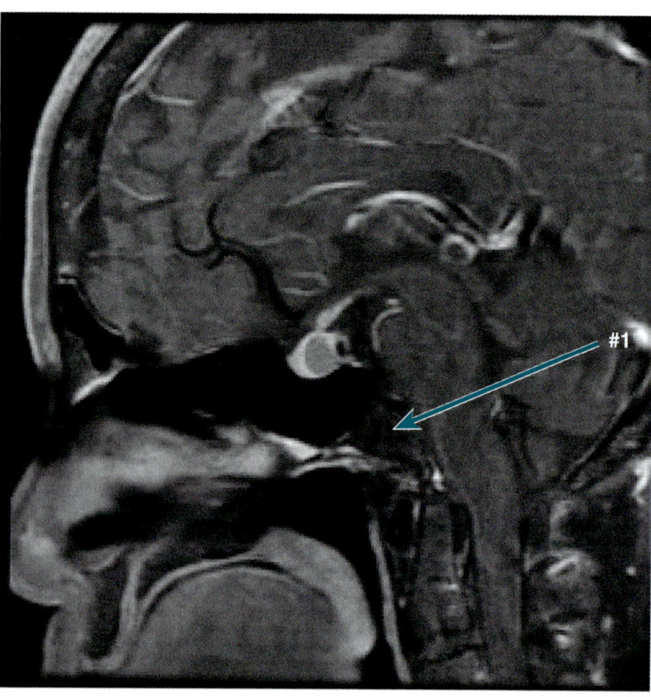

FIGURE 6-47.
(Walter Reed National Military Medical Center)

6-136. What pathology is demonstrated in Figure 6.47?

A. Pituitary mass

B. Multiple sclerosis

C. Thalamus tumor

D. Hemorrhage

6-137. What is the artifact seen through much of Figure 6.47?

A. Arterial pulsatile flow artifact

B. Venous pulsatile flow artifact

C. Gibbs artifact

D. Patient motion

Additional reading:

Evanson J. Radiology of the Pituitary. 2020 Jul 19. In: Feingold KR, Anawalt B, Blackman MR, Boyce A, Chrousos G, Corpas E, de Herder WW, Dhatariya K, Dungan K, Hofland J, Kalra S, Kaltsas G, Kapoor N, Koch C, Kopp P, Korbonits M, Kovacs CS, Kuohung W, Laferrère B, Levy M, McGee EA, McLachlan R, New M, Purnell J, Sahay R, Shah AS, Singer F, Sperling MA, Stratakis CA, Trence DL, Wilson DP, editors. Endotext [Internet]. South Dartmouth (MA): MDText.com, Inc.; 2000–. PMID: 25905384.

6-138. What is the structure labeled #1 in Figure 6.48?

A. Lateral rectus muscle

B. Medial rectus muscle

C. Optic nerve

D. Lacrimal gland

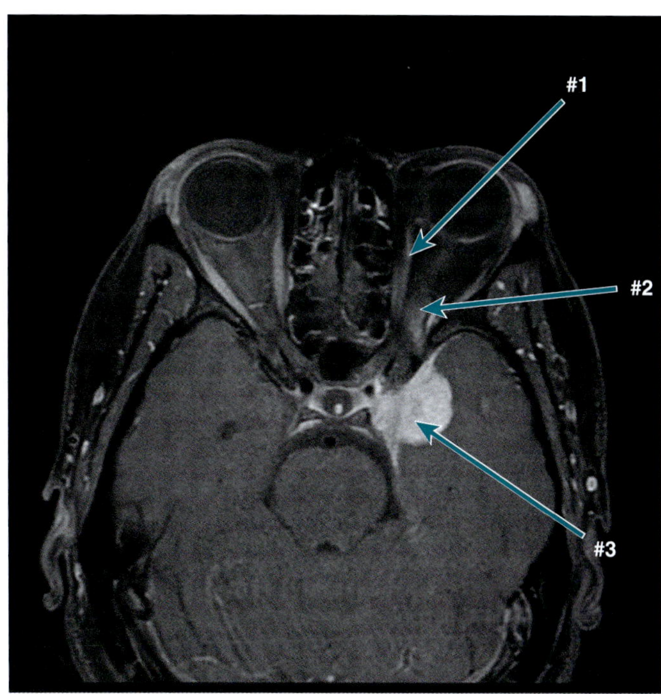

FIGURE 6-48.
(Walter Reed National Military Medical Center)

6-139. What is the structure labeled #2 in Figure 6.48?

A. Lateral rectus muscle

B. Medial rectus muscle

C. Optic nerve

D. Lacrimal gland

6-140. Identify the sequence demonstrated in Figure 6.48.

A. T1

B. FLAIR

C. Diffusion

D. T2

6-141. The mass depicted in Figure 6.48 is most likely what?

- **A.** Temporal lobe stroke
- **B.** **Cavernous sinus tumor**
- **C.** Teratoma
- **D.** AVM

Additional reading:

Nadarajah J, Madhusudhan KS, Yadav AK, Chandrashekhara SH, Kumar A, Gupta AK. MR imaging of cavernous sinus lesions: Pictorial review. J Neuroradiol. 2015 Dec;42(6):305-19. doi: 10.1016/j.neurad.2015.04.010. Epub 2015 Oct 1. PMID: 26421483.

Hoch MJ, Bruno MT, Shepherd TM. Advanced MRI of the Optic Nerve. J Neuroophthalmol. 2017 Jun;37(2):187-196. doi: 10.1097/WNO.0000000000000511. PMID: 28459736.

6-142. What is #1 pointing to in Figure 6.49?

- **A.** Sublingual gland
- **B.** **Parotid gland**
- **C.** Parathyroid gland
- **D.** Submandibular gland

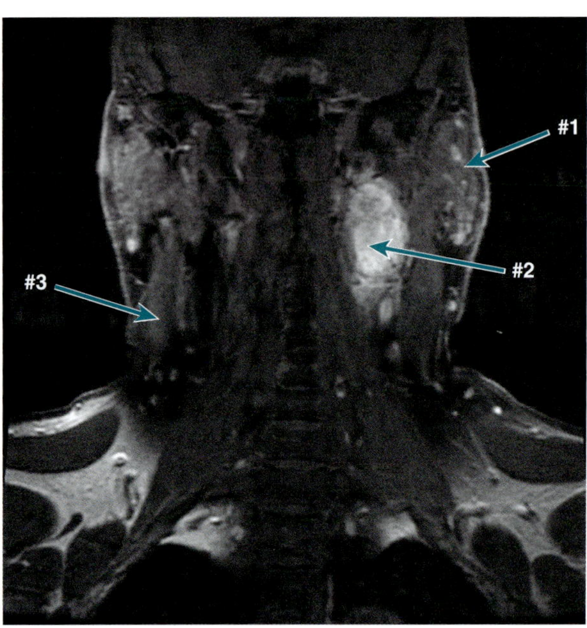

FIGURE 6-49.
(Walter Reed National Military Medical Center)

6-143. What pathology is #2 pointing to in Figure 6.49?

- **A.** Parotid tumor
- **B.** **Paraganglioma**
- **C.** Internal carotid aneurysm
- **D.** Jugular vein distention

6-144. What anatomy is #3 pointing to on Figure 6.49?

- **A.** **Sternocleidomastoid muscle**
- **B.** Semispinalis muscle
- **C.** Stylohyoid muscle
- **D.** Trapezius muscle

Discussion:

The parotid glans is the largest of the salivary glands and is located in the lateral soft tissue neck extending from the zygomatic arch to the inferior border of the mandible, and between the sternocleidomastoid muscle and the masseter muscle.

Additional reading:

http://teachmeanatomy.info/head/organs/salivary-glands/parotid/ Paraganglioma tumors grow in the sympathetic nerve cells on the peripheral nervous system and occur generally near major blood vessels.
Gökçe E. Multiparametric Magnetic Resonance Imaging for the Diagnosis and Differential Diagnosis of Parotid Gland Tumors. J Magn Reson Imaging. 2020 Jul;52(1):11-32. doi: 10.1002/jmri.27061. Epub 2020 Feb 17. PMID: 32065489.

6-145. Figure 6.50 is an image for a study done to show venous flow in what structure?

- **A.** Carotid
- **B.** Liver
- **C.** **Head**
- **D.** Kidneys

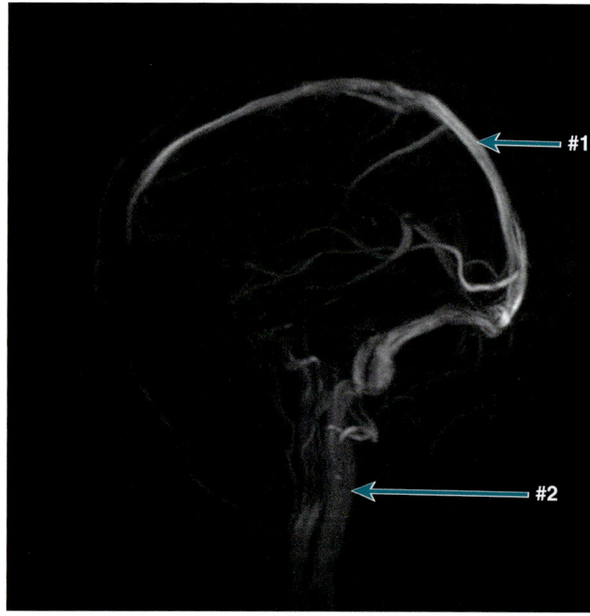

FIGURE 6-50.
(Walter Reed National Military Medical Center)

6-146. What is the structure labeled #1 in Figure 6.50?
- **A.** Sagittal sinus
- **B. Superior sagittal sinus**
- **C.** Internal jugular vein
- **D.** Straight sinus

6-147. What is the structure labeled #2 in Figure 6.50?
- **A.** Sagittal sinus
- **B.** Superior sagittal sinus
- **C. Internal jugular vein**
- **D.** Straight sinus

6-148. What type of sequence produced Figure 6.50?
- **A.** 2-D phase contrast
- **B. 2-D time of flight**
- **C.** 3-D contrast venogram
- **D.** 2-D contrast venogram

Additional reading:

Paoletti M, Germani G, De Icco R, Asteggiano C, Zamboni P, Bastianello S. Intra- and Extracranial MR Venography: Technical Notes, Clinical Application, and Imaging Development. Behav Neurol. 2016;2016:2694504. doi: 10.1155/2016/2694504. Epub 2016 May 31. PMID: 27340338; PMCID: PMC4906191.

Ho JS, Rahmat K, Ramli N, Fadzli F, Chong HT, Tan CT. Cerebral venous sinus thrombosis: Comparison of multidetector computed tomography venogram (MDCTV) and magnetic resonance venography (MRV) of various fi eld strengths. Neuroloyg Asia, 2012; 17(4): 281-291. http://neurologyasia.org/articles/neuroasia-2012-17(4)-281.pdf

6-149. What is the structure labeled #1 in Figure 6.51?
- **A.** Left common carotid artery
- **B. Right common carotid artery**
- **C.** Left vertebral artery
- **D.** Right vertebral artery

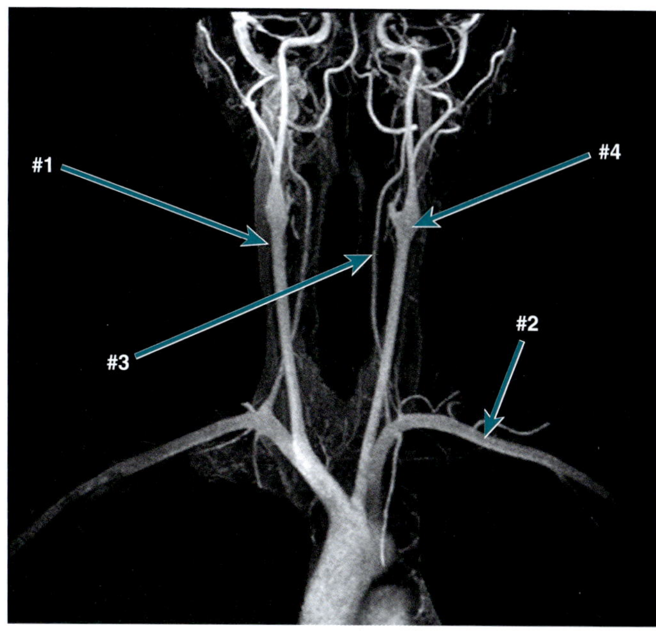

FIGURE 6-51.
(Walter Reed National Military Medical Center)

6-150. What is the structure labeled #2 in Figure 6.51?
- **A. Left subclavian artery**
- **B.** Right subclavian artery
- **C.** Right common carotid artery
- **D.** Left common carotid artery

6-151. What is the structure labeled #3 in Figure 6.51?
- **A.** Left common carotid artery
- **B.** Right common carotid artery
- **C. Left vertebral artery**
- **D.** Right vertebral artery

6-152. What is the structure labeled #4 in Figure 6.51?
- **A.** Carotid Aneurysm
- **B. Carotid Bulb**
- **C.** Vertebral Bulb
- **D.** Carotid Pseudoaneurysm

6-153. Carotid artery contrast-enhanced MRA can use which type of timing run?
- **A.** Automatic detection of bolus arrival
- **B.** Fluoroscopic detection
- **C.** Time resolved
- **D. All of the above**

6-154. MRA of the cerebral arteries in the brain is typically performed?

A. During dynamic injection of a gadolinium-based contrast agent

B. Without a contrast agent

C. With a 60-second delay after the administration of gadolinium-based contrast agent

D. With a 5-minute delay after the administration of gadolinium-based contrast agent

Additional reading:

DeMarco JK, Willinek WA, Finn JP, Huston J 3rd. Current state-of-the-art 1.5 T and 3 T extracranial carotid contrast-enhanced magnetic resonance angiography. Neuroimaging Clin N Am. 2012 May;22(2):235-57, x. doi: 10.1016/j.nic.2012.02.007. PMID: 22548930.

Thurnher SA. MRA of the carotid arteries. Eur Radiol. 2005 Dec;15 Suppl 5:E11-6. doi: 10.1007/s10406-005-0161-2. PMID: 18637226.

Kızılgöz V, Kantarcı M, Kahraman Ş. Evaluation of Circle of Willis variants using magnetic resonance angiography. Sci Rep. 2022 Oct 20;12(1):17611. doi: 10.1038/s41598-022-21833-w. PMID: 36266391; PMCID: PMC9585035.

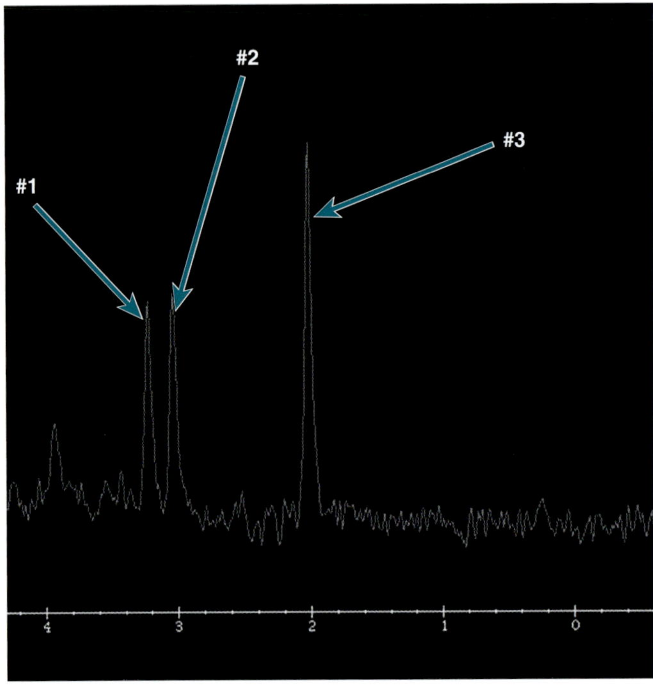

FIGURE 6-52.
(Walter Reed National Military Medical Center)

6-155. What is the peak labeled #1 in this MR Spectroscopy?

A. n-acetyl aspartate (NAA)

B. Glutamate/Glutamine

C. Choline-containing compounds (Cho)

D. Creatine/phosphocreatine (Cr)

6-156. What is the peak labeled #2 in this MR Spectroscopy?

A. n-acetyl aspartate (NAA)

B. Glutamate/Glutamine

C. Choline-containing compounds (Cho)

D. Creatine/phosphocreatine (Cr)

6-157. What is the peak labeled #3 in this MR Spectroscopy?

A. n-acetyl aspartate (NAA)

B. Glutamate/Glutamine

C. Choline-containing compounds (Cho)

D. Creatine/phosphocreatine (Cr)

6-158. MR Spectroscopy is useful at depicting brain chemistry. On most clinical scanners, what type of nuclei is being measured?

A. ^{31}P (phosphorus)

B. ^{1}H (proton)

C. ^{23}Na (sodium)

D. ^{13}C (carbon)

Discussion:

MR spectroscopy is a technique to measure metabolites. Most MR scanners today have proton spectroscopy, with the most common application being assessment of brain tumors and other brain disorders.

Additional Reading:

Oz G, Alger JR, Barker PB, et al; MRS Consensus Group. Clinical proton MR spectroscopy in central nervous system disorders. Radiology. 2014 Mar;270(3):658-79. doi: 10.1148/radiol.13130531.

Manias KA, Peet A. What is MR spectroscopy? Arch Dis Child Educ Pract Ed. 2018 Aug;103(4):213-216. doi: 10.1136/archdischild-2017-312839. Epub 2017 Aug 26. PMID: 28844055.

6-159. What is #1 pointing to in Figure 6.53?

- **A. Cerebellar tonsil**
- B. Lateral cerebellum
- C. Medial cerebellum
- D. Cerebellar floor

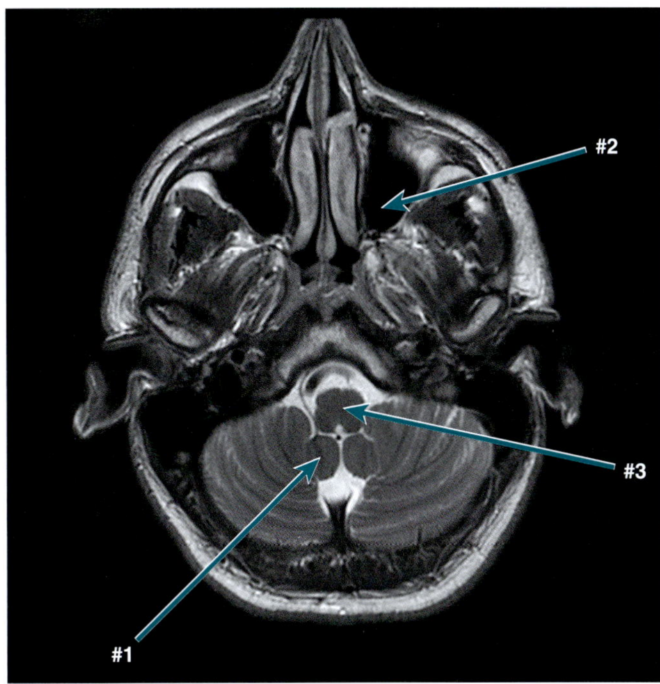

FIGURE 6-53.
(Walter Reed National Military Medical Center)

6-160. What is #2 pointing to in Figure 6.53?

- A. Ethmoid sinus
- **B. Maxillary sinus**
- C. Sagittal sinus
- D. Coronary sinus

6-161. What is #3 pointing to in Figure 6.53?

- A. Cerebral fornix
- **B. Medulla oblongata**
- C. Pons
- D. Cerebral peduncle

Additional reading:

Martin D. Neuroanatomy Text and Atlas, Fifth Edition. New York: McGraw Hill. 2021.

6-162. What is causing the hypointensity in the two round areas being pointed to by the arrow in this T2-weighted image of the midbrain in Figure 6-54?

- A. Ischemia to these areas
- B. Abnormal protein deposition
- **C. Normal iron deposition**
- D. Hemochromatosis

6-163. What is the arrow pointing to in Figure 6.54?

- **A. Red nucleus**
- B. Black nucleus
- C. Hypophysis
- D. Cerebral aqueduct

Discussion:

Red nuclei are easily seen on T2-weighted images as a pair of hypointense round structures located within the midbrain due to low its high iron content.

Additional Reading:

Telford R, Vattoth S. MR Anatomy of Deep Brain Nuclei with Special Reference to Specific Diseases and Deep Brain Stimulation Localization. *The neuroradiology journal.* 2014;27(1):29-43. doi:10.15274/NRJ-2014-10004.

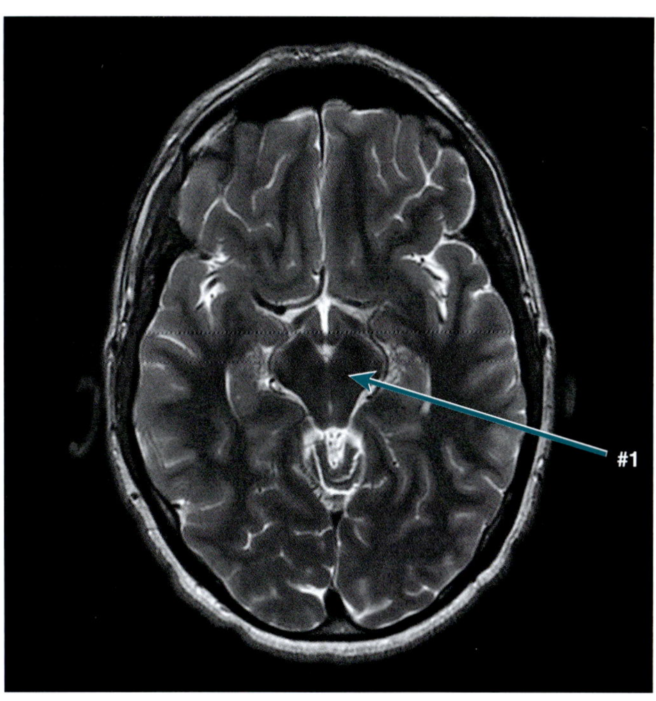

FIGURE 6-54.
(Walter Reed National Military Medical Center)

6-164. The lentiform Nucleus is depicted in the axial image and consists of:

A. Caudate nucleus and putamen

B. Amygdala and globus pallidus

C. Putamen and globus pallidus

D. Putamen and Amygdala

6-165. What structure is #1 pointing to in Figure 6.55?

A. Optic nerve

B. Caudate nucleus

C. Lateral sulcus

D. Cerebral aqueduct

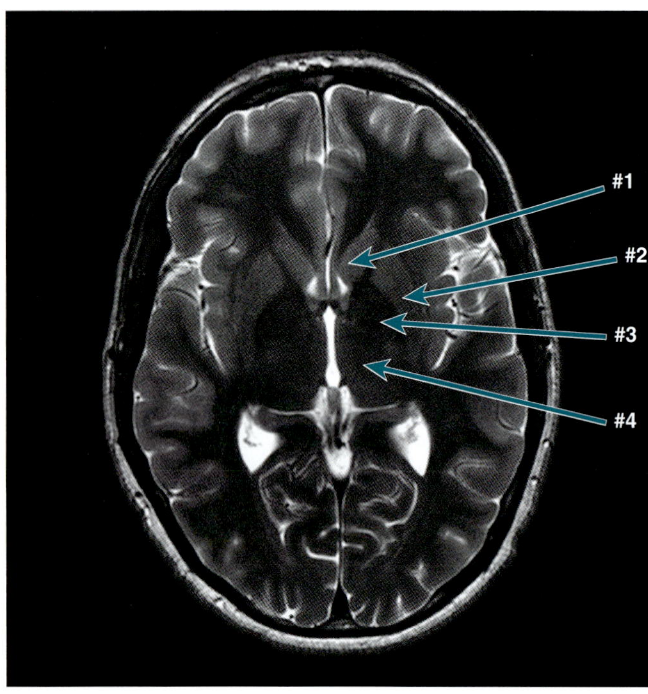

FIGURE 6-55.
(Walter Reed National Military Medical Center)

6-166. The arrows on #1 and 2 in Figure 6.55 is pointing to one of the most easily recognized structures in the deep nuclei of the brain called the Striatum. What is structure #2?

A. Putamen

B. Thalamus

C. Hypothalamus

D. Cerebellar peduncle

6-167. What structure is #3 pointing to in Figure 6.55?

A. Thalamus

B. Globus pallidus

C. Red nuclei

D. Caudate nucleus

6-168. What structure is #4 pointing to in Figure 6.55?

A. Red nuclei

B. Caudate nucleus

C. Thalamus

D. Globus pallidus

Discussion:

The striatum is made up of two easily identifiable nuclei of the deep brain, the caudate and putamen. The globus pallidus is located medial to the putamen. The globus pallidus and putamen together form the lentiform nucleus. On T2-weighted images, the globus pallidus is hypointense compared to the putamen due to iron deposition, but on T1-weighting, the globus pallidus is somewhat hyperintense due to myelination. The thalamus is T2-isointense to gray matter.

Additional Reading:

Bo WJ, Carr JJ, Krueger WA, Wolfman NT, Bowden RL. Basic Atlas of Sectional Anatomy: With Correlated Imaging, 4th Edition. WB Saunders, 2006.

Telford R, Vattoth S. MR Anatomy of Deep Brain Nuclei with Special Reference to Specific Diseases and Deep Brain Stimulation Localization. *The neuroradiology journal.* 2014;27(1):29-43.

6-169. What are the sequences in the two images on T?

A. A is T2-weighted with fat suppression, B is a T2-weighted image

B. A and B are both T2-weighted with fat suppression

C. A and B are both T1-weighted with fat suppression postcontrast injection

D. A and B are both T1-weighted with fat suppression

6-170. What is the arrow pointing to in Figure 6.56?

A. Wide foramen within normal limits

B. Postsurgical scar

C. Tumor

D. CSF

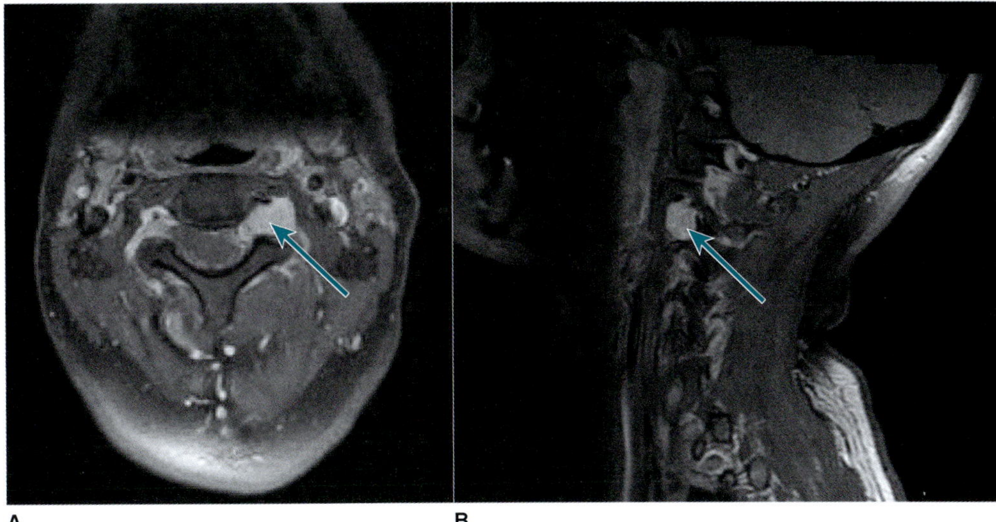

FIGURE 6-56.
(Walter Reed National Military Medical Center)

6-171. What weighting and plane is Figure 6.57?

A. Sagittal T2

B. Coronal T1

C. Axial T1

D. Sagittal T1

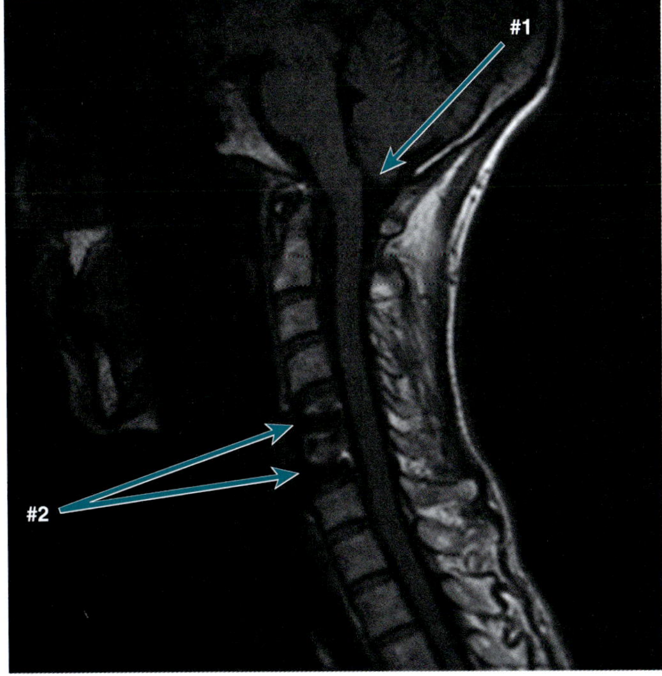

FIGURE 6-57.
(Walter Reed National Military Medical Center)

6-172. What is #1 pointing to in Figure 6.57?

A. Medulla oblongata

B. Pons

C. Cerebellar tonsil

D. Cerebellar capital

6-173. What is #2 pointing to in Figure 6.57?

A. Swallowing artifact

B. Metal artifact from surgical screws

C. Genetic abnormality

D. Gibbs artifact

Additional reading:

Hargreaves BA, Worters PW, Pauly KB, Pauly JM, Koch KM, Gold GE. Metal-induced artifacts in MRI. AJR Am J Roentgenol. 2011 Sep;197(3):547-55. doi: 10.2214/AJR.11.7364. PMID: 21862795; PMCID: PMC5562503.

6-174. This screening spine shown in Figure 6-58 is from what age group?

A. Young pediatric (<10 years of age)

B. Pediatric (12–16 years of age)

C. Adult

D. Elderly (>65 years of age)

6-175. What type of weighting is Figure 6.58?

- **A.** PD weighting
- **B. T1 weighting**
- **C.** T2 weighting
- **D.** T2* weighting

Additional reading:

Ilaslan H, Sundaram M. Pediatric and Adult MRI Atlas of Bone Marrow: Normal Appearances, Variants and Diffuse Disease States. Springer: 2016

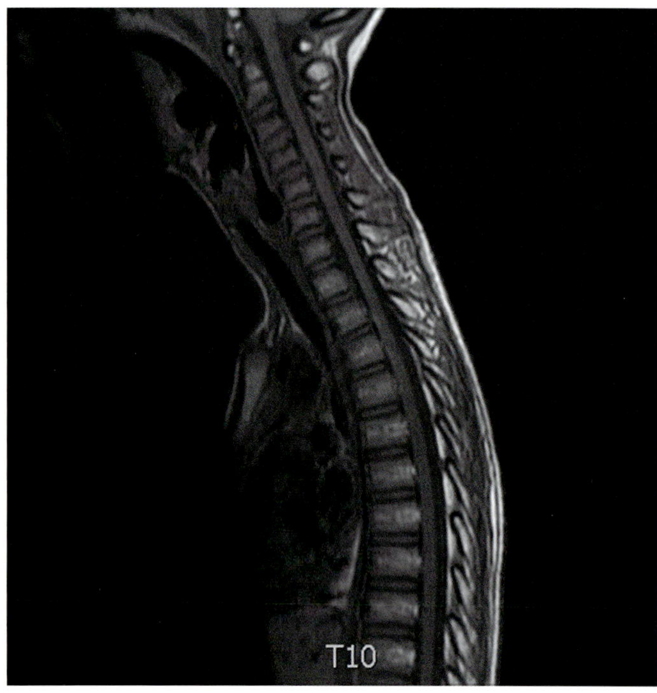

FIGURE 6-58.
(Walter Reed National Military Medical Center)

6-176. Identify the sequence demonstrated in Figure 6.59.

- **A.** T1
- **B.** FLAIR
- **C.** Diffusion
- **D. T2**

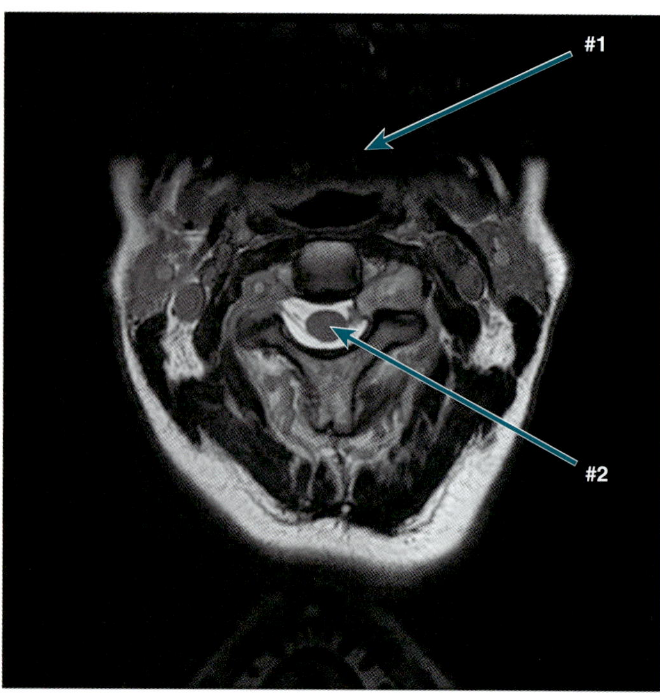

FIGURE 6-59.
(Walter Reed National Military Medical Center)

6-177. Identify the artifact labeled #1 in Figure 6.59.

- **A. Sat band**
- **B.** Metal
- **C.** Pulse band
- **D.** Dentures

6-178. What is the structure labeled #2 in Figure 6.59?

- **A.** Ligamentum flavum
- **B.** Cerebrospinal fluid
- **C.** Lamina
- **D. Spinal cord**

Additional reading:

Ozhinsky E, Vigneron DB, Nelson SJ. Improved spatial coverage for brain 3D PRESS MRSI by automatic placement of outer-volume suppression saturation bands. J Magn Reson Imaging. 2011 Apr;33(4):792-802. doi: 10.1002/jmri.22507. PMID: 21448942; PMCID: PMC3071575.

6-179. Identify the sequence demonstrated in Figure 6.60.

- **A.** T1
- **B.** FLAIR
- **C.** Diffusion
- **D. T1 with contrast**

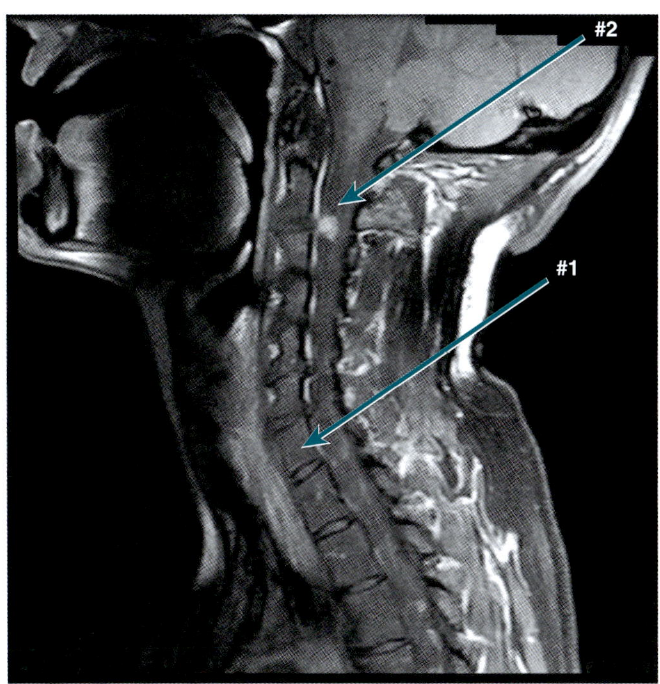

FIGURE 6-60.
(Walter Reed National Military Medical Center)

6-180. What pathology is demonstrated in Figure 6.60, #2?

A. Tumor
B. Multiple sclerosis
C. Herniated nucleus pulposis
D. Hemorrhage

6-181. What imaging plane is pictured in Figure 6.60?

A. Coronal
B. Oblique
C. Transverse
D. Sagittal

6-182. What is the structure labeled #1 in Figure 6.60?

A. Body of C7
B. Body of C5
C. Body of T1
D. Spinal cord

Additional reading:

Rossi A, Gandolfo C, Morana G, Tortori-Donati P. Tumors of the spine in children. Neuroimaging Clin N Am. 2007 Feb;17(1):17-35. doi: 10.1016/j.nic.2006.11.004. PMID: 17493537.

Fatterpekar GM. Spine Tumors: An Overview. https://www.youtube.com/watch?v=P4g8mwrLI8Q

6-183. The coil used to acquire Figure 6.61 would be:

A. Head coil
B. Head and neck coil
C. Body coil
D. Spine coil

6-184. What is the structure labeled #1 in Figure 6.61?

A. Ala; wing of sacrum
B. L sacral iliac joint
C. R sacral iliac joint
D. Sacral base

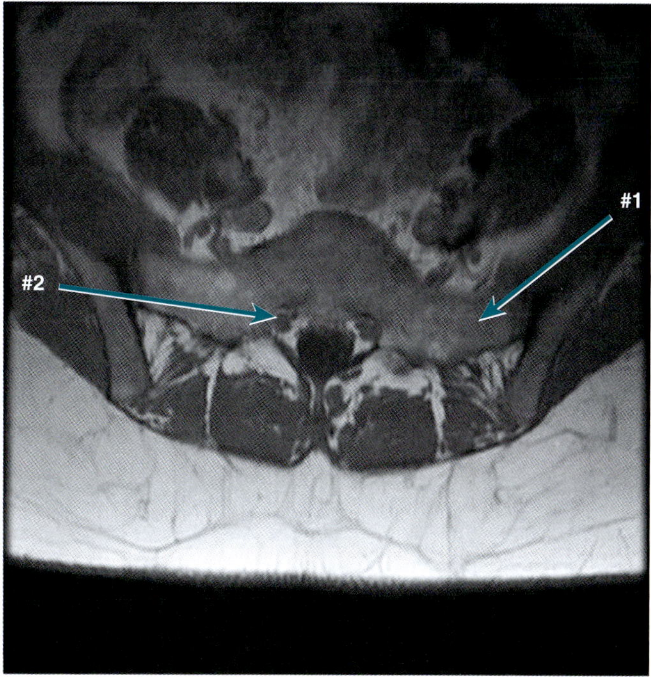

FIGURE 6-61.
(Walter Reed National Military Medical Center)

6-185. What is the structure labeled #1 in Figure 6.61?

A. Spinal cord
B. Nerve root
C. Sacral artery
D. Lumbosacral canal

Additional reading:

Roudsari B, Jarvik JG. Lumbar spine MRI for low back pain: indications and yield. AJR Am J Roentgenol. 2010 Sep;195(3):550-9. doi: 10.2214/AJR.10.4367. PMID: 20729428.

6-186. What is the abnormality in Figure 6.62?

- **A.** Syrinx
- **B.** Nerve root tumor
- **C.** Drop mets
- **D.** **Chiari I**

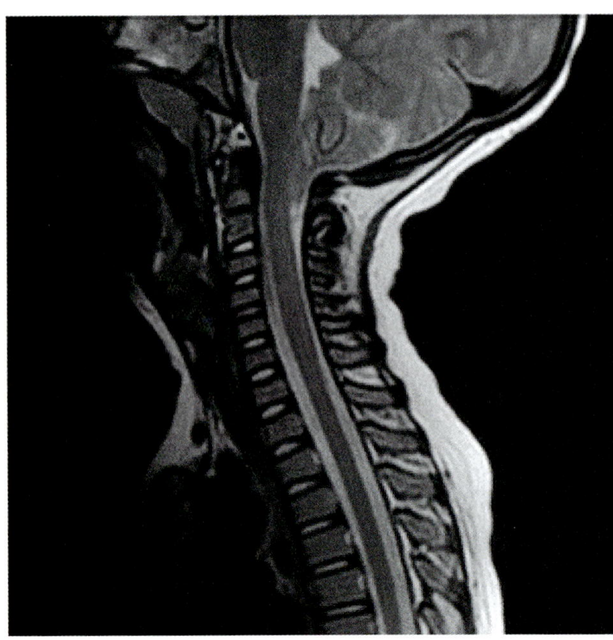

FIGURE 6-62.
(Walter Reed National Military Medical Center)

6-187. What is the sequence of Figure 6.62?

- **A.** T2 sagittal of an adult
- **B.** **T2 sagittal of a child**
- **C.** FLAIR sagittal of an adult
- **D.** Flair sagittal of a child

Discussion:

Chiari malformation is a type of hind brain anomaly that often presents with spinal cord syringohydromyelia (syrinx), intracranial hypertension, and other abnormalities. It is important to be able to see the cerebellar tonsil and how far down it extends.

Additional reading:

Rosenblum JS, Pomeraniec IJ, Heiss JD. Chiari Malformation (Update on Diagnosis and Treatment). Neurol Clin. 2022 May;40(2):297-307. doi: 10.1016/j.ncl.2021.11.007. Epub 2022 Mar 31. PMID: 35465876; PMCID: PMC9043468.

Talamonti G, Marcati E, Gribaudi G, Picano M, D'Aliberti G. Acute presentation of Chiari 1 malformation in children. Childs Nerv Syst. 2020 May;36(5):899-909. doi: 10.1007/s00381-020-04540-7. Epub 2020 Feb 13. PMID: 32055974.

6-188. What is arrow #1 pointing to in Figure 6.63 on this sagittal?

- **A.** Normal spinal cord
- **B.** **Spinal cord tumor**
- **C.** Spinal cord infarct
- **D.** Tethered cord

6-189. What are arrows #2 and 3 pointing to in Figure 6.63 on this sagittal?

- **A.** Normal spinal cord
- **B.** Multiple sclerosis plaques
- **C.** **Syrinx**
- **D.** Tethered cord

6-190. What is arrow #4 pointing to in Figure 6.63?

- **A.** Sternal body
- **B.** **Sternal manubrium**
- **C.** Sternal xiphoid
- **D.** Sternal notch

Additional reading:

Kobayashi K, Ando K, Kato F, Sato K, Kamiya M, Tsushima M, Machino M, Ota K, Morozumi M, Tanaka S, Kanbara S, Ito S, Ishiguro N, Imagama S. Variety of preoperative MRI changes in spinal cord ependymoma of WHO grade II: a case series. Eur Spine J. 2019 Feb;28(2):426-433. doi: 10.1007/s00586-018-5760-4. Epub 2018 Sep 12. PMID: 30209583.

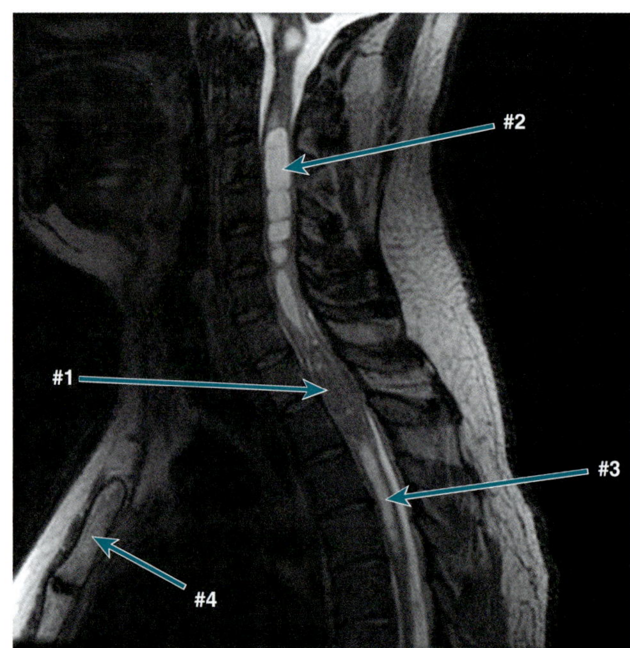

FIGURE 6-63.
(Walter Reed National Military Medical Center)

6-191. What is plane and weighting is Figure 6.64?

- **A.** Axial T1
- **B. Axial T2**
- **C.** Axial PD
- **D.** Axial T1 post contrast

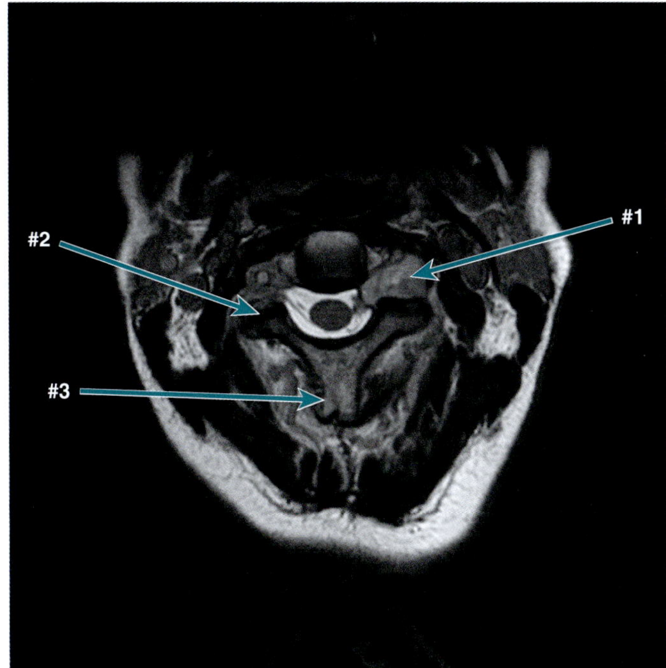

FIGURE 6-64.
(Walter Reed National Military Medical Center)

6-192. What is arrow #1 pointing to in Figure 6.64?

- **A.** Nerve root
- **B. Tumor**
- **C.** Herniated nucleus pulposus
- **D.** Hemorrhage

6-193. What is arrow #2 pointing to in Figure 6.64?

- **A.** Pedicle
- **B.** Lamina
- **C.** Spinous process
- **D. Inferior articular process or facet joint**

6-194. What is arrow #3 pointing to in Figure 6.64?

- **A.** Pedicle
- **B.** Lamina
- **C. Spinous process**
- **D.** Inferior articular process or facet joint

Additional reading:

Jain N, Verma R, Garga UC, Baruah BP, Jain SK, Bhaskar SN. CT and MR imaging of odontoid abnormalities: A pictorial review. Indian J Radiol Imaging. 2016 Jan-Mar;26(1):108-19. doi: 10.4103/0971-3026.178358. PMID: 27081234; PMCID: PMC4813060. "https://www.ncbi.nlm.nih.gov/pmc/articles/PMC4813060/" CT and MR imaging of odontoid abnormalities: A pictorial review - PMC (nih.gov)

6-195. Arrow #1 point to what in Figure 6-65?

- **A.** Conus terminalis
- **B. Intradural extramedullary hypointense mass**
- **C.** Degenerative conus
- **D.** Infection of the conus medullaris

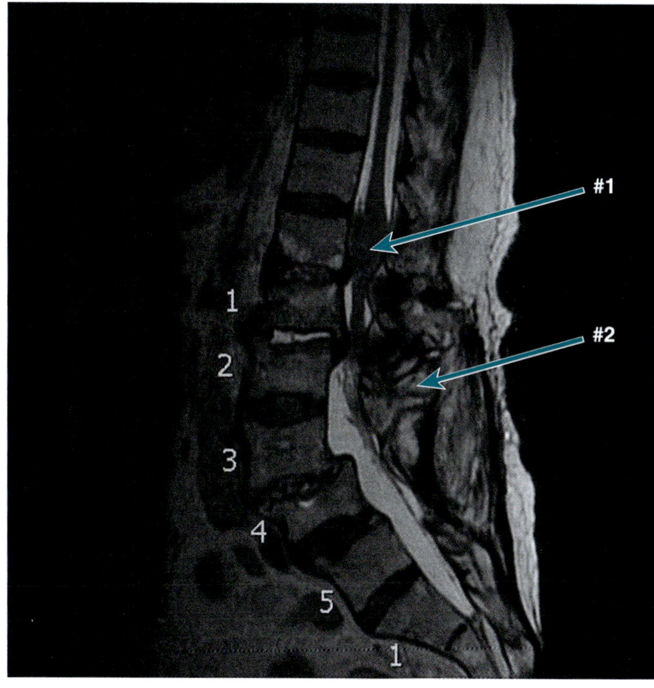

FIGURE 6-65.
(Walter Reed National Military Medical Center)

6-196. What has most likely caused the anatomic changes in the general area of arrow #2 in Figure 6.65?

- **A.** Trauma
- **B. Surgery**
- **C.** Degenerative changes
- **D.** Normal anatomy

6-197. What is the most likely happening in the area between L1 and L2 in Figure 6.65?

A. Degenerative changes

B. Disc injection

C. Cancerous bone

D. Slipped disc

Additional reading:

Herrera Herrera I, Moreno de la Presa R, González Gutiérrez R, Bárcena Ruiz E, García Benassi JM. Evaluation of the postoperative lumbar spine. Radiologia. 2013 Jan-Feb;55(1):12-23. English, Spanish. doi: 10.1016/j.rx.2011.12.004. Epub 2012 Apr 19. PMID: 22520556.

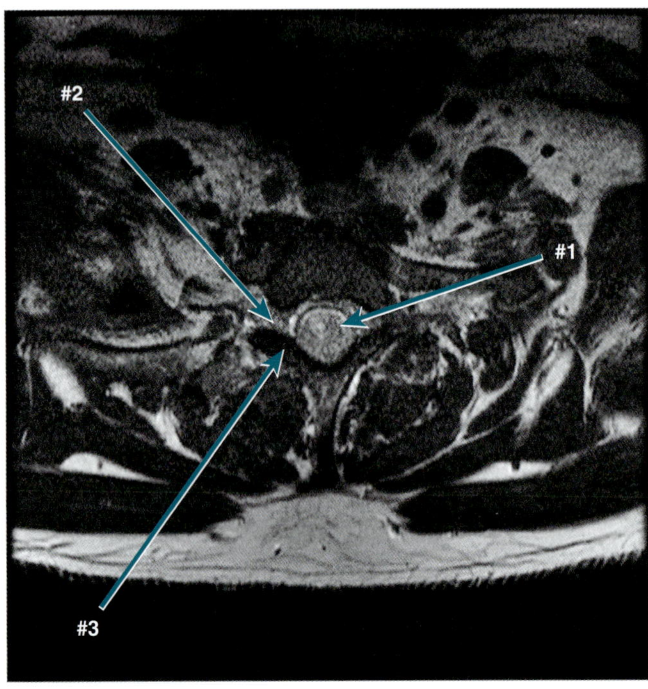

FIGURE 6-66.
(Walter Reed National Military Medical Center)

6-198. What is arrow #1 pointing to in Figure 6.66?

A. Normal spinal cord

B. Spinal cord tumor

C. Spinal cord infarct

D. Tethered cord

6-199. What is arrow #2 pointing to in Figure 6.66?

A. Foramen

B. Intervertebral disc

C. Spinous process

D. Lamina

6-200. What is arrow #3 pointing to in Figure 6.66?

A. Foramen

B. Intervertebral disc

C. Spinous process

D. Lamina

Discussion:

When imaging the spinal cord, pay attention to abnormal signal in the cord.

Additional reading:

N'da H, Dauleac C, Toquart A, Afathi M, Meyronet D, Barrey C. Thoracic spine intra- and extradural dumbbell-shaped meningioma: Case report and extensive review of the literature with 21 cases. Neurochirurgie. 2018 Jun;64(3):206-210. doi: 10.1016/j.neuchi.2018.03.001. Epub 2018 May 3. PMID: 29730052.

Samartzis D, Gillis CC, Shih P, O'Toole JE, Fessler RG. Intramedullary Spinal Cord Tumors: Part I-Epidemiology, Pathophysiology, and Diagnosis. Global Spine J. 2015 Oct;5(5):425-35. doi: 10.1055/s-0035-1549029.

6-201. What is the artifact in Figure 6.67?

A. Air caused by severe disc disease

B. Metal artifact from orthopedic screws

C. Flow artifact from abdominal aorta

D. Machine artifact

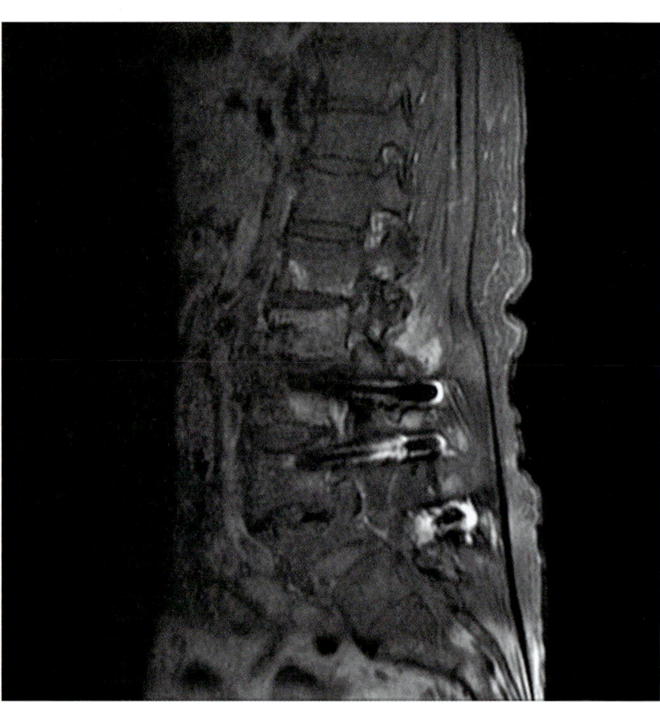

FIGURE 6-67.
(Walter Reed National Military Medical Center)

6-202. What is the artifact that can mimic a syrinx down the length of a spinal cord?

A. Ghosting artifact

B. Truncation artifact

C. Motion artifact

D. Swallowing artifact

Discussion:

A band of low or high signal intensity can occur along the length of tissue along the phase encoding direction when the number of phase encodings is too low. This can be confused with a number of pathologic entities such as dilated central canal or syrinx. This occurs in areas that have abrupt tissue signal changes such as between CSF and a spinal cord.

Additional reading:

Taber KH, Herrick RC, Weathers SW, Kumar AJ, Schomer DF, Hayman LA. Pitfalls and artifacts encountered in clinical MR imaging of the spine. Radiographics. 1998 Nov-Dec;18(6):1499-521.

6-203. Identify the sequence demonstrated in A and B in Figure 6.68.

A. T1

B. T1 fat sat with contrast

C. Diffusion

D. T2

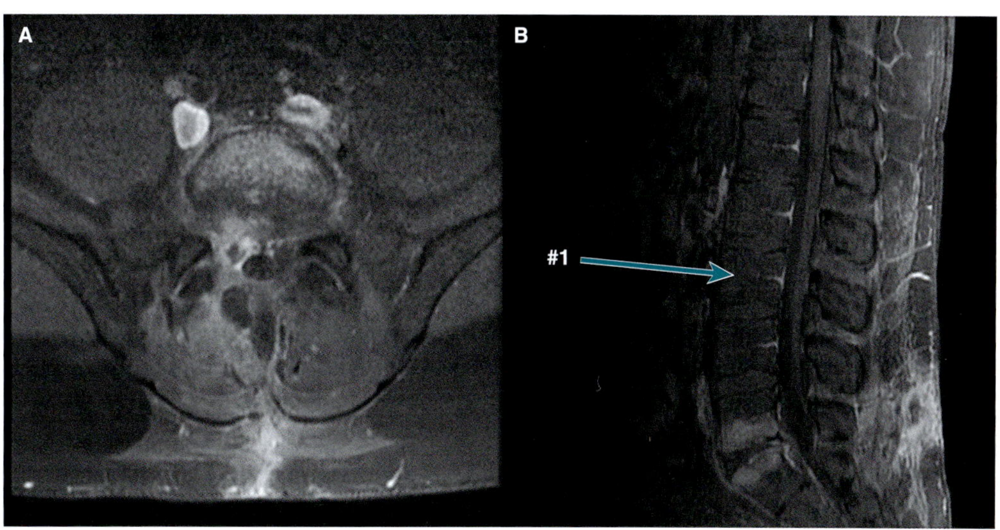

FIGURE 6-68.
(Walter Reed National Military Medical Center)

6-204. What pathology is demonstrated in #L1 and #L2 in Figure 6.68?

A. Discitis/osteomyelitis

B. Herniated nucleus pulposus

C. Compression fracture

D. Postsurgical hemorrhage

6-205. What plane is image L1 in Figure 6.68?

A. Sagittal

B. Axial

C. Coronal

D. Oblique reconstruction

6-206. What is the structure labeled #1 in Figure 6.68?

A. Body of T12

B. Body of L2

C. Body of L3

D. Body of L4

Additional reading:

Zimmerli W. Clinical practice. Vertebral osteomyelitis. N Engl J Med. 2010 Mar 18;362(11):1022-9. doi: 10.1056/NEJMcp0910753. PMID: 20237348.

6-207. What is the structure labeled #1 in Figure 6.69?

A. Intervertebral disc

B. Body of L3

C. Tumor

D. Infection

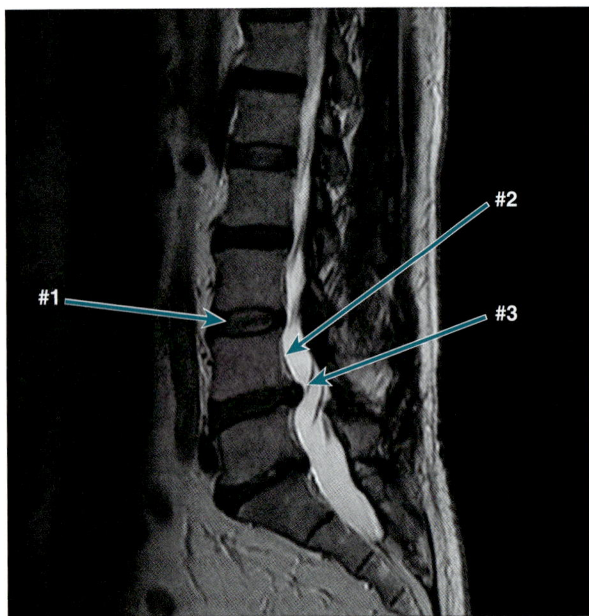

FIGURE 6-69.
(Walter Reed National Military Medical Center)

6-208. What structure (the dark line) is #2 pointing at in Figure 6.69?

A. Spinal sac

B. Posterior longitudinal ligament

C. Longitudinal tendon

D. Neural sac

6-209. What is #3 pointing at in Figure 6.69?

A. Ruptured nucleus pulposus

B. Herniated nucleus pulposus

C. Large osteophyte

D. Spondylolisthesis

Additional reading:

Smithuis R. Lumbar Disc Herniation and other causes of nerve compression. https://radiologyassistant.nl/neuroradiology/spine/lumbar-disc-herniation

Aryal V, Jimenez A. Anatomy, Back, Posterior Longitudinal Ligament. [Updated 2022 Jul 25]. In: StatPearls [Internet]. Treasure Island (FL): StatPearls Publishing; 2023 Jan. Available from: https://www.ncbi.nlm.nih.gov/books/NBK560691/

6-210. What is the structure labeled #1 in Figure 6.70?

A. Superior vena cava

B. Inferior vena cava

C. Abdominal aorta

D. Femoral artery

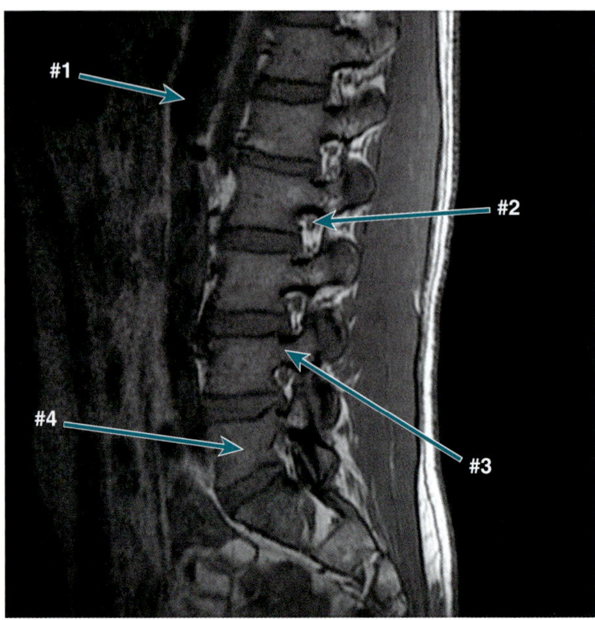

FIGURE 6-70.
(Walter Reed National Military Medical Center)

6-211. What is the structure labeled #2 in Figure 6.70?

A. Chemical shift artifact

B. Loose body

C. Aliasing artifact from CSF flow

D. Nerve root

6-212. What is the structure labeled #3 in Figure 6.70?

A. Pedicle

B. Body

C. Intervertebral disc

D. Lamina

6-213. What is the structure labeled #4 in Figure 6.70?

A. Pedicle

B. Body

C. Intervertebral disc

D. Lamina

Additional reading:

Khanna AJ. MRI Essentials for the Spine Specialist. Thieme Medical Publishers, Inc.: New York. 2014

6-214. Match the structures in Figure 6.71.

A. Ilium_____3_____

B. Ala of sacrum_____2_____

C. Psoas major muscle_____1_____

D. Multifidus muscle_____4_____

Additional reading:

Fortin M, Macedo LG. Multifidus and paraspinal muscle group cross-sectional areas of patients with low back pain and control patients: a systematic review with a focus on blinding. Phys Ther. 2013 Jul;93(7):873-88. doi: 10.2522/ptj.20120457.

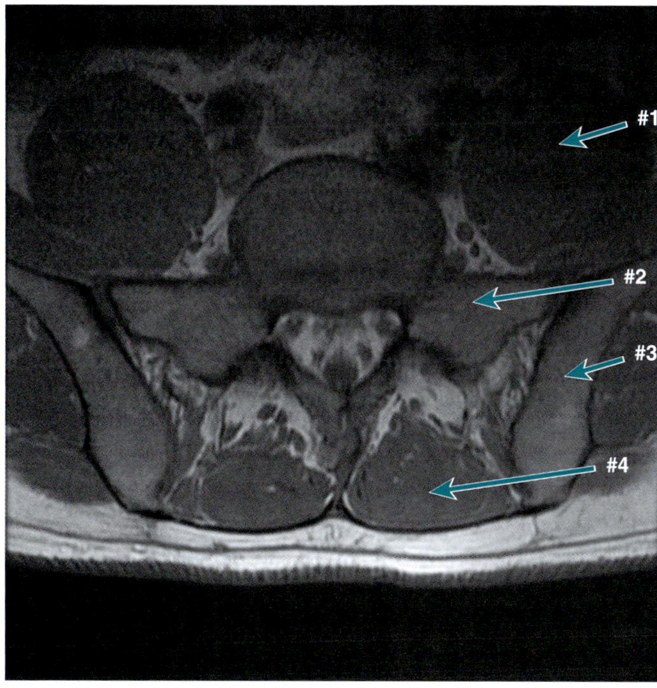

FIGURE 6-71.
(Walter Reed National Military Medical Center)

6-215. What is the structure labeled #1 in Figure 6.72?

A. Normal lumbar disc

B. Lumbar disc protrusion

C. Enlarged nerve root

D. Compression fracture

6-216. What is the structure labeled #2 in Figure 6.72?

A. Disc fragments

B. CSF pulsation artifacts

C. Nerve root

D. Cauda equina

6-217. What is the structure labeled #3 in Figure 6.72?

A. Disc fragment

B. Nerve root

C. Lamina

D. Lateral spinous process

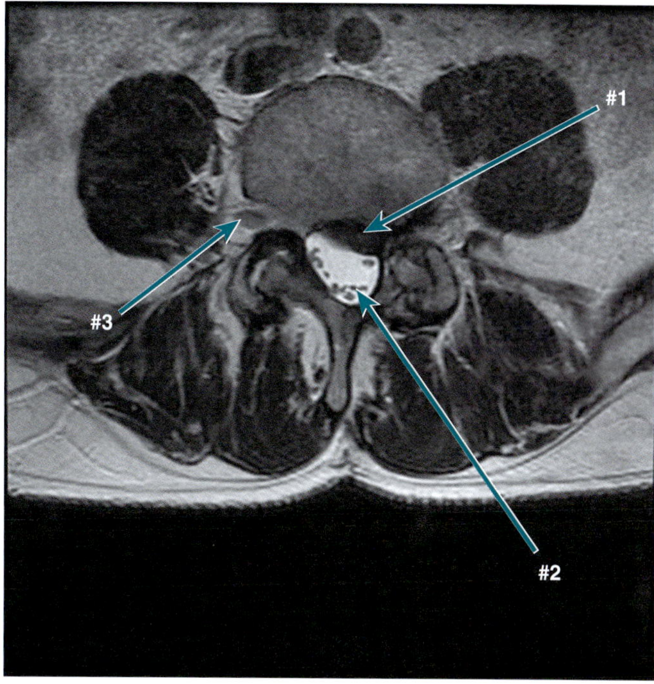

FIGURE 6-72.
(Walter Reed National Military Medical Center)

6-218. What is the pathology most likely doing in Figure 6.72?

A. Buffering the thecal sac from damage

B. Pressing upon the left intervertebral nerve root

C. Pressing upon the spinal cord

D. Pressing on the posterior spinal process

Additional reading:

http://casemed.case.edu/clerkships/neurology/Web%20Neurorad/MRI_Spine/nl%20ls%20anatomy.htm

Roudsari B, Jarvik JG. Lumbar spine MRI for low back pain: indications and yield. AJR Am J Roentgenol. 2010 Sep;195(3):550-9. doi: 10.2214/AJR.10.4367

6-219. What is the structure labeled #1 in Figure 6.73?

A. Esophagus

B. Inferior vena cava

C. Aorta

D. Femoral artery

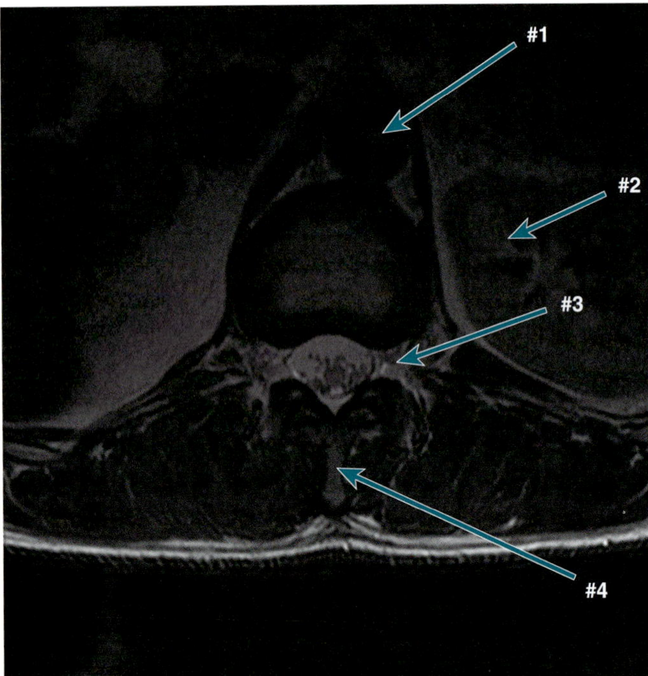

FIGURE 6-73.
(Walter Reed National Military Medical Center)

6-220. What is the structure labeled #2 in Figure 6.73?

A. Spleen

B. Kidney

C. Stomach

D. Bowel

6-221. What is the structure labeled #3 in Figure 6.73?

A. Lateral foramen

B. Lateral artery

C. Cauda equina

D. Lamina

6-222. What is the structure labeled #4 in Figure 6.73?

A. Spinous process

B. Body

C. Cauda equina

D. Lamina

Additional reading:

Khanna AJ. MRI Essentials for the Spine Specialist. Thieme Medical Publishers, Inc.: New York. 2014

6-223. What is the weighting, plane, and age group of Figure 6.74?

A. Sagittal T2, pediatric

B. Sagittal T1, adult

C. Sagittal SWI, pediatric

D. Sagittal T2, adult

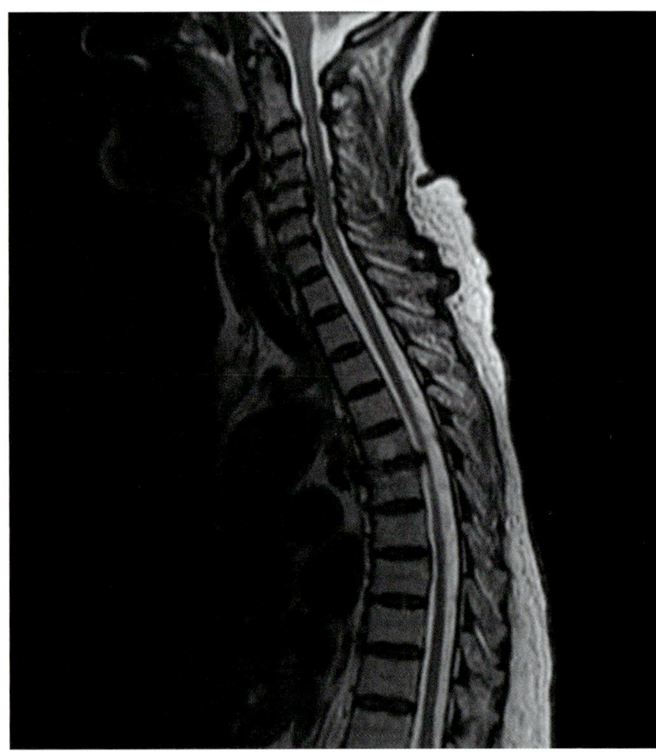

FIGURE 6-74.
(Walter Reed National Military Medical Center)

6-224. What coil was most likely used to acquire this image in figure 6-74?

A. Cervical spine surface coil

B. C, T, L, or spine surface coil

C. Body coil

D. Cardiac surface coil

6-225. What is the age range of the person in Figure 6.75?

A. Neonate (0–1 years of age)
B. Pediatric (2–16 years of age)
C. Adult (18–50 years of age)
D. Elderly (>65 years of age)

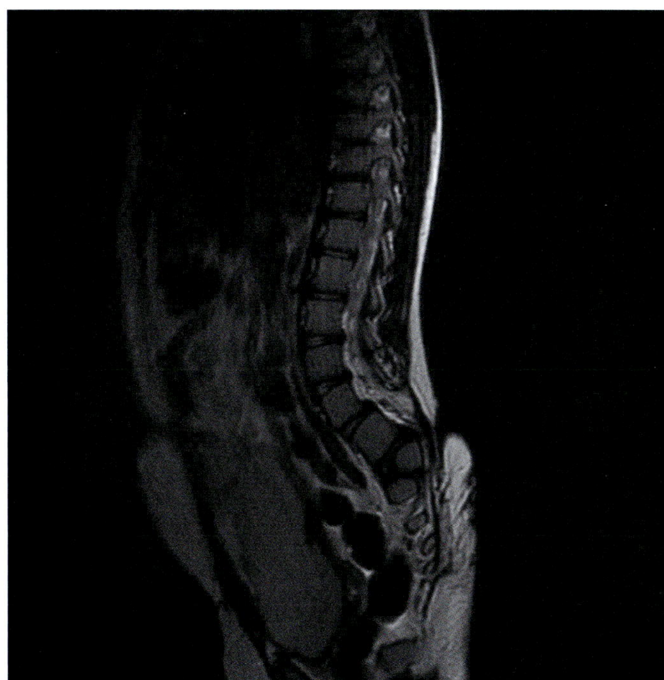

FIGURE 6-75.
(Walter Reed National Military Medical Center)

6-226. What is the abnormality most likely in this image in Figure 6-75?

A. Postsurgical repair of myelomeningocele
B. Postsurgical repair of lumbosacral fracture
C. Postsurgical repair of congenital scoliosis
D. Postsurgical repair of simple neural tube deformity

Discussion:

Congenital abnormalities of the spine and spinal cord are referred to as myelomeningoceles, the most serious form of spina bifida. These children may also have other problems such as hydrocephalus, syringomyelia, tethered cord, problems with movement, lack of sensation, and bowel and bladder problems.

Additional reading:

Kumar J, Afsal M, Garg A. Imaging spectrum of spinal dysraphism on magnetic resonance: A pictorial review. World J Radiol. 2017;9(4):178-190.

6-227. What is the structure labeled #1 in Figure 6.76?

A. Spinal canal
B. Sacral canal
C. Spinal fistula
D. Spinal foramen sacrum

6-228. What is the structure labeled #2 in Figure 6.76?

A. Sacrum
B. Coccyx
C. Ilium
D. Ischium

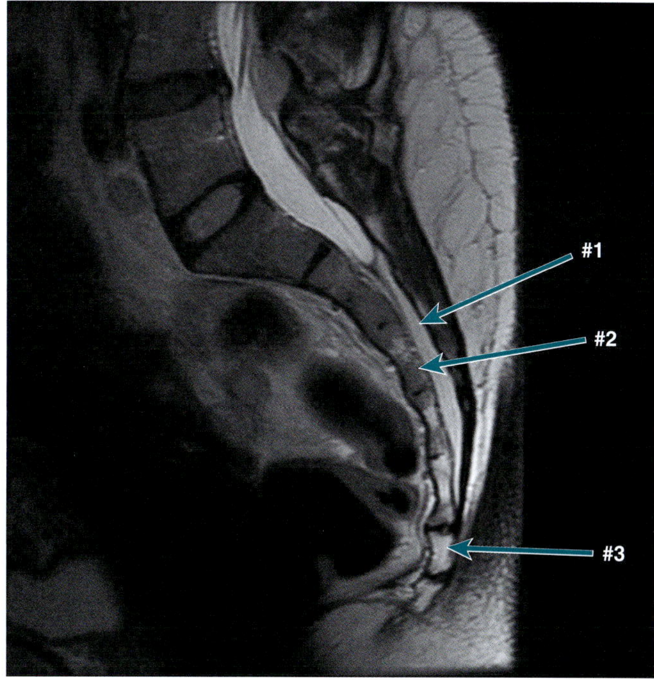

FIGURE 6-76.
(Walter Reed National Military Medical Center)

6-229. What is the structure labeled #3 in Figure 6.76?

A. Sacrum
B. Coccyx
C. Ilium
D. Ischium

6-230. What is the dark band angled across the anterior portion of the Figure 6.76?

A. Gas in the rectum
B. Saturation band
C. Contrast in the bladder
D. Motion artifact from the bowel

MSK Section

6-231. Match the anatomy on Figure 6-77:

A. Mandibular Condyle_____5_____

B. Articular Disc_____3_____

C. Articular Fossa_____2_____

D. External acoustic meatus_____4_____

E. Mandibular ramus_____1_____

6-232. The arrows points to what on these open and closed TMJ images (Figure 6.78)?

A. Anterior displacement of disc

B. Posterior displacement of disc

C. Normal movement of disc

D. Abnormal displacement of the mandibular condyle

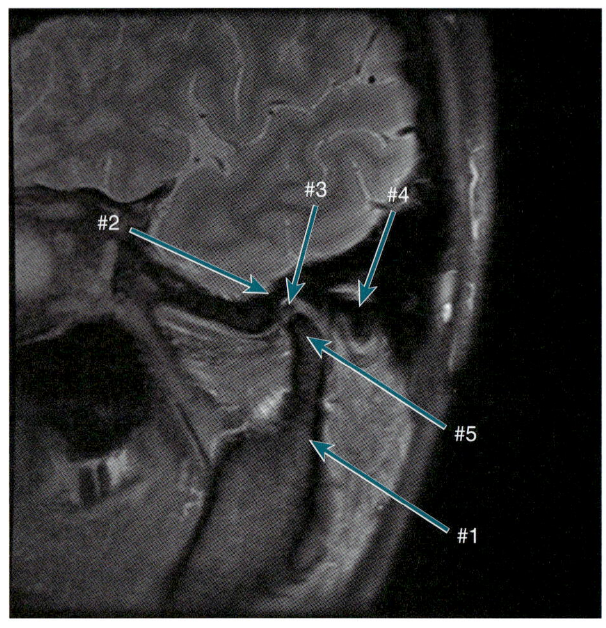

FIGURE 6-77.
(Walter Reed National Military Medical Center)

6-233. What is this imaging plane being shown on these open and closed TMJ images (Figure 6.78)?

A. Oblique sagittal

B. Oblique coronal

C. Oblique axial

D. Orthogonal axial

Additional reading:

Behzadi F, Mandell JC, Smith SE, Guenette JP. Temporomandibular joint imaging: current clinical applications, biochemical comparison with the intervertebral disc and knee meniscus, and opportunities for advancement. Skeletal Radiol. 2020 Aug;49(8):1183-1193. doi: 10.1007/s00256-020-03412-0. Epub 2020 Mar 11. PMID: 32162049.

Tomas X, Pomes J, Berenguer J, Quinto L, Nicolau C, Mercader JM, Castro V. MR imaging of temporomandibular joint dysfunction: a pictorial review. Radiographics. 2006 May-Jun;26(3):765-81.

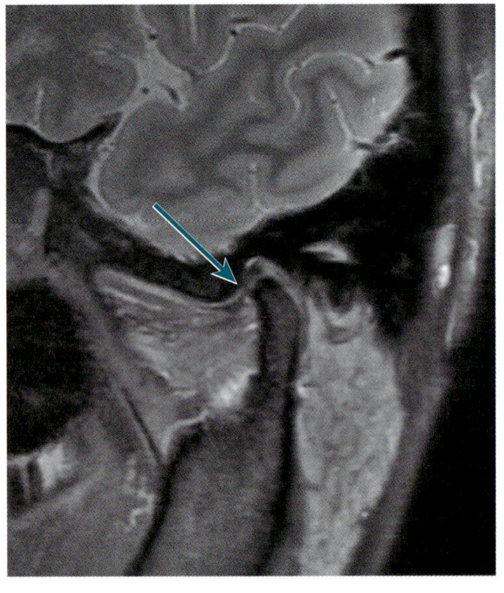

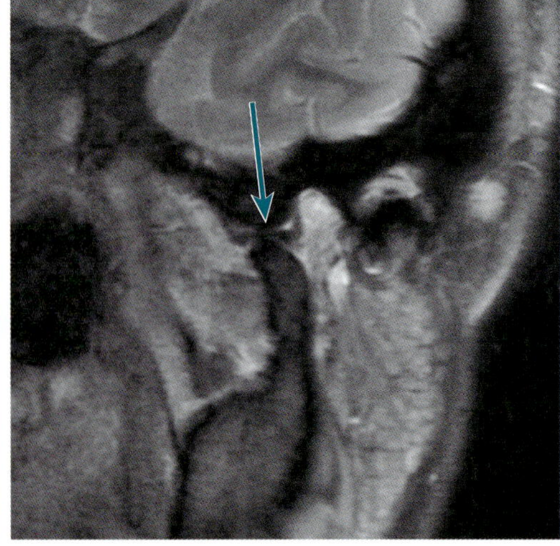

FIGURE 6-78.
(Walter Reed National Military Medical Center)

6-234. Figure 6.79 anatomy of the shoulder. #1 points to what?

- **A. Supraspinatus tendon**
- B. Trapezius muscle
- C. Biceps tendon
- D. Teres minor tendon

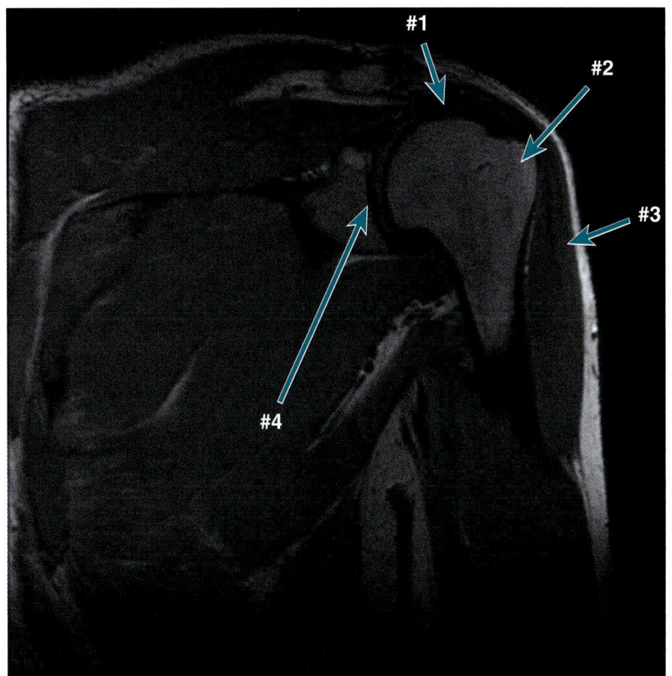

FIGURE 6-79.
(Walter Reed National Military Medical Center)

6-235. Figure 6.79 anatomy of the shoulder. #2 points to what?

- A. Acromion
- **B. Greater tuberosity**
- C. Clavicle
- D. Glenoid

6-236. Figure 6.79 anatomy of the shoulder. #3 points to what?

- A. Trapezius muscle
- B. Biceps muscle
- **C. Deltoid muscle**
- D. Triceps muscle

6-237. Figure 6.79 anatomy of the shoulder. #4 points to what?

- A. Acromion
- B. Clavicle
- C. Greater tuberosity
- **D. Glenoid**

6-238. Figure 6.80 anatomy of the shoulder. #1 points to what?

- A. Infraspinatus tendon
- **B. Supraspinatus tendon**
- C. Trapezius muscle
- D. Biceps tendon

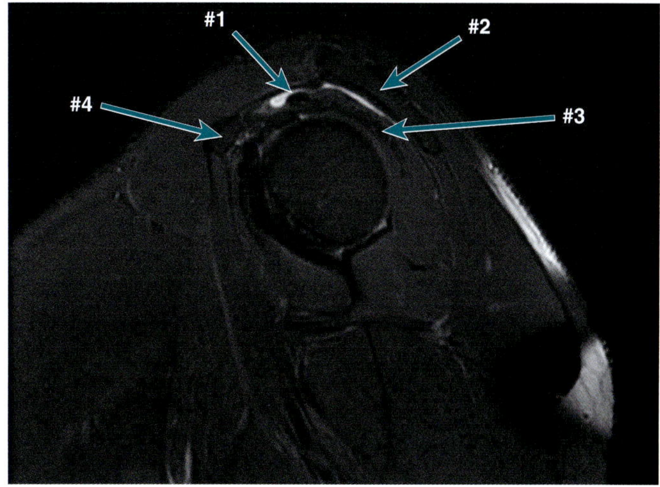

FIGURE 6-80.
(Walter Reed National Military Medical Center)

6-239. Figure 6.80 anatomy of the shoulder. #2 points to what?

- A. Trapezius muscle
- B. Glenoid
- **C. Acromion**
- D. Coracoid process

6-240. Figure 6.80 anatomy of the shoulder. #3 points to what?

- **A. Infraspinatus tendon**
- B. Supraspinatus tendon
- C. Trapezius muscle
- D. Biceps tendon

6-241. Figure 6.80 anatomy of the shoulder. #4 points to what?

A. Trapezius muscle

B. Glenoid

C. Acromion

D. **Coracoid process**

6-242. Figure 6.80 is depicting what plane in the shoulder?

A. **Sagittal**

B. Coronal

C. Axial

D. Planar

Additional reading:

Cook TS, Stein JM, Simonson S, Kim W. Normal and variant anatomy of the shoulder on MRI. Magn Reson Imaging Clin N Am. 2011 Aug;19(3):581-94. doi: 10.1016/j.mric.2011.05.005. PMID: 21816332.

Petchprapa CN, Beltran LS, Jazrawi LM, Kwon YW, Babb JS, Recht MP. The rotator interval: a review of anatomy, function, and normal and abnormal MRI appearance. AJR Am J Roentgenol. 2010 Sep;195(3):567-76. doi: 10.2214/AJR.10.4406. PMID: 20729432.

6-243. The arrow is pointing to what abnormality in Figure 6.81?

A. Annular ligament tear

B. Triceps brachii ligament tear

C. **Biceps brachii ligament tear**

D. Ulnar collateral ligament tear

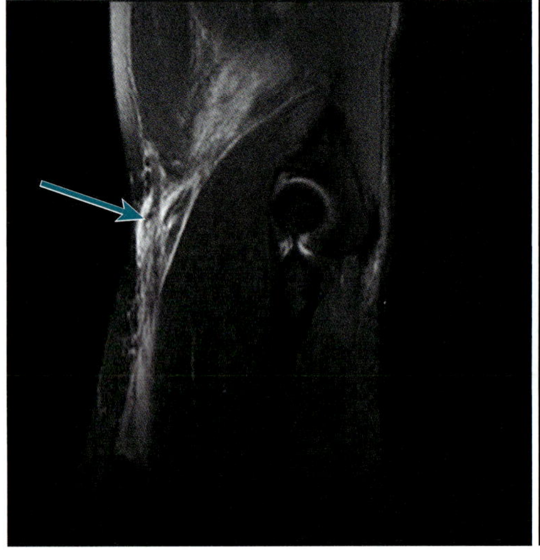

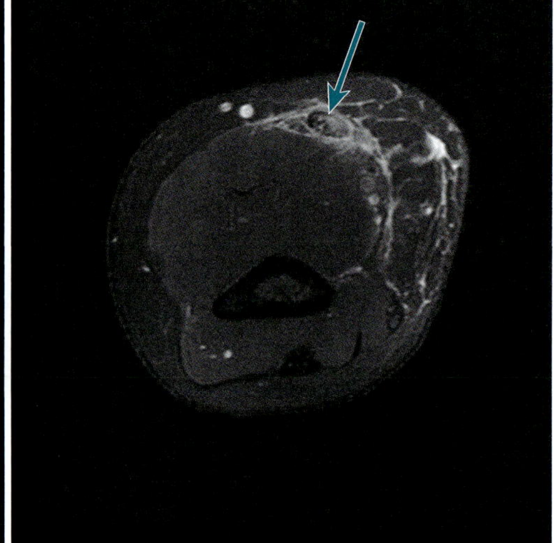

FIGURE 6-81.
(Walter Reed National Military Medical Center)

6-244. Figure 6.82 anatomy of the elbow. #1 points to what?

A. Trapezius muscle

B. **Biceps brachii muscle**

C. Triceps muscle

D. Brachioradialis muscle

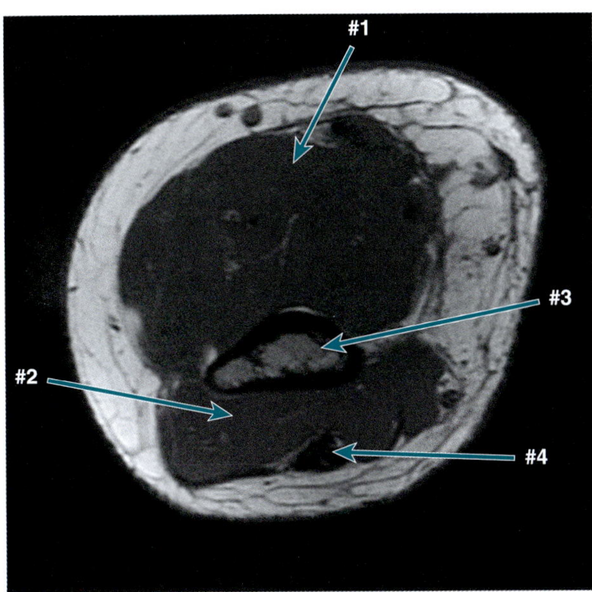

FIGURE 6-82.
(Walter Reed National Military Medical Center)

6-245. Figure 6.82 anatomy of the elbow. #2 points to what?

- **A.** Trapezius muscle
- **B.** Biceps brachii muscle
- **C. Triceps muscle**
- **D.** Brachioradialis muscle

6-246. Figure 6.82 anatomy of the elbow. #3 points to what?

- **A. Humerus**
- **B.** Radius
- **C.** Ulna
- **D.** Fibula

6-247. Figure 6.82 anatomy of the elbow. #4 points to what?

- **A. Triceps tendon**
- **B.** Trapezius tendon
- **C.** Biceps brachii tendon
- **D.** Brachioradialis tendon

Additional reading:

Binaghi D. MR Imaging of the Elbow. Magn Reson Imaging Clin N Am. 2015 Aug;23(3):427-40. doi: 10.1016/j.mric.2015.04.005.

Hauptfleisch J, English C, Murphy D. Elbow magnetic resonance imaging: imaging anatomy and evaluation. Top Magn Reson Imaging. 2015 Apr;24(2):93-107. doi: 10.1097/RMR.0000000000000047. PMID: 25835585.

6-248. Figure 6.83 is depicting what plane?

- **A.** Sagittal
- **B. Coronal**
- **C.** Axial
- **D.** Planar

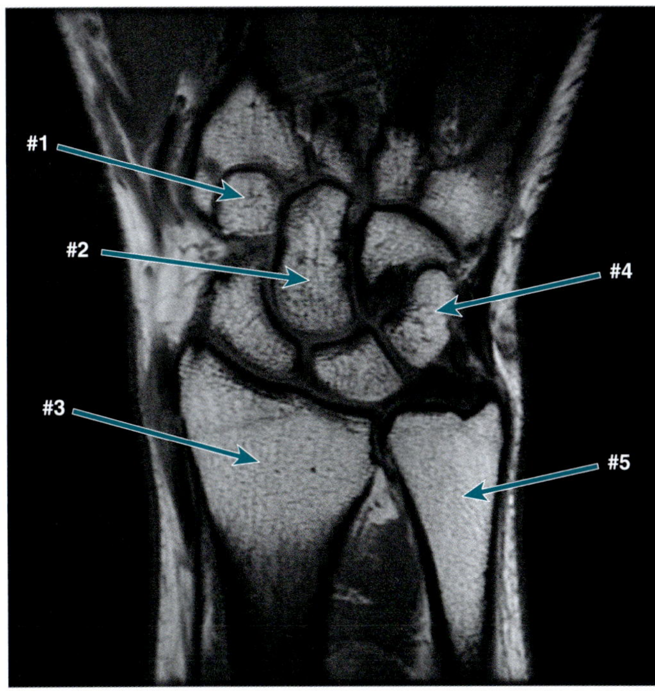

FIGURE 6-83.
(Walter Reed National Military Medical Center)

6-249. Identify Figure 6.83 anatomy.

- **A.** Hamate_____2_____
- **B.** Radius_____3_____
- **C.** Ulna_____5_____
- **D.** Trapezoid_____1_____
- **E.** Triquetrum_____4_____

6-250. Figure 6.84 anatomy of the wrist. #1 points to what?

- **A. Extensor digitorum tendons**
- B. Flexor digitorum tendons
- C. Extensor carpi radialis longus tendon
- D. Ulnar artery and nerve

6-251. Figure 6.84 anatomy of the wrist. #2 points to what?

- A. Extensor digitorum tendons
- **B. Flexor digitorum tendons**
- C. Extensor carpi radialis longus tendon
- D. Ulnar artery and nerve

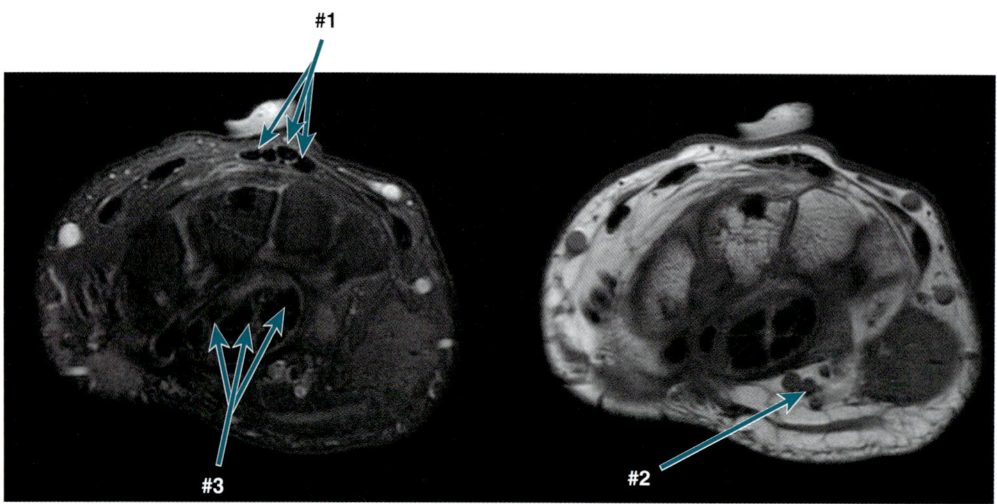

FIGURE 6-84.
(Walter Reed National Military Medical Center)

6-252. Figure 6.84 anatomy of the wrist. #3 points to what?

- A. Extensor digitorum tendons
- B. Flexor digitorum tendons
- C. Extensor carpi radialis longus tendon
- **D. Ulnar artery and nerve**

Additional reading:

Stein JM, Cook TS, Simonson S, Kim W. Normal and variant anatomy of the wrist and hand on MR imaging. Magn Reson Imaging Clin N Am. 2011 Aug;19(3):595-608; ix. doi: 10.1016/j.mric.2011.05.007. PMID: 21816333.

Meraj S, Gyftopoulos S, Nellans K, Walz D, Brown MS. MRI of the Extensor Tendons of the Wrist. AJR Am J Roentgenol. 2017 Nov;209(5):1093-1102. doi: 10.2214/AJR.17.17791. Epub 2017 Aug 31. PMID: 28858545.

6-253. Name the structure labeled by #1 in Figure 6.85.

- **A.** Middle interphalangeal joint
- **B. Interphalangeal joint**
- **C.** Distal phalange
- **D.** Proximal phalange

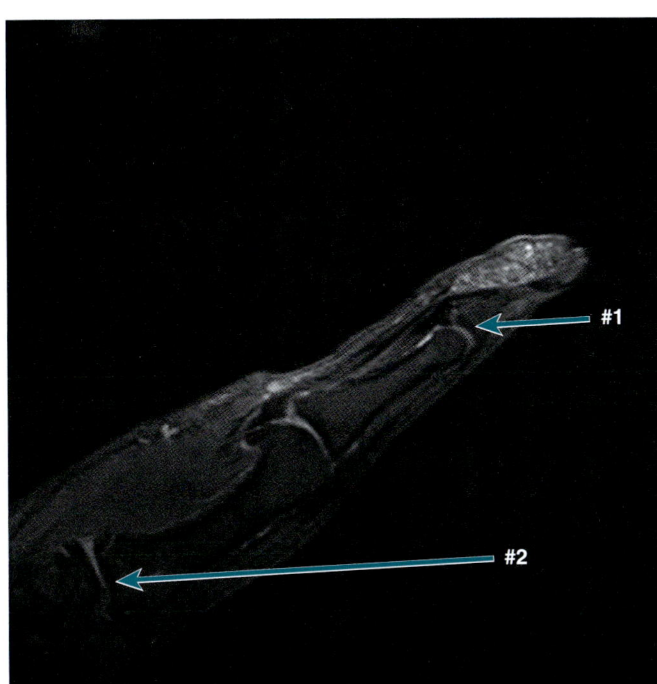

FIGURE 6-85.
(Walter Reed National Military Medical Center)

6-254. Name the structure labeled by #2 in Figure 6.85.

- **A. Carpometacarpal joint**
- **B.** Metacarpophalangeal joint
- **C.** Interphalangeal joint
- **D.** Distal interphalangeal joint

6-255. Identify the sequence demonstrated in Figure 6.85.

- **A.** T1
- **B.** T1 postcontrast
- **C. STIR**
- **D.** T2

6-256. Name the structure pointed to be the yellow arrow in Figure 6.86.

- **A.** Bone spur
- **B. Sesamoid bone**
- **C.** Distal tuberosity phalange
- **D.** Proximal tuberosity phalange

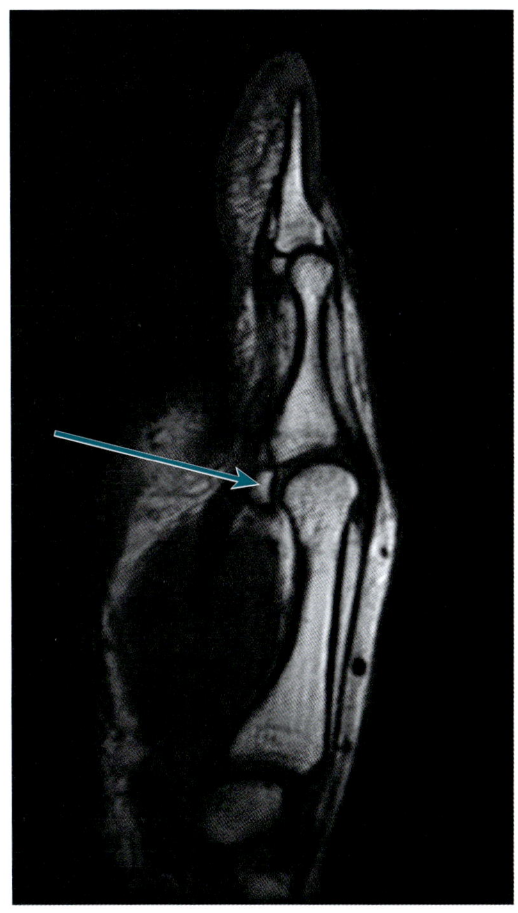

FIGURE 6-86.
(Walter Reed National Military Medical Center)

6-257. What is important about imaging the coronal view of the thumb?

A. Coronal should be coronal in respect to the hand not the thumb

B. Need coronals to be coronal when the hand is not also being imaged

C. Coronal should be coronal in respect to the thumb not the hand

D. Need coronals only when the hand images cut off anatomy

Additional reading:

Hirschmann A, Sutter R, Schweizer A, Pfirrmann CW. MRI of the thumb: anatomy and spectrum of findings in asymptomatic volunteers. AJR Am J Roentgenol. 2014 Apr;202(4):819-27. doi: 10.2214/AJR.13.11397. PMID: 24660712.

Stein JM, Cook TS, Simonson S, Kim W. Normal and variant anatomy of the wrist and hand on MR imaging. Magn Reson Imaging Clin N Am. 2011 Aug;19(3):595-608; ix. doi: 10.1016/j.mric.2011.05.007. PMID: 21816333.

6-258. Axial Hip, arrow #1 points to the area of what in Figure 6.87?

A. Acetabular ligament

B. Ligament of head of femur

C. Ligament of the base of the pelvis

D. Hip ligament

6-259. Axial Hip, arrow #2 points to what in Figure 6.87?

A. Spine of the ischium

B. Spine of the pubis

C. Ischial tuberosity

D. Iliac tuberosity

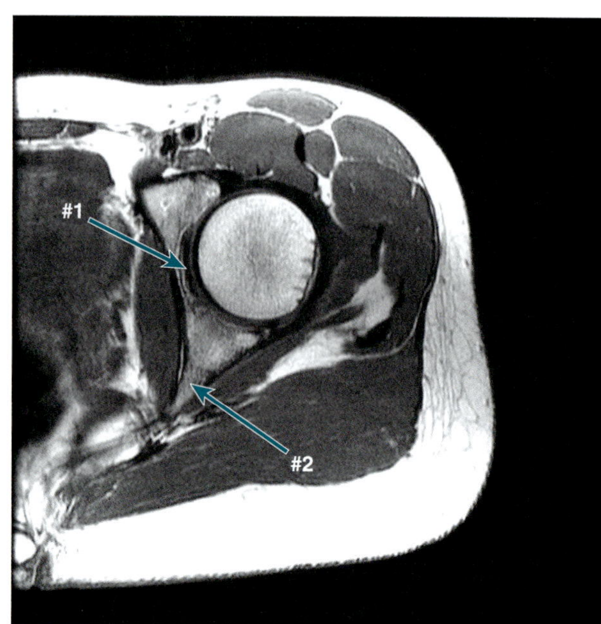

FIGURE 6-87.
(Walter Reed National Military Medical Center)

6-260. Hip MRI is best positioned:

A. Patient supine, pillow under head and knees for comfort, center about 4 inches below iliac crest

B. Patient supine, pillow under head and knees for comfort, center about 4 inches below umbilicus

C. Patient supine, legs flat, feet secured parallel with straps and pad, pillow under head for comfort, center about 4 inches below iliac crest

D. Patient supine, legs flat, pillow under head for comfort, center about 4 inches above iliac crest

6-261. What is the arrow pointing to in the images shown in Figure 6.88?

A. Excessive synovial fluid in the left hip

B. Dilute gadolinium contrast injection into the left hip

C. Edema from a torn ligament

D. Infection of the left hip

Additional reading:

Osinski T, Malfair D, Steinbach L. Magnetic resonance arthrography. Orthop Clin North Am. 2006 Jul;37(3):299-319, vi. doi: 10.1016/j.ocl.2006.04.002. PMID: 16846763.

Jose J. MRI Anatomy of the hip. https://www.youtube.com/watch?v=Fm8VnKRdNL4

Mak MS, Teh J. Magnetic resonance imaging of the hip: anatomy and pathology. Pol J Radiol. 2020 Sep 4;85:e489-e508. doi: 10.5114/pjr.2020.99414. PMID: 33101554; PMCID: PMC7571513.

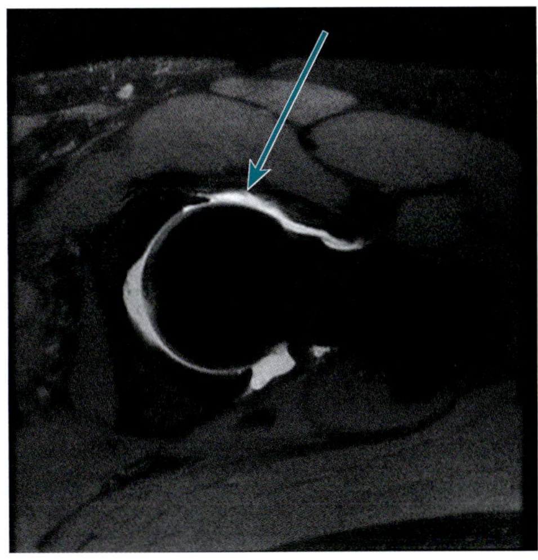

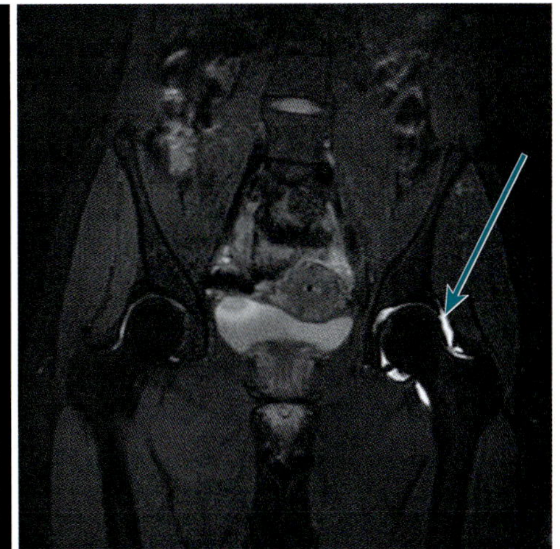

FIGURE 6-88.
(Walter Reed National Military Medical Center)

6-262. What is the arrow pointing to in the images shown in Figure 6.89?

A. Excessive synovial fluid in the left hip

B. Dilute gadolinium contrast injection into the left hip

C. Edema from a torn ligament

D. Infection of the left hip

Additional reading:

Mitchell DG, Rao V, Dalinka M, Spritzer CE, Gefter WB, Axel L, Steinberg M, Kressel HY. MRI of joint fluid in the normal and ischemic hip. AJR Am J Roentgenol. 1986 Jun;146(6):1215-8. doi: 10.2214/ajr.146.6.1215. PMID: 3486565.

Annabell L, Master V, Rhodes A, Moreira B, Coetzee C, Tran P. Hip pathology: the diagnostic accuracy of magnetic resonance imaging. J Orthop Surg Res. 2018 May 29;13(1):127. doi: 10.1186/s13018-018-0832-z. PMID: 29843749; PMCID: PMC5975565.

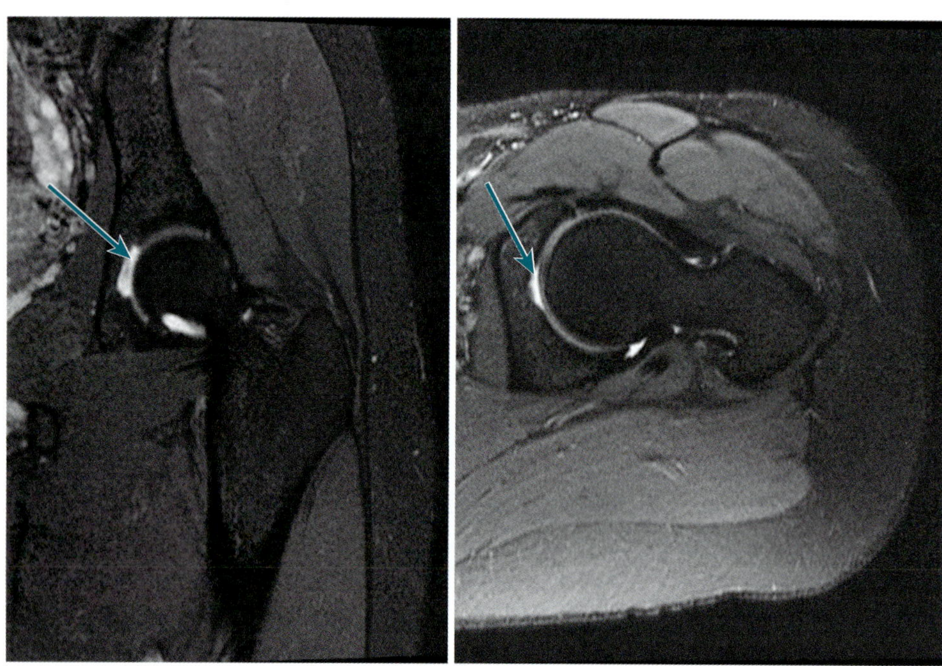

FIGURE 6-89.
(Walter Reed National Military Medical Center)

6-263. Match the anatomy pointed to in Figure 6.90.

A. Achilles tendon_____4_____

B. Peroneus Tendon_____3_____

C. Flexor Digitorum Longus Tendon_____1_____

D. Tibialis Posterior Tendon_____2_____

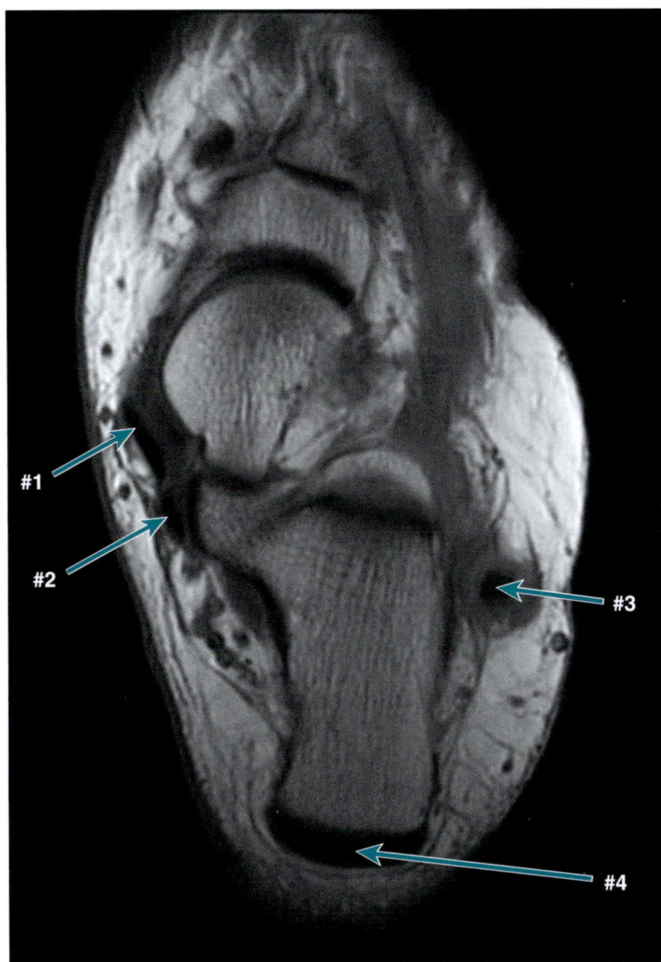

FIGURE 6-90.
(Walter Reed National Military Medical Center)

6-264. The best position for an Ankle MRI is

A. Place in coil and immobilize foot plantarflexed so the dorsal aspect of foot is in a roughly 90-degree angle to the leg

B. Place in coil and immobilize foot dorsiflexed so the dorsal aspect of foot is in a roughly 90-degree angle to the leg

C. Place in coil and immobilize foot in a comfortable position to minimize motion

D. Place in coil and immobilize foot rolled in eversion to minimize motion

6-265. When imaging the entire Achilles tendon, you must include:

A. From bottom of foot to just above lateral malleolus

B. From bottom of foot to just above medial malleolus

C. From bottom of foot to distal gastrocnemius muscle

D. From bottom of foot to distal soleus muscle

6-266. Name the anatomy pointed to in #1 in Figure 6.91.

A. Calcaneus

B. Talus

C. Navicular

D. Medial cuneiform

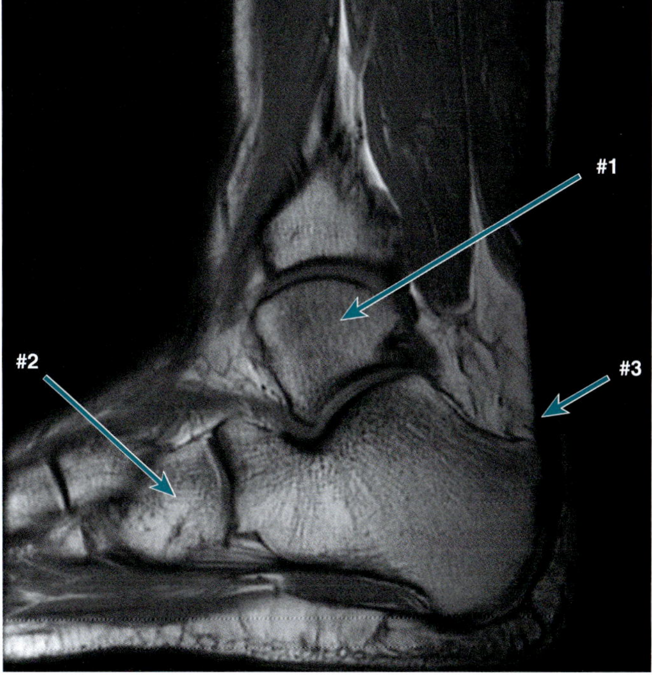

FIGURE 6-91.
(Walter Reed National Military Medical Center)

6-267. Name the anatomy pointed to in #2 in Figure 6.91.

A. Calcaneus

B. Talus

C. Navicular

D. Medial cuneiform

6-268. Name the anatomy pointed to in #3 in Figure 6.91.

- **A. Achilles tendon**
- **B.** Calcaneal tendon
- **C.** Posterior tibial tendon
- **D.** Peroneus tendon

Additional reading:

Schweitzer ME, Karasick D. MRI of the ankle and hindfoot. Semin Ultrasound CT MR. 1994 Oct;15(5):410-22. doi: 10.1016/s0887-2171(05)80007-1. PMID: 7803075.

Smithuis F, Smithuuis R. MRI Examination of the ankle. https://radiologyassistant.nl/musculoskeletal/ankle/mri-examination

Szaro P, Nilsson-Helander K, Carmont M. MRI of the Achilles tendon-A comprehensive pictorial review. Part one. Eur J Radiol Open. 2021 Mar 26;8:100342. doi: 10.1016/j.ejro.2021.100342. PMID: 33850971; PMCID: PMC8039565.

6-269. What abnormality is depicted in Figure 6.92?

- **A.** Subluxation of the patella
- **B. Anterior crucial ligament tear**
- **C.** Posterior cruciate tear
- **D.** Patellar ligament tear

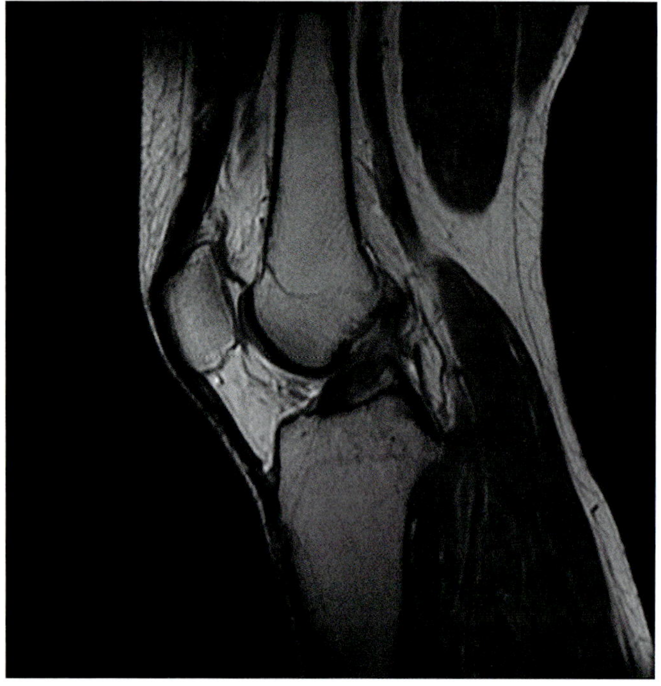

FIGURE 6-92.
(Walter Reed National Military Medical Center)

6-270. Match the anatomy from Figure 6.93.

- **A.** Anterior cruciate ligament_____2_____
- **B.** Meniscus_____1_____
- **C.** Tibial tuberosity_____5_____
- **D.** Collateral ligament_____4_____
- **E.** Posterior cruciate ligament_____3_____

Additional reading:

Farshad-Amacker NA, Potter HG. MRI of knee ligament injury and reconstruction. J Magn Reson Imaging. 2013 Oct;38(4):757-73. doi: 10.1002/jmri.24311. PMID: 24129921.

Vohra S, Arnold G, Doshi S, Marcantonio D. Normal MR imaging anatomy of the knee. Magn Reson Imaging Clin N Am. 2011 Aug;19(3):637-53, ix-x. doi: 10.1016/j.mric.2011.05.012. Epub 2011 Jun 22. PMID: 21816336.

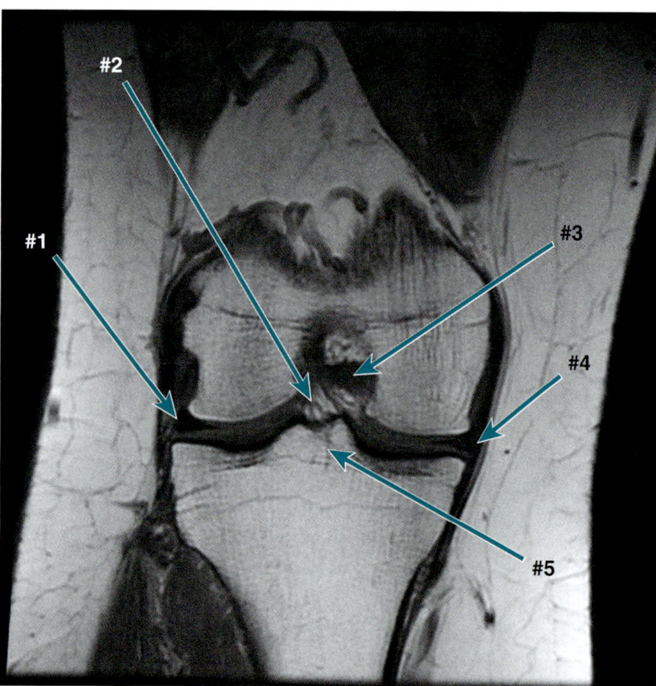

FIGURE 6-93.
(Walter Reed National Military Medical Center)

6-271. What is the most likely pathology depicted on the T1 and T2 with fat saturation weighted images in Figure 6.94?

A. Nonspecific dorsal subcutaneous fluid collection

B. Nonspecific plantar subcutaneous fluid collection

C. Nonspecific tissue fibrosis

D. Nonspecific foot ulcer

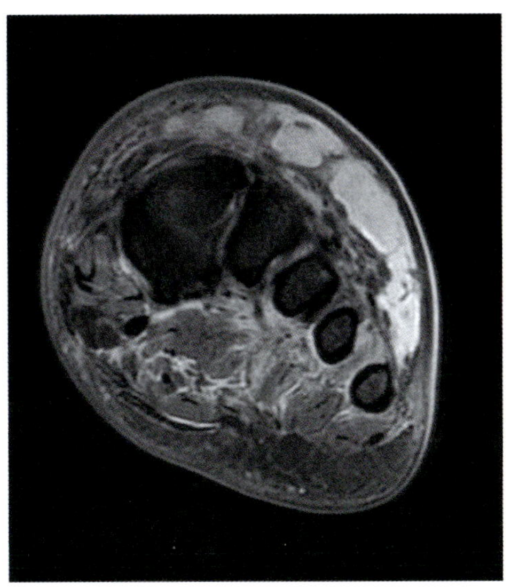

FIGURE 6-94.
(Walter Reed National Military Medical Center)

6-272. What is being pointed to in Figure 6.95 of a foot?

A. Bone spurs on the calcaneus

B. Fractured bone fragments on the posterior metatarsal

C. Sesamoid bones of the great toe

D. Bone spurs on the great toe

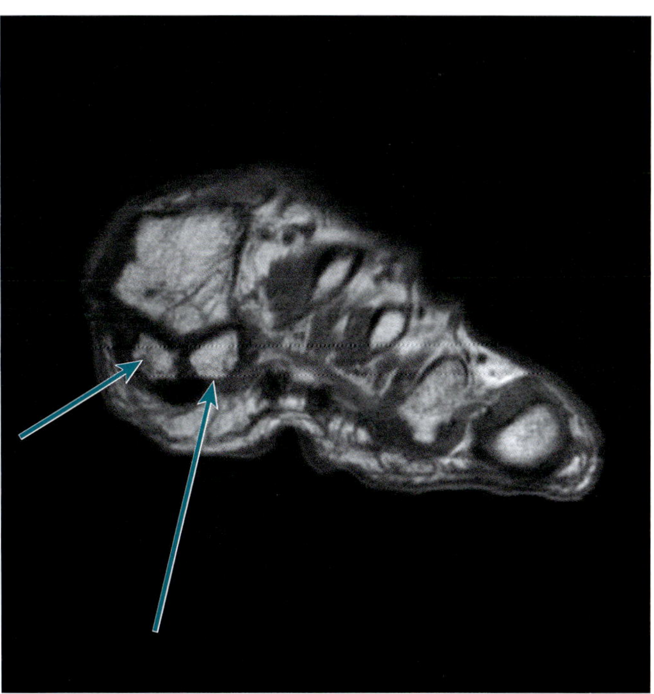

FIGURE 6-95.
(Walter Reed National Military Medical Center)

Additional reading:

Weaver JS, Omar IM, Mar WA, Klauser AS, Winegar BA, Mlady GW, McCurdy WE, Taljanovic MS. Magnetic resonance imaging of musculoskeletal infections. Pol J Radiol. 2022 Mar 5;87:e141-e162. doi: 10.5114/pjr.2022.113825. PMID: 35505859; PMCID: PMC9047866.

Chan BY, Markhardt BK, Williams KL, Kanarek AA, Ross AB. Os Conundrum: Identifying Symptomatic Sesamoids and Accessory Ossicles of the Foot. AJR Am J Roentgenol. 2019 Aug;213(2):417-426. doi: 10.2214/AJR.18.20761. Epub 2019 Apr 11. PMID: 30973781.

McCarthy E, Morrison WB, Zoga AC. MR Imaging of the Diabetic Foot. Magn Reson Imaging Clin N Am. 2017 Feb;25(1):183-194. doi: 10.1016/j.mric.2016.08.005. Epub 2016 Oct 20. PMID: 27888847.

6-273. What patient population is Figure 6.96 from?

A. Adult cancer patient

B. Pediatric cancer patient

C. Healthy adult

D. Adult athlete

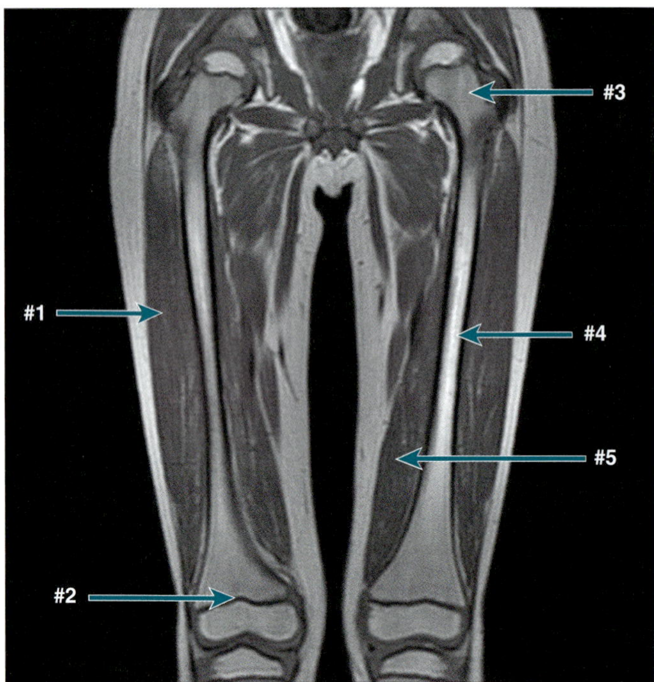

FIGURE 6-96.
(Walter Reed National Military Medical Center)

6-274. Label the identified anatomy in Figure 6–96

A. Femoral Shaft_____4_____

B. Femoral Neck_____3_____

C. Distal femoral epiphysis_____2_____

D. Vastus lateralis_____1_____

E. Vastus medialis_____5_____

Additional reading:

Foster K, Chapman S, Johnson K. MRI of the marrow in the paediatric skeleton. Clin Radiol. 2004 Aug;59(8):651-73. doi: 10.1016/j.crad.2004.02.001. PMID: 15262540.

6-275. Bilateral leg MRI/MRA require that the legs be positioned how to be able to acquire all three planes equivocally for each leg?

A. Patient supine, legs flat, ankles/feet taped together with a foam block between the limbs

B. Patient supine, legs with small sponge under knees, ankles/feet taped together with a foam block between the limbs

C. Patient supine, legs flat, ankles/feet angled outward at a 45-degree angle

D. Patient supine, legs with small sponge under knees, ankles/feet angled outward at a 45-degree angle

6-276. What anatomy is #1 pointing to in Figure 6.97?

A. Popliteal artery

B. Iliac artery

C. Femoral artery

D. Popliteal vein

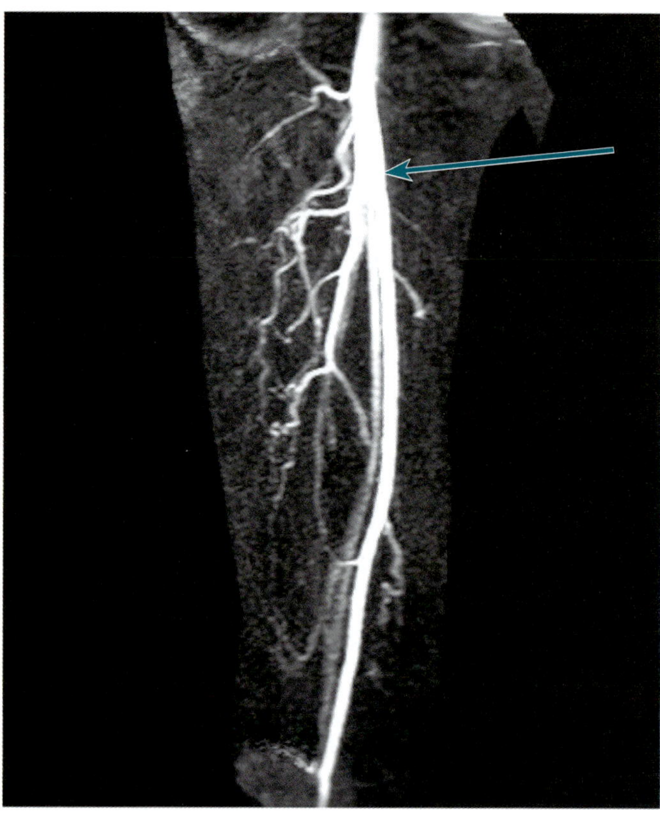

FIGURE 6-97.
(Walter Reed National Military Medical Center)

6-277. What anatomy is #1 pointing to in Figure 6.98?

- **A.** Popliteal artery
- **B.** Posterior tibial artery
- **C. Anterior tibial artery**
- **D.** Peroneal artery

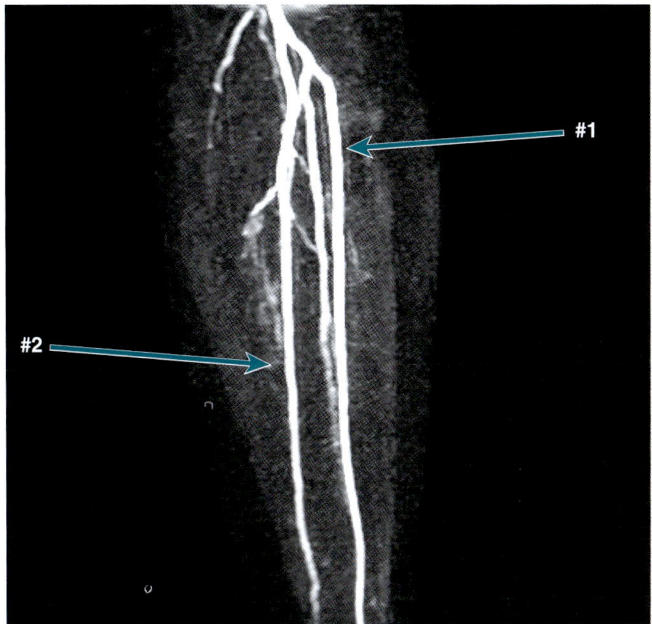

FIGURE 6-98.
(Walter Reed National Military Medical Center)

6-278. What anatomy is #2 pointing to in Figure 6.98?

- **A.** Popliteal artery
- **B. Posterior tibial artery**
- **C.** Anterior tibial artery
- **D.** Peroneal artery

Additional reading:

Kramer JH, Grist TM. Peripheral MR Angiography. Magn Reson Imaging Clin N Am. 2012 Nov;20(4):761-76. doi: 10.1016/j.mric.2012.08.002. Epub 2012 Sep 25. PMID: 23088949.

Cavallo AU, Koktzoglou I, Edelman RR, Gilkeson R, Mihai G, Shin T, Rajagopalan S. Noncontrast Magnetic Resonance Angiography for the Diagnosis of Peripheral Vascular Disease. Circ Cardiovasc Imaging. 2019 May;12(5):e008844. doi: 10.1161/CIRCIMAGING.118.008844. PMID: 31088154.

Yadav MK, Mohammed AKM, Puramadathil V, Geetha D, Unni M. Lower extremity arteries. Cardiovasc Diagn Ther. 2019 Aug;9(Suppl 1):S174-S182. doi: 10.21037/cdt.2019.07.08. PMID: 31559162; PMCID: PMC6732106.

6-279. What is the most likely pathology depicted on Figure 6.99?

- **A.** Nonspecific fluid collection
- **B. Dermatomyositis**
- **C.** Pulled muscle
- **D.** Hematoma

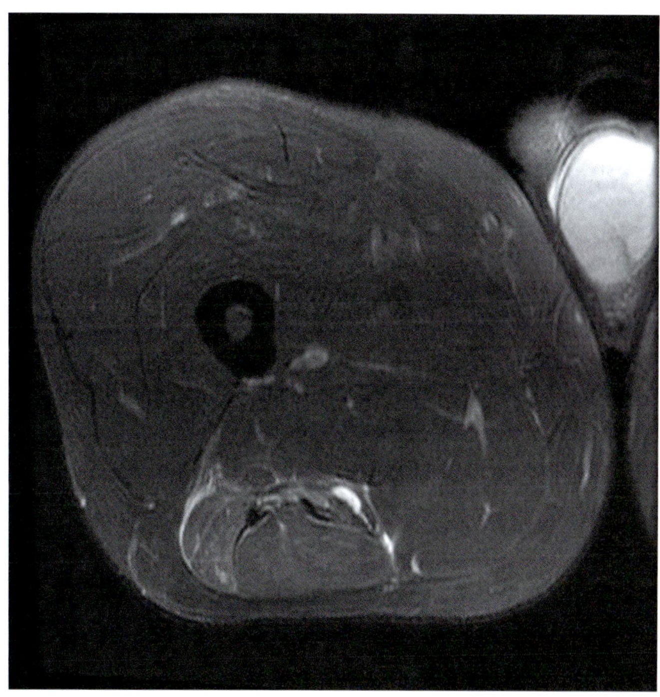

FIGURE 6-99.
(Walter Reed National Military Medical Center)

6-280. What is the body part on Figure 6.99?

- **A.** Lower leg
- **B.** Upper arm
- **C. Upper leg**
- **D.** Lower arm

Discussion:

Juvenile dermatomyositis is a common idiopathic inflammatory myopathy in children. MRI is the gold standard imaging modality for detecting inflammatory myopathy.

Additional reading:

Ladd PE, Emery KH, Salisbury SR, Laor T, Lovell DJ, Bove KE. Juvenile dermatomyositis: correlation of MRI at presentation with clinical outcome. AJR Am J Roentgenol. 2011 Jul;197(1):W153-8. doi: 10.2214/AJR.10.5337.

6-281. What is the anatomy pointing to in #1 on Figure 6.100?

A. Obturator externus muscle

B. Obturator internus muscle

C. Vastus lateralis muscle

D. Adductor magus muscle

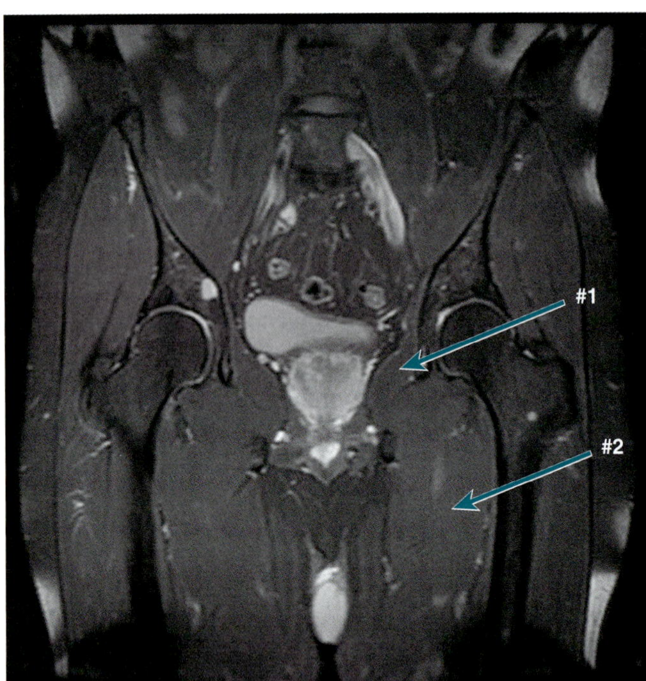

FIGURE 6-100.
(Walter Reed National Military Medical Center)

Department of Defense Disclaimer:

The views expressed in this book chapter are those of the author and do not reflect the official policy of the Department of Army/Navy/Air Force, Department of Defense, or U.S. Government.

6-282. What is the anatomy pointing to in #2 on Figure 6.100?

A. Obturator externus muscle

B. Obturator internus muscle

C. Vastus lateralis muscle

D. Adductor magus muscle

Additional reading:

Stanford MSK MRI Atlas. http://xrayhead.com/

MRI Questions—Anatomy and Pathology

7-1. What imaging plane is pictured in Figure 7-1?

- **A.** Coronal
- **B.** Oblique
- **C.** Transverse
- **D.** **Sagittal**

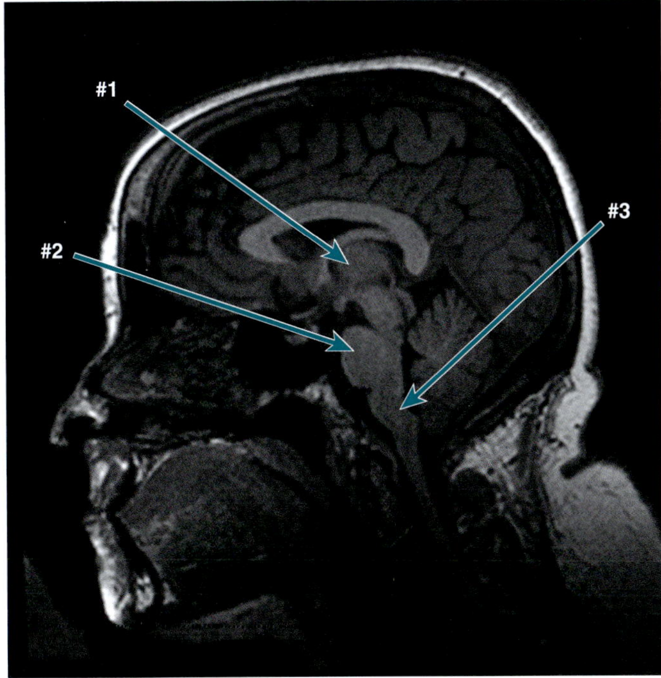

FIGURE 7-1.
(Walter Reed National Military Medical Center)

7-2. What is the structure labeled #1 in Figure 7-1?

- **A.** **Thalamus**
- **B.** Body of the corpus callosum
- **C.** Thalamus
- **D.** Splenium of the corpus callosum

7-3. Identify the structure labeled #2 in Figure 7-1?

- **A.** Cerebral peduncle
- **B.** **Pons**
- **C.** Corpora quadrigemina
- **D.** Medulla oblongata

7-4. Identify the structure labeled #3 in Figure 7-1?

- **A.** Cerebral peduncle
- **B.** Pons
- **C.** Corpora quadrigemina
- **D.** **Medulla oblongata**

Additional reading:

Learning Neuorology. "https://learningneurology.com/diagnostic-tests/approach-to-mri-brain/" Approach to MRI brain | LearningNeurology.com

The Whole brain atlas. "https://www.med.harvard.edu/aanlib/home.html" The Whole Brain Atlas (harvard.edu)

7-5. What pathology is demonstrated in Figure 7-2?

A. Bleed

B. Multiple sclerosis

C. Tuberculosis

D. Brain metastasis

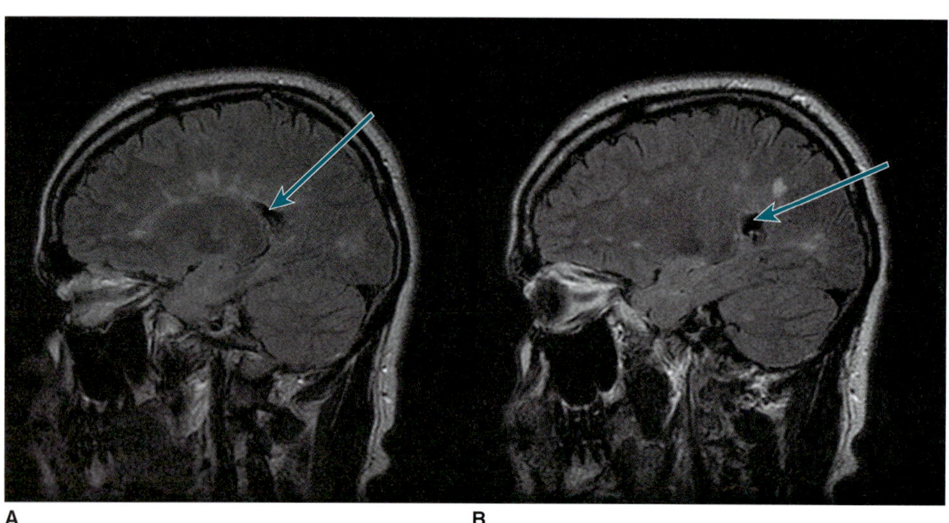

FIGURE 7-2.
(Walter Reed National Military Medical Center)

7-6. Identify the structure the blue arrow is pointing to in Figure 7-2.

A. Third ventricle

B. Lateral ventricle

C. Hemorrhage

D. Central sinus

Additional reading:

Healy GM, Redmond CE, Gaughan M, Fleming H, Carroll AG, Purcell YM, McGuigan C, McNeill G, Killeen RP. The accuracy of standard multiple sclerosis MRI brain sequences for the diagnosis of optic neuropathy. Mult Scler Relat Disord. 2020 Feb;38:101521. doi: 10.1016/j.msard.2019.101521. Epub 2019 Nov 12. PMID: 3175660

7-7. What area is #1 pointing to Figure 7-3?

A. Inferior frontal

B. Temporal

C. Occipital

D. Post central

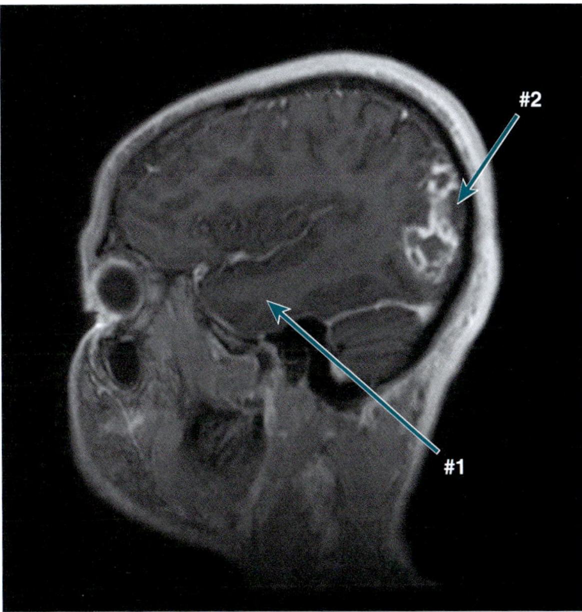

FIGURE 7-3.
(Walter Reed National Military Medical Center)

7-8. What pathology is #2 pointing to Figure 7-3?

A. Stroke

B. Multiple sclerosis

C. Tuberculosis

D. Brain metastasis

Additional reading:

Vilela P. Acute stroke differential diagnosis: Stroke mimics. Eur J Radiol. 2017 Nov;96:133-144. doi: 10.1016/j.ejrad.2017.05.008. Epub 2017 May 5. PMID: 28551302.

7-9. What is the structure labeled #1 in Figure 7-4?

A. Internal carotid artery

B. Right common carotid artery

C. Left vertebral artery

D. Right vertebral artery

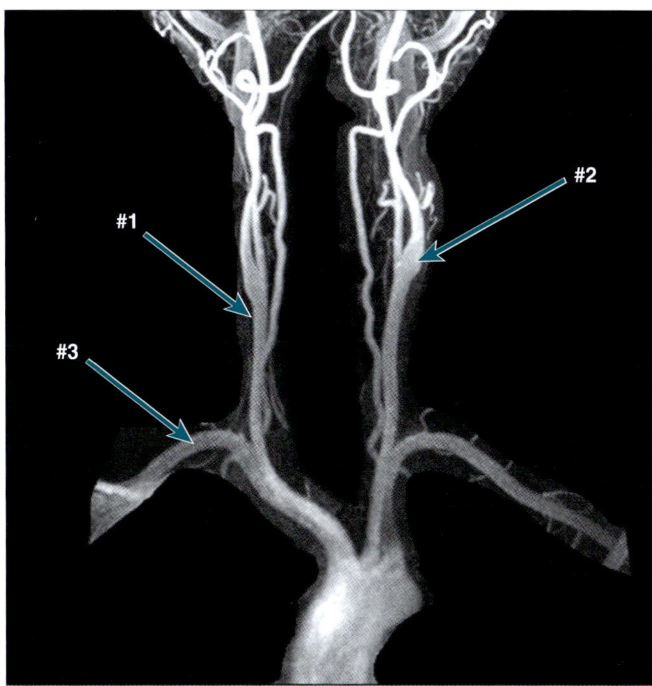

FIGURE 7-4.
(Walter Reed National Military Medical Center)

7-10. What is the structure labeled #2 in Figure 7-4?

A. Carotid bifurcation

B. Right subclavian artery

C. Vertebral artery

D. Left common carotid artery

7-11. What is the structure labeled #3 in Figure 7-4?

A. Left common carotid artery

B. Right common carotid artery

C. Left subclavian artery

D. Right subclavian artery

Additional reading:

Ota H, Reeves MJ, Zhu DC, Majid A, Collar A, Yuan C, DeMarco JK. Sex differences of high-risk carotid atherosclerotic plaque with less than 50% stenosis in asymptomatic patients: an in vivo 3T MRI study. AJNR Am J Neuroradiol. 2013 May;34(5):1049-55, S1. doi: 10.3174/ajnr.A3399. Epub 2012 Nov 29. PMID: 23194832; PMCID: PMC5506561.

Lim RP, Shapiro M, Wang EY, Law M, Babb JS, Rueff LE, Jacob JS, Kim S, Carson RH, Mulholland TP, Laub G, Hecht EM. 3D time-resolved MR angiography (MRA) of the carotid arteries with time-resolved imaging with stochastic trajectories: comparison with 3D contrast-enhanced Bolus-Chase MRA and 3D time-of-flight MRA. AJNR Am J Neuroradiol. 2008 Nov;29(10):1847-54. doi: 10.3174/ajnr.A1252. Epub 2008 Sep 3. PMID: 18768727; PMCID: PMC8118944.

7-12. What is the age of the patient pictured in Figure 7-5?

A. Geriatric

B. Middle age

C. Pediatric

D. Bariatric

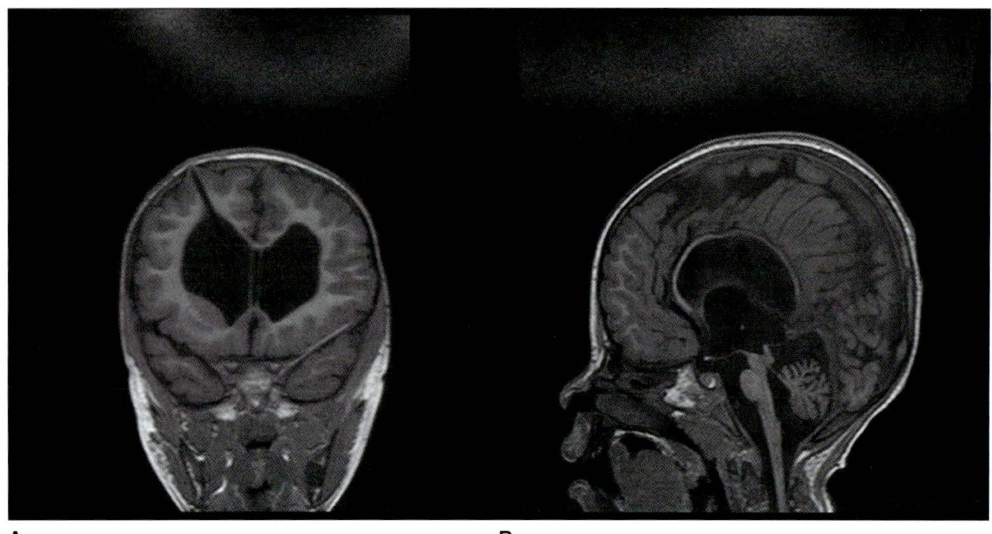

A B

FIGURE 7-5.
(Walter Reed National Military Medical Center)

7-13. What pathology is demonstrated in Figure 7-5?

A. Bleed

B. Hydrocephalus

C. Tuberculosis

D. Brain metastasis

7-14. Identify the sequence demonstrated in Figure 7-5.

A. T1

B. FLAIR

C. Diffusion

D. T2

Additional reading:

Krishnan P, Raybaud C, Palasamudram S, Shroff M. Neuroimaging in Pediatric Hydrocephalus. Indian J Pediatr. 2019 Oct;86(10):952-960. doi: 10.1007/s12098-019-02962-z. Epub 2019 May 10. PMID: 31077004.

7-15. Identify the sequence demonstrated in Figure 7-6.

A. T1

B. FLAIR

C. Diffusion

D. T2

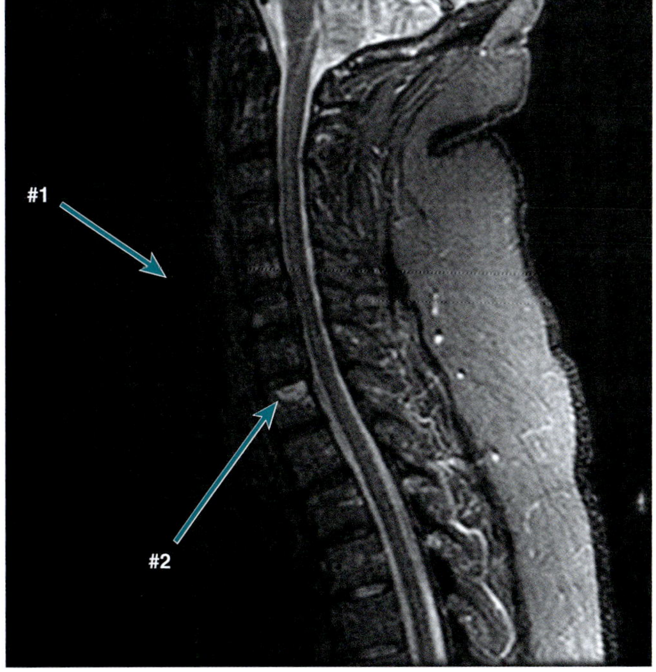

A

FIGURE 7-6.
(Walter Reed National Military Medical Center)

7-16. Identify the artifact labeled #1 in Figure 7-6.

A. Sat band

B. Metal

C. Pulse band

D. Dentures

Additional reading:

Abbas J, Slon V, Stein D, Peled N, Hershkovitz I, Hamoud K. In the quest for degenerative lumbar spinal stenosis etiology: the Schmorl's nodes model. BMC Musculoskelet Disord. 2017 Apr 20;18(1):164. doi: 10.1186/s12891-017-1512-6. PMID: 28424050; PMCID: PMC5397788.

7-17. What is the structure labeled #2 in Figure 7-6.

A. Metastatic lesion

B. Schmorl's node

C. Osteoporosis

D. Spinal degeneration

7-18. Identify the sequence demonstrated in Figure 7-7A&B.

A. T1

B. FLAIR

C. Diffusion

D. T2

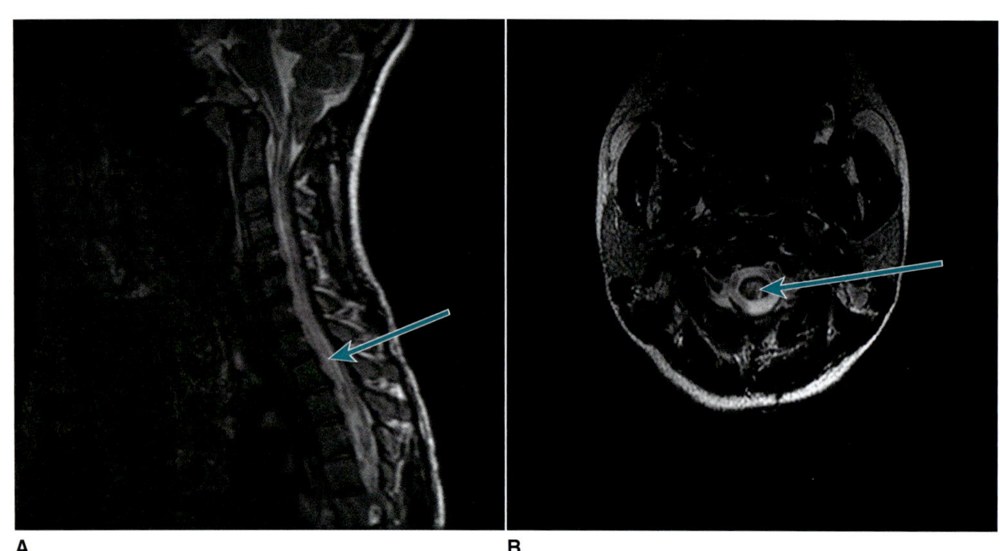

FIGURE 7-7.
(Walter Reed National Military Medical Center)

7-19. What pathology is demonstrated in Figure 7-7A&B?

A. Syringomyelia

B. Multiple sclerosis

C. Herniated nucleus pulposus

D. Hemorrhage

Additional reading:

Although syringohydromyelia are usually considered as a chronic process, acute syringohydromyelia can also occur. Sudden loss of movement post-operatively needs to be assessed quickly via MRI to ascertain the need for surgery.

Rao KS, Balasubramaniam C, Subramaniam K. Acute onset of postoperative syringohydromyelia. J Pediatr Neurosci. 2015 Jul-Sep;10(3):240-3. doi: 10.4103/1817-1745.165671. PMID: 26557165; PMCID: PMC4611893.

7-20. What imaging plane is pictured in Figure 7-7A?

A. Coronal

B. Oblique

C. Transverse

D. Sagittal

7-21. Figure 7-8 is an image for a study done to show venous flow in what structure?

A. Carotid

B. Liver

C. **Head**

D. Kidneys

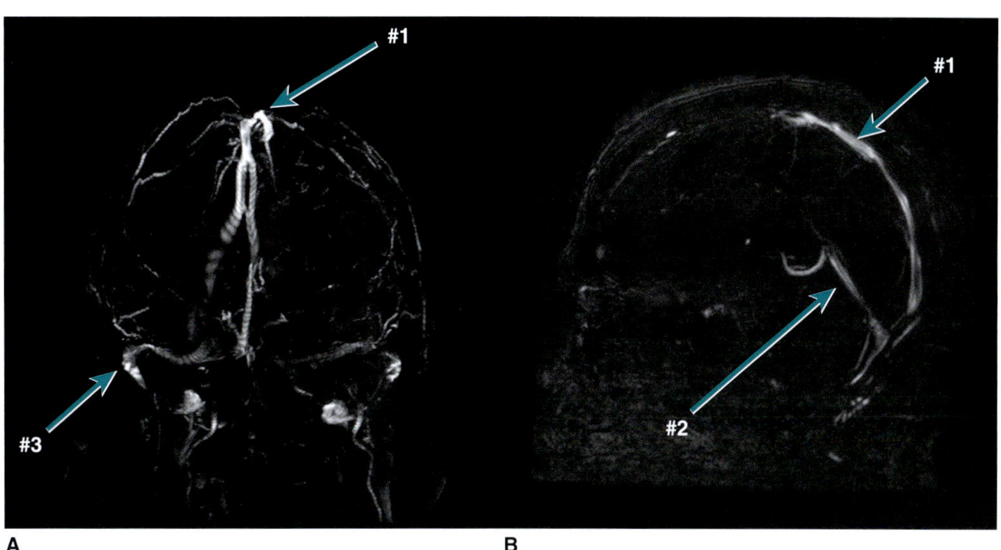

FIGURE 7-8.
(Walter Reed National Military Medical Center)

7-22. What is the structure labeled #1 in Figure 7-8?

A. Sagittal sinus

B. **Superior sagittal sinus**

C. Internal jugular vein

D. Straight sinus

7-23. What is the structure labeled #2 in Figure 7-8?

A. Sagittal sinus

B. Superior sagittal sinus

C. Internal jugular vein

D. **Straight sinus**

7-24. What is the structure labeled #3 in Figure 7-8?

A. Sagittal sinus

B. Superior sagittal sinus

C. **Sigmoid sinus**

D. Straight sinus

Additional reading:

Bozzao A, Finocchi V, Romano A, Ferrante M, Fasoli F, Trillò G, Ferrante L, Fantozzi LM. Role of contrast-enhanced MR venography in the preoperative evaluation of parasagittal meningiomas. Eur Radiol. 2005 Sep;15(9):1790-6. doi: 10.1007/s00330-005-2788-8. Epub 2005 May 20. PMID: 15906036.

Cerebral venous thrombosis: a practical guide. "https://pn.bmj.com/content/20/5/356" Cerebral venous thrombosis: a practical guide | Practical Neurology (bmj.com)

7-25. What is the structure labeled #1 in Figure 7-9?

- **A.** **Pituitary mass**
- **B.** Infundibulum
- **C.** Pituitary gland
- **D.** Optic chiasm

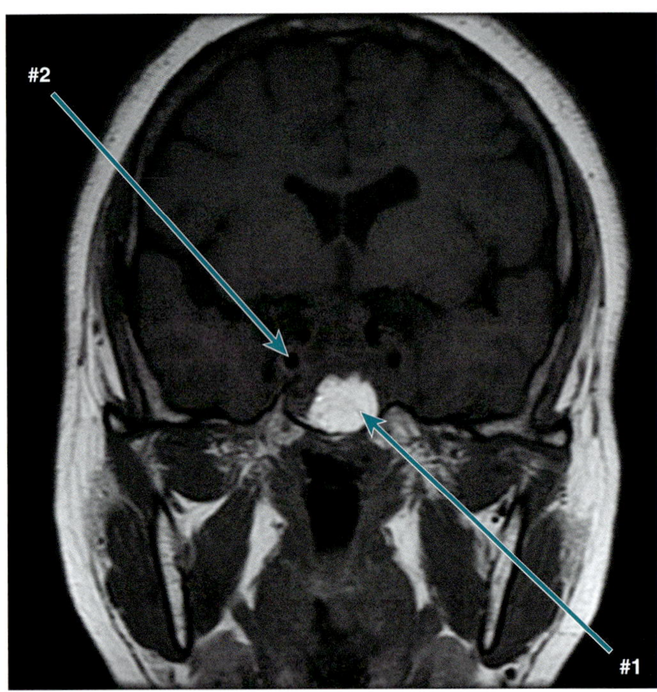

FIGURE 7-9.
(Walter Reed National Military Medical Center)

7-26. What is the structure labeled #2 in Figure 7-9?

- **A.** Middle cerebral artery
- **B.** Central cerebral artery
- **C.** **Internal carotid artery**
- **D.** Vertebral artery

7-27. What is the structure labeled #1 in Figure 7-10?

- **A.** Optic chiasm
- **B.** **Aqueduct of Silvius**
- **C.** Fourth ventricle
- **D.** Basilar artery

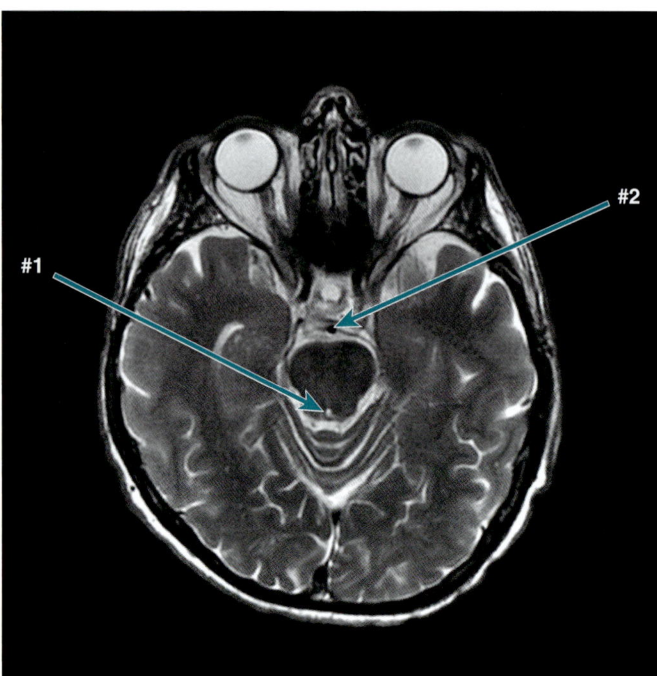

FIGURE 7-10.
(Walter Reed National Military Medical Center)

7-28. What is the structure labeled #2 in Figure 7-10?

- **A.** Optic chiasm
- **B.** Aqueduct of Silvius
- **C.** Fourth ventricle
- **D.** **Basilar artery**

7-29. What is the structure labeled #1 in Figure 7-11?

A. Lateral rectus muscle

B. Medial rectus muscle

C. Optic nerve

D. Lacrimal gland

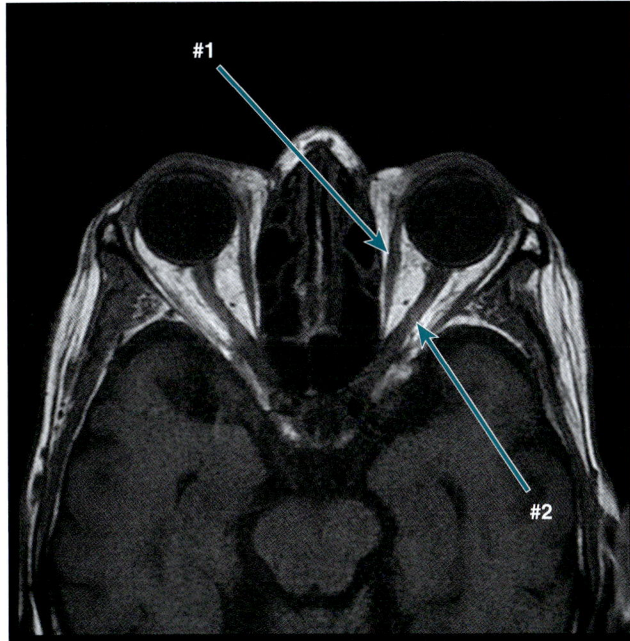

FIGURE 7-11.
(Walter Reed National Military Medical Center)

7-30. What is the structure labeled #2 in Figure 7-11?

A. Lateral rectus muscle

B. Medial rectus muscle

C. Optic nerve

D. Lacrimal gland

7-31. The sequence in Figure 7-11 was most likely done using what slice thickness?

A. 1–2 mm

B. 3–5 mm

C. 5–7 mm

D. 7–10 mm

7-32. What are the structures labeled #1 in Figure 7-12?

A. Vestibulocochlear nerve and the hypoglossal nerve

B. Vestibulocochlear nerve and the facial nerve

C. Cranial nerve VII and cranial nerve VIII

D. Both B and C

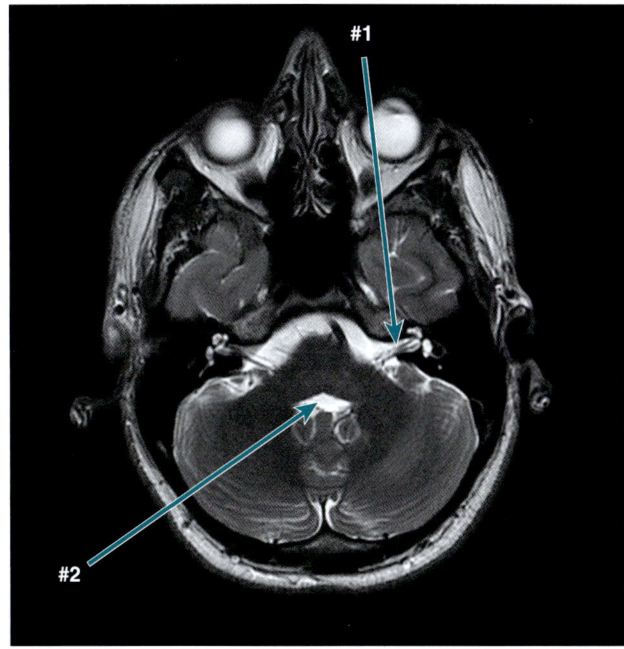

FIGURE 7-12.
(Walter Reed National Military Medical Center)

7-33. What is the structure labeled #2 in Figure 7-12?

A. Crus cerebri

B. Substantia nigra

C. Fourth ventricle

D. Red nucleus

7-34. The sequence in Figure 7-12 was most likely done using what slice thickness?

A. 1–2 mm

B. 3–5 mm

C. 5–7 mm

D. 7–10 mm

7-35. Identify the sequence demonstrated in Figure 7-12.

A. T1

B. FLAIR

C. Diffusion

D. T2

7-36. What is the bone shown in Figure 7-13?

A. Femur

B. Humerus

C. Greater trochanter

D. Tibia

7-37. What is the pathology labeled #1 in Figure 7-13A?

A. Long bone tumor

B. Pathological fracture

C. Dislocation

D. Ewing's sarcoma

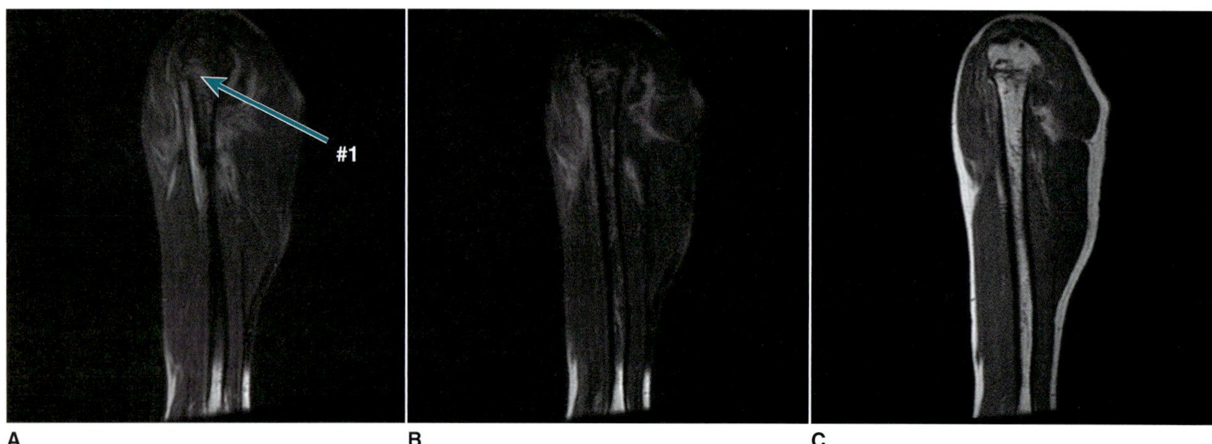

FIGURE 7-13.
(Walter Reed National Military Medical Center)

7-38. What is being displayed in the bone in Figure 7-13 B&C?

A. Normal bone

B. Periosteal edema

C. T1 hypointense and T2 hyperintense line at the epiphyseal line

D. Both B and C

7-39. What pathology is being pointed at by #1 in Figure 7-14A?

A. Vertebral body burst fracture in a 20-year-old

B. Spinal metastasis

C. Spondylolisthesis

D. Degenerative disease in an 80-year-old

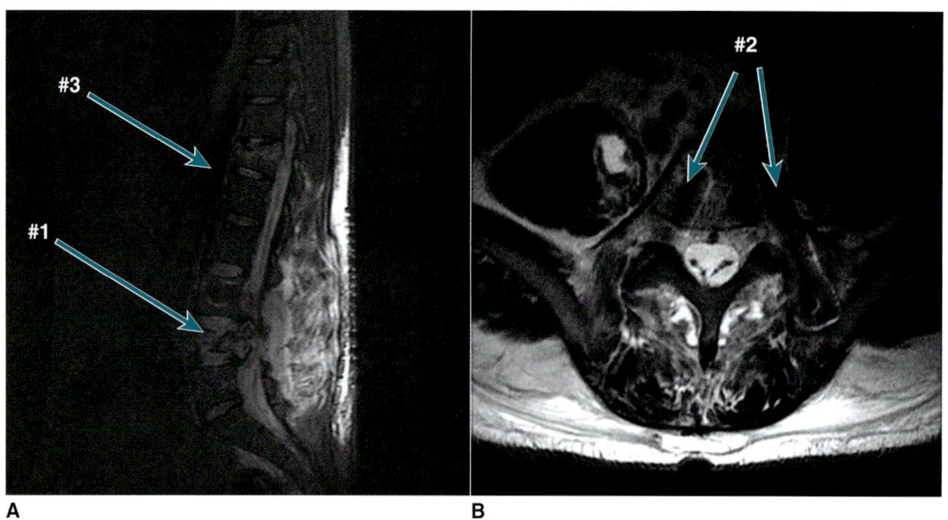

FIGURE 7-14.
(Walter Reed National Military Medical Center)

7-40. What is the artifact labeled #2 caused by in Figure 7-14B?

A. Motion

B. Air in the bowel

C. Metal

D. Body of L4

7-41. What is the structure labeled #3 in Figure 7-14A?

A. Lumbar nerve

B. Abdominal aorta

C. Iliac artery

D. Straightening rod

Discussion:

Traumatic injury can result in burst fractures. Plain radiographs and CT can assess the bony structures well, but MRI in important for the disc and ligament assessment for stability.

Additional reading:

Mi J, Sun XJ, Zhang K, Zhao CQ, Zhao J. Prediction of MRI findings including disc injury and posterior ligamentous complex injury in neurologically intact thoracolumbar burst fractures by the parameters of vertebral body damage on CT scan. Injury. 2018 Feb;49(2):272-278. doi: 10.1016/j.injury.2017.12.011. Epub 2017 Dec 15. PMID: 29290375.

Cicala D, Briganti F, Casale L, Rossi C, Cagini L, Cesarano E, Brunese L, Giganti M. Atraumatic vertebral compression fractures: differential diagnosis between benign osteoporotic and malignant fractures by MRI. Musculoskelet Surg. 2013 Aug;97 Suppl 2:S169-79. doi: 10.1007/s12306-013-0277-9. Epub 2013 Aug 15. PMID: 23949939.

7-42. In Figure 7-15, what MRA technique is being depicted?

A. Traditional non-contrast-enhanced 3D MRA

B. Traditional non-contrast-enhanced 2D MRA

C. Fluoro-triggered contrast-enhanced 3D MRA

D. Time-resolved contrast-enhanced 3D MRA

7-43. In Figure 7-15, what is arrow #1 pointing to?

A. Anterior cerebral artery

B. Middle cerebral artery

C. Basilar artery

D. Internal carotid artery

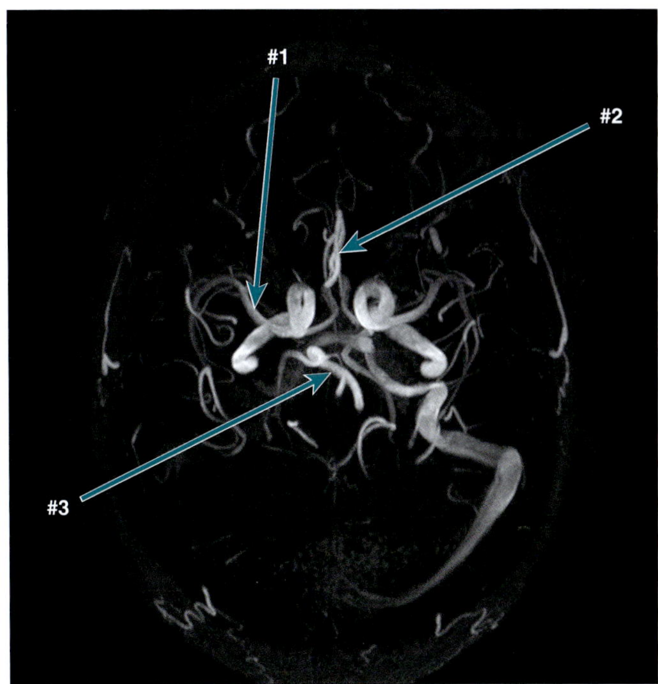

FIGURE 7-15.
(Walter Reed National Military Medical Center)

7-44. In Figure 7-15, what is arrow #2 pointing to?

A. Anterior cerebral artery

B. Middle cerebral artery

C. Basilar artery

D. Anterior communicating artery

7-45. In Figure 7-15, what is arrow #3 pointing to?

A. Anterior cerebral artery

B. Middle cerebral artery

C. Basilar artery

D. Posterior cerebral artery

Additional reading:

Naveen SR, Bhat V, Karthik GA. Magnetic resonance angiographic evaluation of circle of Willis: A morphologic study in a tertiary hospital set up. Ann Indian Acad Neurol. 2015 Oct-Dec;18(4):391-7. doi: 10.4103/0972-2327.165453. PMID: 26713008; PMCID: PMC4683875.

7-46. Identify the sequence demonstrated in Figure 7-16.

A. PD

B. T1

C. STIR

D. T2

7-47. What pathology is demonstrated in Figure 7-16, #1?

A. Mass

B. Cyst

C. Lipoma

D. Hematoma

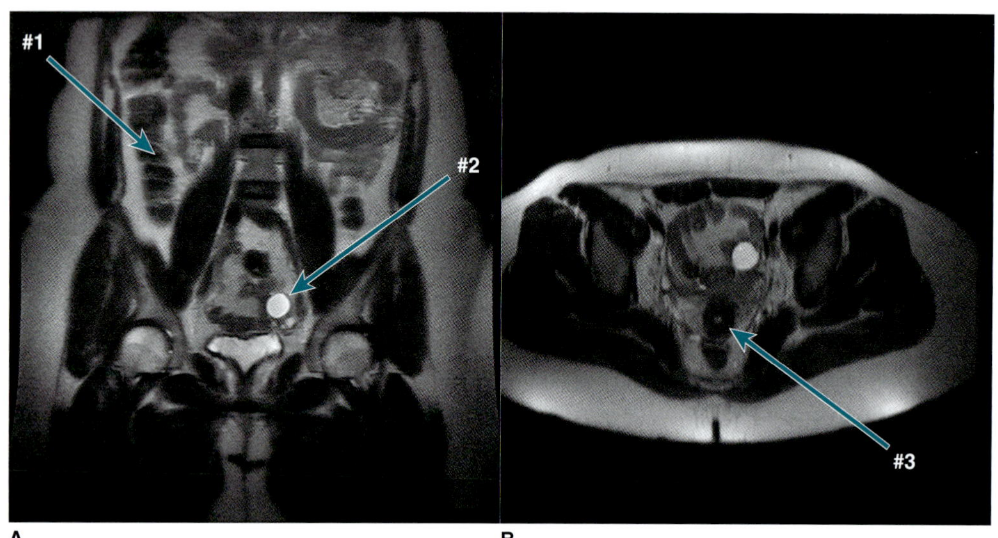

FIGURE 7-16.
(Walter Reed National Military Medical Center)

7-48. What is the structure labeled #2 in Figure 7-16?

A. Uterus

B. Prostate gland

C. Rectum

D. Anal canal

Additional reading:

Canellas R, Rosenkrantz AB, Taouli B, Sala E, Saini S, Pedrosa I, Wang ZJ, Sahani DV. Abbreviated MRI Protocols for the Abdomen. Radiographics. 2019 May-Jun;39(3):744-758. doi: 10.1148/rg.2019180123. Epub 2019 Mar 22. PMID: 30901285.

7-49. Name the structure labeled by #1 in Figure 7-17.

- **A.** Middle interphalangeal joint
- **B.** Interphalangeal joint
- **C. Distal phalanx**
- **D.** Proximal phalange

7-50. Name the structure labeled by #2 in Figure 7-17.

- **A.** Carpometacarpal joint
- **B. Metacarpophalangeal joint**
- **C.** Interphalangeal joint
- **D.** Distal interphalangeal joint

7-51. Name the structure labeled by #3 in Figure 7-17.

- **A. Carpometacarpal joint**
- **B.** Metacarpophalangeal joint
- **C.** Interphalangeal joint
- **D.** Distal interphalangeal joint

Additional reading:

Zbojniewicz AM. MRI anatomy and injuries of the fingers. Pediatr Radiol. 2023 Jul;53(8):1562-1575. doi: 10.1007/s00247-023-05624-7. Epub 2023 Feb 18. PMID: 36808525.

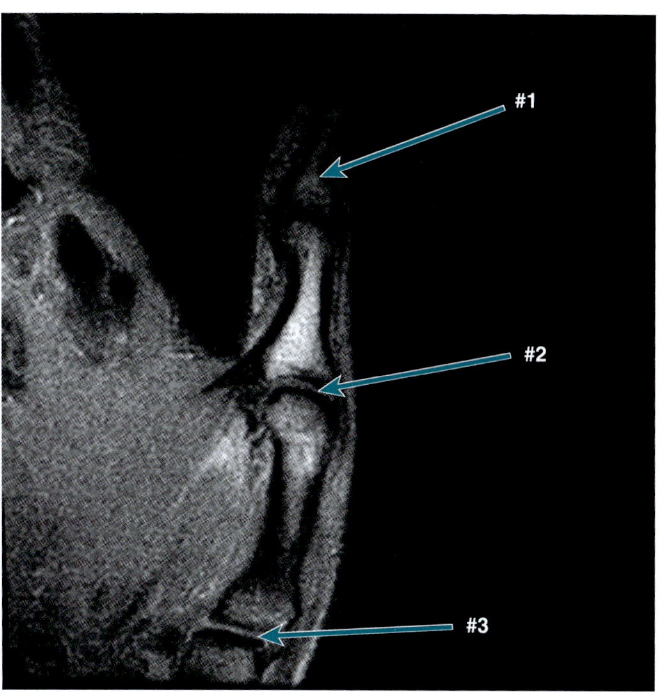

FIGURE 7-17.
(Walter Reed National Military Medical Center)

7-52. What is the probable age range of the person shown in Figure 7-18A?

A. 8–12 years of age

B. 12–16 years of age

C. 16–25 years of age

D. Over 25 years of age

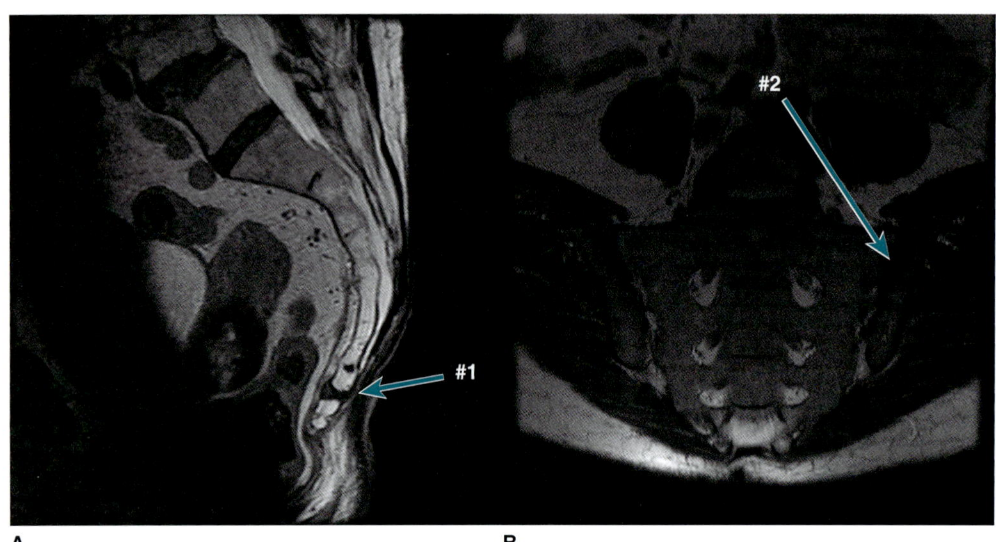

FIGURE 7-18.
(Walter Reed National Military Medical Center)

7-53. What is the structure pointed to by the arrow labeled #1 in Figure 7-18A?

A. Sacrococcygeal joint

B. Intercoccygeal joint

C. Intercoccygeal tumor

D. Intercoccygeal cyst

7-54. In what plane is the image shown in Figure 7-18B?

A. Oblique sagittal

B. Oblique transaxial

C. Oblique coronal

D. Planar

Additional reading:

Woon JT, Stringer MD. Clinical anatomy of the coccyx: A systematic review. Clin Anat. 2012 Mar;25(2):158-67. doi: 10.1002/ca.21216. Epub 2011 Jul 7. PMID: 21739475.

Castillo S, Joodi R, Williams LE, Pezeshk P, Chhabra A. Sacrum magnetic resonance imaging for low back and tail bone pain: A quality initiative to evaluate and improve imaging utility. World J Methodol. 2021 Jul 20;11(4):110-115. doi: 10.5662/wjm.v11.i4.110. PMID: 34322363; PMCID: PMC8299904

7-55. What is the structure pointed to by the arrow labeled #2 in Figure 7-18B?

A. Sacrococcygeal joint

B. Sacroiliac joint

C. Sacral fracture

D. Lumbosacral joint

7-56. What is the structure pointed to by arrow #1 in Figure 7-19A?

A. Xyphoid

B. Manubrium

C. Body

D. Costal cartilage

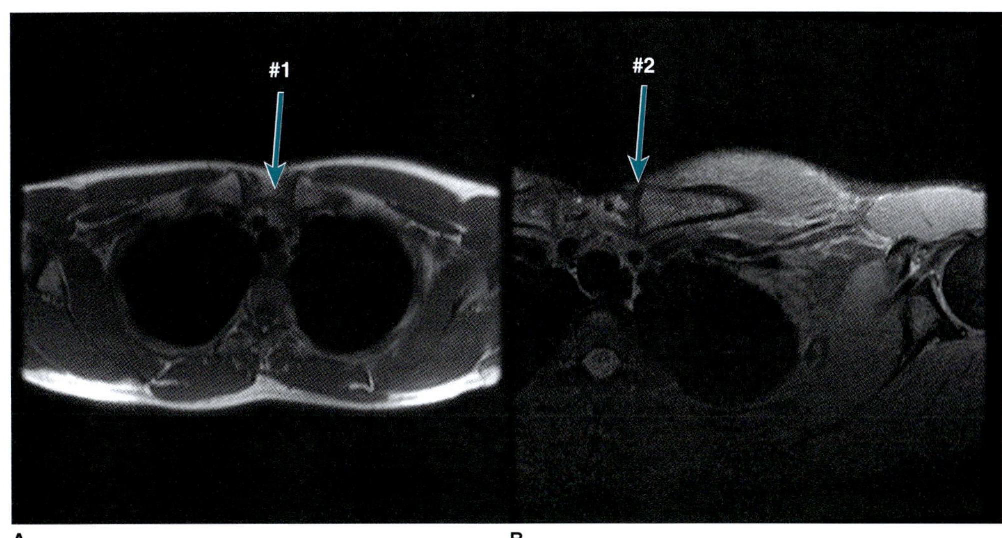

FIGURE 7-19.
(Walter Reed National Military Medical Center)

7-57. What is the structure pointed to by arrow #1 in Figure 7-19A?

A. Sternoclavicular joint

B. Manubrioclavicular joint

C. Acromioclavicular joint

D. Costoclavicular joint

Additional reading:

https://radsource.us/sternoclavicular-joint-pathology/

Sternoclavicular Joint Pathology | Radsource

Kang BS, Shim HS, Kwon WJ, Lim S, Park GM, Lee TY, Bang M. MRI findings for unilateral sternoclavicular arthritis: differentiation between infectious arthritis and spondyloarthritis. Skeletal Radiol. 2019 Feb;48(2):259-266. doi: 10.1007/s00256-018-3023-4. Epub 2018 Jul 5. PMID: 29978244.

7-58. What is the structure pointed to by arrow #1 in Figure 7-20A?

A. Intervertebral foramen

B. Pedicle

C. Lamina

D. Spinous process

7-59. What is the structure pointed to by arrow #2 in Figure 7-20B?

A. Right superior articular process

B. Lamina

C. Intervertebral foramen

D. Spinous process

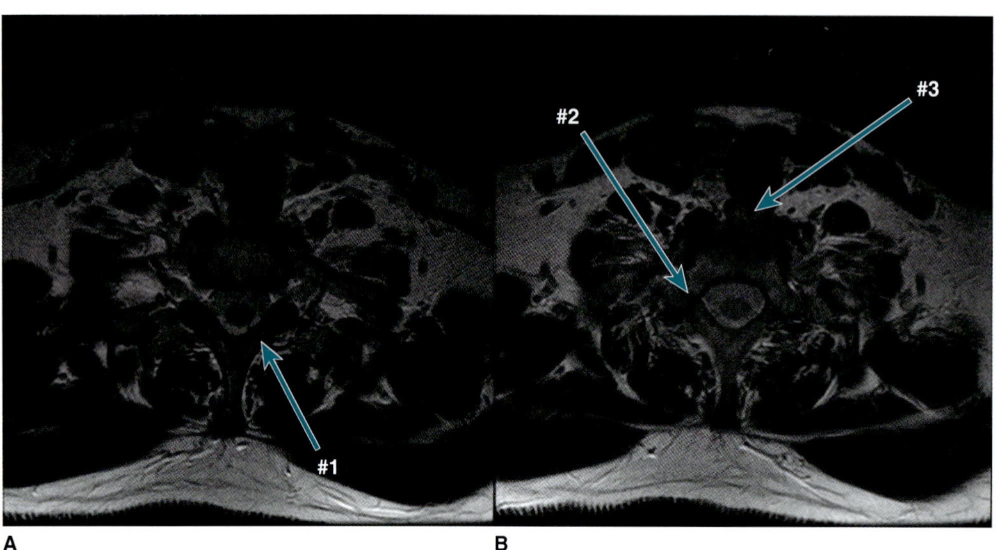

FIGURE 7-20.
(Walter Reed National Military Medical Center)

7-60. What is the structure pointed to by arrow #3 in Figure 7-20B?

A. Bronchial tube

B. Lamina

C. Esophagus

D. Tumor

Additional reading:

Winegar BA, Kay MD, Taljanovic M. Magnetic resonance imaging of the spine. Pol J Radiol. 2020 Sep 25;85:e550-e574. doi: 10.5114/pjr.2020.99887. PMID: 33101557; PMCID: PMC7571515.

7-61. What is the structure pointed to by the arrow in Figure 7-21 A&B?

A. Blood vessels in the brachial plexus

B. Tendons of the brachial plexus

C. Nerves of the brachial plexus

D. Ligaments of the brachial plexus

Discussion:

Imaging the brachial plexus is challenging because it is difficult to see and follow the complex anatomy in this region in order to see and follow the nerves when the anatomy is normal or the pathology is subtle. The imaging is better at higher field strengths such as 3T in order to get better SNR with thinner slices. When the nerves are inflamed, it is much easier to see the brachial plexus.

Additional reading:

van Es HW, Bollen TL, van Heesewijk HP. MRI of the brachial plexus: a pictorial review. Eur J Radiol. 2010 May;74(2):391-402. doi: 10.1016/j.ejrad.2009.05.067. Epub 2010 Mar 11. PMID: 20226609.

Szaro P, McGrath A, Ciszek B, Geijer M. Magnetic resonance imaging of the brachial plexus. Part 1: Anatomical considerations, magnetic resonance techniques, and non-traumatic lesions. Eur J Radiol Open. 2021 Dec 20;9:100392. doi: 10.1016/j.ejro.2021.100392. PMID: 34988263; PMCID: PMC8695258.

Gilcrease-Garcia BM, Deshmukh SD, Parsons MS. Anatomy, Imaging, and Pathologic Conditions of the Brachial Plexus. Radiographics. 2020 Oct;40(6):1686-1714. doi: 10.1148/rg.2020200012. PMID: 33001787.

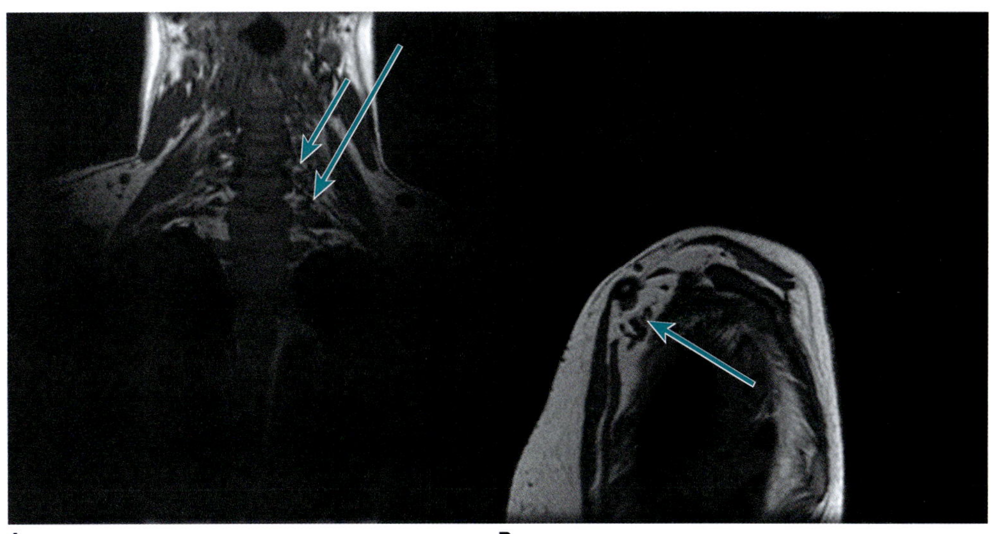

FIGURE 7-21.
(Walter Reed National Military Medical Center)

7-62. What is the pathology pointed to by arrow #1 in Figure 7-22?

A. Blood

B. Normal synovial fluid

C. Excess synovial fluid

D. Tumor

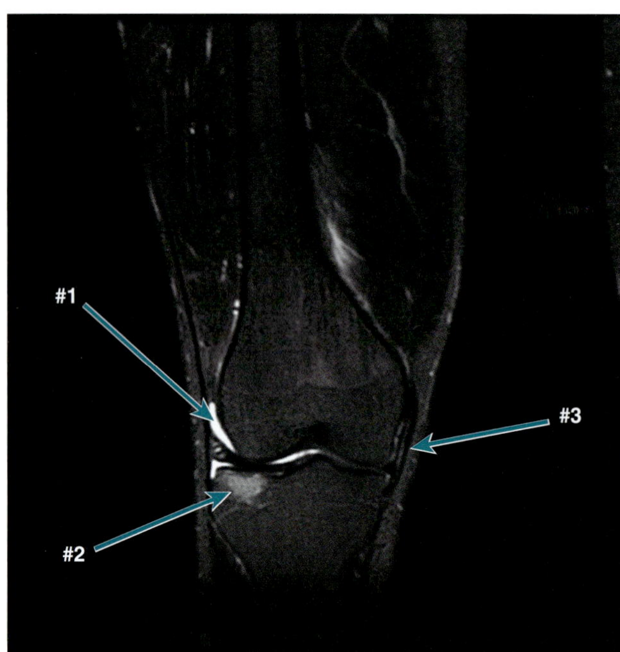

FIGURE 7-22.
(Walter Reed National Military Medical Center)

7-63. What is the pathology pointed to by arrow #2 in Figure 7-22?

A. Tibial plateau metastatic tumor

B. Femoral plateau bone contusion

C. Tibial plateau bone contusion

D. Fibular plateau bone contusion

7-64. What is the structure pointed to by arrow #3 in Figure 7-22?

A. Anterior cruciate ligament

B. Lateral collateral ligament

C. Medial collateral ligament

D. Anterior collateral ligament

Additional reading:

Chien A, Weaver JS, Kinne E, Omar I. Magnetic resonance imaging of the knee. Pol J Radiol. 2020 Sep 11;85:e509-e531. doi: 10.5114/pjr.2020.99415. PMID: 33101555; PMCID: PMC7571514.

Department of Defense Disclaimer:

The views expressed in this chapter are those of the author and do not reflect the official policy of the Department of Army/Navy/Air Force, Department of Defense, or U.S. Government.

INDEX

Note: Page numbers followed by f indicate figures.

J

K

L

M

Q

R